Developmentally Disabled Infants and Toddlers: Assessment and Intervention

Developmentally Disabled Infants and Toddlers: Assessment and Intervention

RAEONE S. ZELLE, R.N., M.N.
MATERNAL-CHILD HEALTH CONSULTANT
YOLO COUNTY HEALTH DEPARTMENT
WOODLAND, CALIFORNIA
CONSULTANT, CHILD DEVELOPMENT AND
DEVELOPMENTAL DISABILITIES
PRIVATE PRACTICE

ATHLEEN B. COYNER, R.N., M.S., F.A.A.N.
NURSE CONSULTANT, PRIVATE PRACTICE
FORMERLY, DIRECTOR, INFANT DEVELOPMENT PROGRAM
DIVISION OF FAMILY HEALTH SERVICES
UTAH DEPARTMENT OF HEALTH
SALT LAKE CITY, UTAH

CONTRIBUTING AUTHOR

JOYCE E. SHIGEKAWA, R.N., M.N.
NANI PROJECT, HIGH-RISK INFANT FOLLOWUP
UNIVERSITY OF CALIFORNIA DAVIS MEDICAL CENTER
SACRAMENTO, CALIFORNIA

ILLUSTRATED BY JUDY WATTS

FOREWORD BY KATHRYN BARNARD, PH.D.

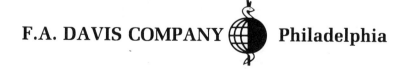

F.A. DAVIS COMPANY　Philadelphia

Printed in the United States of America

Library of Congress Cataloging in Publication Data

Zelle, Raeone S., 1934–
  Developmentally disabled infants and toddlers.

  Bibliography: p.
  Includes index.
  1. Developmental disabilities. 2. Developmentally disabled children—Rehabilitation. I. Coyner, Athleen B., 1934. II.Title. [DNLM: 1. Child development disorders—Diagnosis. 2. Child development disorders—Therapy. 3. Handicapped. 4. Infant, Newborn, Diseases—Diagnosis. 5. Infant, Newborn, Diseases—Therapy. WS 350.6 Z51d]
  RJ135.Z44   1983   618.92   83-1423 ISBN 0-8036-9775-9

FOREWORD

Knowledge is the basis of professional practice. The information used in health care comes from a broad base of biological and behavioral sciences. The contribution of knowledge gained through a blending of scientific principles and the testing of these laws and concepts in everyday practice provides the building blocks of one's professional knowledge. Such is the case with the contribution that Raeone Zelle, Athleen Coyner, and Joyce Shigekawa are making in this book. The authors have woven together strands of developmental theories, biological axioms of neurodevelopmental function, affiliative concepts of human interaction and relationships, the nursing process, and principles of habilitation.

This is a clinician's book in the most scholarly sense; the authors, all sharing a professional background in nursing, have written from the experience of their countless days, months, and years of professional practice with children and their families. The integrated knowledge they present will be helpful to many clinicians practicing in the field of developmental disabilities. The text goes beyond a recital of the normal principles of development to a dynamic focus on cognitive, motor, and affective function in everyday living. The descriptive case studies are reminders that the child is not just a motorically functioning individual or just a biological machine that needs a certain number of calories, but rather a whole dynamic being, interacting with and influencing his environment in a manner we failed to recognize just a short twenty years ago.

Because each clinician, whether nurse, physician, physical therapist, occupational therapist, speech therapist, nutritionist, social worker, or educator, must eventually practice at a level of dynamic integration of the biological, behavioral, and environmental interfaces, this template of professional knowledge will offer much guidance.

Rightfully so, a major emphasis of the book is on assessment. Prominent attention is given to motor function, which is a common area of difficulty with infants and young children who have some type of developmental problem. The pragmatic approach that Raeone Zelle uses in her presentation of developmental appraisal is precisely indicative of the careful observations that the clinician must make about present function before deciding what the developmental problems are and how the infant is functioning given the problem and making further observations that will serve as the basis for therapeutic measures.

At least half of our professional acts in clinical work involve, in my estimation, skills of assessment. The approach used here is one of comprehensive assessment of the developmental function of the child in the motor, cognitive, and relationship domains. The assessment relies on professional knowledge and judgment. The assessment process outlined is not a systematic assessment that allows you to fill out a checklist of symptoms, but rather it is a nonstandardized guide to the appraisal of how the infant and young child use body motion and thinking to accomplish the mastery of goals and interact with the environment. This text can be used as a handbook that deals first with topics of familiarity, and as that schema becomes understood and expanded, then goes on to other dimensions of assessment and intervention as you apply the knowledge in your practice.

From the results of the health and developmental appraisal comes information that helps both the clinician and the family to know best how to structure the child's environment to maximize the child's mastery, whether it be taking in calories, grasping for a ball, or bringing about a more effective respiratory exchange. In thinking about the environment, the importance of feedback loops is as evident in considering functioning of the internal pathways of the central nervous system as it is in understanding parent-child interaction or in promoting the learning of new behavior. All recent evidence of mastery in cognitive or social realms points to the critical nature of contingent feedback in promoting optimum development and function. A major frame of reference is to intervene in directions that create additional positive contingent feedback for the child and, likewise, positive contingent feedback to the parent from the child.

For parents with children who have developmental problems, often the child's feedback to the parent is less than needed. Our studies of premature infants, specifically infants born prior to 34 weeks of gestation, have documented that prematurely born infants tend to be less responsive and less organized in their behavioral acts. For instance, on the Brazelton Neonatal Assessment Scale, when matched for conceptual age with their newborn term counterparts, the prematurely born infants are less responsive to auditory and visual stimuli and have fewer self-quieting behaviors. This lack of coordinated motor responses and less effective quieting behaviors make self-control more difficult for the infant and result in the infant's behavior being harder for the parent to understand and handle. Likewise, the feature of being less responsive has an effect on the parent or caregiver, since most investigations report that parents of premature infants are superparents in the early months; they are attentive and responsive, and they provide a growth-fostering environment; they are talking to, smiling, touching, and moving the baby.

As Shigekawa and Zelle have reported in this book, the preterm infant, however, is not as responsive. It may be, as they describe, that the infant has more difficulty with sensory processing, since a common behavior is for the infant to turn away from the caregiver. Over time the evidence shows that the majority of the preterm infants deal better with their environment. They develop the ability to regulate state, to habituate more rapidly, and to attend to meaningful stimuli. However, it is also becoming evident that those early months when the infant is not very responsive and is sometimes very irritable and hard to console have the effect of making the parents less sensitive and responsive, so that by eight months of age, the interactive system is out of regulation because of the parents' lack of responsiveness.

The situation of caring for the preterm infant illustrates an application of social learning theory. The parents' efforts were not reinforced by the infant's responsiveness, and over long months of interaction the parents learned not to be as sensitive or to provide as much stimulation. In many respects this illustration of the parent-child interaction regulation is what this book is all about. Feedback is critical to the maintenance of the caregiving role, either directly, from the responsiveness of the child, or indirectly, by seeing developmental changes and growth. Through the use of health and developmental assessments the caregiver can be guided to understand the responses and, in many instances, to channel the infant's efforts into more successful mastery.

Intervention with health and developmental problems involves giving clients new information, validating their thinking, assisting them in adopting new roles, and generally giving support. It is important to realize that with the child who has developmental problems the intervention will be with the family, parents, and/or other caregivers. Even at the assessment phase, the clinician will be dependent on the family for input about typical responses and behaviors from a broader range of situations than it is possible to observe during limited contact. The assessment phase enables the clinician to establish a relationship in which the family members feel respected and cared about. Since parents seldom have the opportunity to discuss observations about their child or their child rearing with someone they respect as an authority, the clinician, by listening in the beginning, will establish a transactional approach that will bring the parents and clinician to the same level of awareness of the child's health and developmental status. This transactional approach leads to mutual goal-setting by the family and clinician, which in the final analysis, is the only therapeutic approach associated with positive change. The parents are the mediators of the child's environment; therefore, any approaches not enlisting their full participation are inappropriate.

Giving the parents equal status is frustrating at times to the clinician, especially when it means sacrificing what the clinician thinks is best for the child's eventual function. It is well to remember the emotional turmoil that the parent is dealing with and the demanding job of balancing family resources for all members. It may well be that the therapeutic device, the visit to the orthopedic clinic, or the exercises to accompany diapering need to be put aside at times to facilitate other family goals.

Even in the rearing of normal children, the importance of giving support to the major caregiver is being documented. Especially in families with less educational and financial resources, the support each parent gives to the other is being recognized as associated with the best developmental progress for the child. The husband has an important role in supporting his wife when she has a major caregiving role with young children, and vice versa if the husband is assuming the major caregiving role. The concept of buffering has been introduced as central to how the parenting figure accomplishes refueling and dealing with the demanding job of caring for children. This partnership is even more essential with parents whose child has health and/or developmental problems. It is therefore essential that the clinician focus on both parents.

An important aspect of caregiving emphasized by the authors is the facilitation of internal stabilization through promoting good physical health and normal neuromuscular responses. Based on available evidence, these biological factors can either facilitate or impede development. For the infant with sensory motor disturbances, the basic matter of state modulation can be problematic. The parents will profit from as many tips as possible on how to help quiet an irritable baby, how to recognize stimulus overload before it happens, and how to help the baby achieve an optimal level of responsiveness. All these aspects of state modulation deal with how the central nervous system processes incoming stimuli.

The integration of health, developmental, and interactional components in this book reflects an increasing trend. Clinicians representing varied disciplines share responsibility for the knowledge base and assessment and intervention approaches that address the developmentally disabled child's multifaceted needs. It is reasonable that the focus be centered on a home-oriented program, as it is customary and best for infants to be cared for in their own homes and by their parents. Although we recognize the responsibility of the parents to care for the child, at the same time society must accept its responsibility to support the family. The recent report of the Select Panel on Children's Health, entitled *Better Health for our Nation's Children: A National Strategy*, emphasizes the important role that the family plays as the basic health care unit. As health providers it is our task to aid in the appraisal of health, to give information to improve or promote health, to validate the family's observations and behaviors, and to provide the emotional support, respect, and encouragement that will promote mastery of the family's responsibility in the care of its members. The authors of this volume have provided a significant body of knowledge to assist clinicians in working with developmentally disabled infants and toddlers and their families.

Kathryn Barnard, Ph.D.
University of Washington
Seattle, Washington

PREFACE

Health, education, and therapy services for the developmentally disabled infant and child have expanded, and the concept of early intervention has evolved. Interdisciplinary, multidisciplinary, and transdisciplinary teams have been organized privately and within existing community service agencies to enhance the level of wellness and development of handicapped infants and children and to help parents cope with the multiple, complex problems and stresses often precipitated by a member with special needs. Thus, a holistic approach has evolved.

There has been an infusion of federal and state funds to develop these programs and support research during the last decade. The framework for early intervention has dynamically changed in response to the expansion of knowledge and the wisdom of experience. More and more questions have also been raised, which has had a humbling effect.

We have recognized the need to synthesize and integrate theories, constructs, research findings, and our own longitudinal experience into a working-level framework for professional persons in the allied health and educational fields who sense a need to expand and deepen their practice. In the process, the intervener will gain a more adaptive and flexible perspective, which can accommodate to any child functioning at the infant or toddler level who has normal or atypical patterns with habilitative implications. The content will also help the graduate student begin to develop a more in-depth framework for assessment and intervention. Generic students may use portions of the content and the overall philosophy as a reference, under the direction of a member of the faculty or a preceptor.

Since there is an interaction between health and development, with the expression of either phenomenon mutually influencing the other, each chapter in the book is part of a whole. The content is meant to be read and reread, because some aspects may be readily assimilated into the practitioner's or graduate student's framework, whereas other aspects of the content may have to be studied with the support of other references. A holistic approach insures that the theoretical and practical base is developed in an interrelated rather than a compartmentalized way.

Chapter 1 introduces concepts of traditional versus current wellness-oriented health management for handicapped infants. A new model illustrates the cyclical nature of the effects of health problems in handicapped infants and discusses the origin of these problems, their interrelationships, and appropriate interventions that can prevent, reduce, or ameliorate health problems secondary to the primary handicapping condition. Although written from a nursing perspective, this information can assist other health and nonhealth professionals understand and appreciate the necessity of health management as the foundation for effective early intervention services.

In Chapter 2, the emphasis is on the underlying process of development and the functional relationship of patterns. This serves as the substrate for assessing the adequacy of the overall environment in terms of the core needs of all infants and toddlers as we now know them. The framework also serves as the basis for identifying subtle qualitative differences in behaviors and more obvious aberrant developmental patterns that have functional significance. There is a carry-over of the interrelated model in the framework for habilitation. The approaches have a multidimensional focus for the most part to support the complex interaction of the infant or toddler with his natural environment.

Chapter 3 underscores the interdependence of health and development by providing a more in-depth description of regulatory mechanisms that determine the infant's or child's capacity to respond to stimuli in the environment. This capacity is determined by the organization and regulation of physiologic and behavioral parameters. Disorders can occur reflected by too high or too low a threshold to sensory input and/or too high or too low muscle tone. The last section of this chapter provides a framework for mediating sensory input to compensate for deviances in internal regulatory mechanisms and normalize these mechanisms to the extent possible.

Chapter 4 complements and builds upon the content in Chapters 1 and 2 relative to oral and language patterns. The authors emphasize the importance of maintaining a balance between affective and technical components in the assessment and habilitation of aberrant oral and feeding patterns. Thus, the chapter has a philosophical bent, while it also provides practical suggestions that the caregiver can blend with her interactive style to promote the development of oral control and progressively more independent feeding behaviors.

The framework in the above chapters provides the basis for recognizing the contrasts and similarities in the evolvement of development in the intrauterine and extrauterine environment. In Chapter 5, the authors provide a provisional model for assessing the unique development of the embryo and fetus and mediating the extrauterine environment in ways that support the preterm infant's development when he is born at risk.

RSZ
ABC

ACKNOWLEDGMENTS

This book is an outgrowth of our association with handicapped children and their families, colleagues in varied disciplines, and the integrated effort of a number of very dedicated persons. Lyle Waters served in the role of principal typist over the months, with the backup of Valerie Larzelere. Gail Knudsen responded to an emergent request to type a preliminary manuscript of most of the book. Charly Price provided consultation during the development of the figures and tables and designed the comparison layout for some of the figures. Wilma Bryant provided much needed respite for the illustrator, Judy Watts, by creating some of the figures in the last stage of Chapter 2. Zsanenn Zelle, daughter of one of the authors, assumed the role of Girl Friday throughout the project. A special thanks is extended to all members of the team and our supportive families. The authors also appreciate the assistance that the staff at the F.A. Davis Company provided over the months.

RSZ
ABC

CONTENTS

Chapter 1

MEETING HEALTH NEEDS OF HANDICAPPED INFANTS

Athleen B. Coyner

The first year of life is characterized by rapid change in size and physiologic function. Physical growth is dramatic: weight is tripled and height is increased by 50 percent. Physical growth and changes in physiologic functions occur simultaneously, although they are not always correlated. Every body system experiences increases in numbers of cells, increases in cell size, and ongoing differentiation of function. Hence, newborn levels of renal, cardiovascular, metabolic, digestive, and neuromotor function evolve rapidly towards a more mature status during infancy. Measures of height, weight, head circumference, limb lengths, and so forth, validate easily visible manifestations of growth and are well known parameters of health.

Changes in the functions of cells and body systems, as well as the significance of these changes, are less well recognized by parents and nonhealth professionals. Differences between infant and adult (or mature) levels of physiologic function are significant to the health status and special health needs of children under one year. Significant differences that affect the health of infants are:

1. Body Composition. Fluid and electrolyte ratios differ for infants; a larger percentage of the infant's body weight is water. The proportion of body fat and muscle tissue changes during the second half of the first year, reflecting the increased production of body tissue.

2. Skeletal System. Growth of the head and trunk precedes the later rapid growth of the long bones (extremities). By the end of the first year, growth of the mandible catches up, and the discrepancy between biting surfaces of the anterior jaw is decreased. Closure of the fontanels and fusion of skull bones parallel brain growth, and the head will be about two thirds of its adult size by the end of the first year.

3. Teeth. Tooth eruption normally begins at about four months of age, and dentition proceeds rapidly during the first two years.

4. Skin. The newborn skin loses its propensity to peel, and older infants secrete more lubricating sebum. Sweat glands begin to secrete after the first or second month and assist the infant in regulation of his body temperature. Rashes and skin irritations are common during the first year.

5. Nervous System. As myelinization of the brain and nervous system occurs, neuromotor function is observed in proximal-distal, ventral-dorsal, and cephalocaudal directions. The maturation process is observable in the form of changes in motor, sensory, cognitive, and social responses and functions.

6. Cardiovascular and Pulmonary Systems. The transition from fetal to infant circulation results in corresponding changes in respiratory function; the lungs increase in size and respiratory rates decrease. The heart/pulse rate remains labile during infancy, and blood pressure is approximately 85/60 mm Hg during this period.

7. Renal System. The ability of the infant to regulate the composition, volume, and pH of body fluids through selective excretion and maintain endocrine functions is limited and attains adult levels by one year.

8. Hematologic System. During the first year there are notable shifts in the quantities of cellular elements that circulate in the peripheral blood. These shifts correlate with the use of specific elements and metabolites required to support the rapid growth and maturation at the systems and cellular levels.

9. Lymphatic System. The lymph tissue, including lymph nodes and vessels and tonsils and adenoids, grow rapidly the first year; however, this system does not reach full function until around school age. Hypertrophy is a common response of lymph tissue to infection in infants and young children.

Improved health practices during the past century have made the first year of life safer for babies. The infant mortality rates of the early 1900s have decreased sharply owing to better prenatal, obstetric, perinatal, and pediatric care and better nutrition and housing. Despite this progress, *Healthy People: The Surgeon General's Report on Health Promotion and Disease Prevention*[1] reports that the first year of life is the most hazardous period, until age 65. Mortality rates due to the incidence of birth defects and other handicapping conditions have received much attention, and the health professional's responsibilities to those with handicapping disorders termed the new morbidity has been addressed in medical and health literature.[2] Less information has been available concerning the health problems associated with or secondary to the major handicapping conditions seen during infancy.

The purpose of this chapter is to review aspects of health care and promotion for nurses and other health professionals serving handicapped infants through various early intervention programs. In their zeal to promote the developmental advancements of handicapped and high-risk infants, many otherwise excellent early intervention services have overlooked the health needs and rights of this vulnerable population. Health services available in early intervention programs often consist of a loosely defined affiliation with a diagnostic agency. However, in some programs the local public health nurse is a member of the intervention team and is a resource person who is responsible for liaison with physicians. Diagnostic data sent to early intervention programs provide information about medical diagnosis and therapy needs, as well as the results of psychological and family evaluations. Very seldom is information about well-child care needs transmitted to or sought by early intervention programs. Well-child care (prevention and health promotion services) seems to be the component that is lacking in a comprehensive care design for many early intervention programs.

Usually, the role of the public health nurse or school nurse who is associated with an early intervention program involves interpreting medical data, facilitating receipt of diagnostic data for use by the intervention team, checking immunization status, teaching selected first aid measures to intervention team members, initiating referrals for additional medical diagnosis, making contact with the family when a health or medical emergency arises, and arranging on-going screenings for clients of the intervention program. Once again, well-child care needs might be overlooked if staff and parents assume that the expert diagnostic services and comprehensive intervention services directed to the identification and amelioration of the handicapping condition are adequate to meet the infant's health needs. In these instances pediatric care often consists of irregular visits to a local family physician for treatment of acute illness only, and there may be no single health professional overseeing a total health care plan for the handicapped infant. Fragmentation, duplication, and gaps in health services occur, which ultimately worsen the outlook for the infant's health and development.

This chapter begins with an overview of the role of the nurse who is affiliated with early intervention programs or who specializes in the care of high-risk or handicapped infants. This assessment and intervention information subsequently presented should be useful to nurses and other health professionals associated with early intervention services to handicapped children in coordinating their services with other nurses and physicians to promote optimal health.

HEALTH APPRAISAL AND INTERVENTIONS

The promotion and maintenance of physical and mental health have been primary goals for physicians, nurses, and other health professionals for many years. These goals have been a central focus for nursing management of the young handicapped child in the hospital, home, and community setting. The advent of a specialized area of nursing practice to work with handicapped and high-risk infants has resulted in a shifting of goals and has increased the emphasis on a developmental approach to nursing interventions.[3,4] During the mid- and late 1970s nurse specialists sought to expand their role in caring for normal and atypical infants by adding developmental interventions to their practice in hospital maternity and pediatric units, in clinics, and other community health settings, and in schools. In some instances, this shift in focus to developmental intervention lessened the emphasis on interventions related to the physical and mental health needs of the handicapped infant and his family.

As a member of a multidisciplinary, interdisciplinary, or transdisciplinary team, the nurse has often withheld or deferred judgments relating to the infant's physical and health needs, acquiescing to the proposed interventions of other team members who might or might not have considered health needs in prescribing developmental interventions. Unfortunately, in these same team settings the nurse and other staff members have assumed that, because the family has a physician for the infant and on-going regular medical care, his health needs were being met.

One outcome of the above factors has been confusion by the nurse and others about the role of nursing in early intervention services, regardless of whether the services have been provided in ambulatory care centers, public health agencies, schools, or other special settings. The role of nurses in these programs has not been well defined. The major responsibilities assigned have been similar to school nursing and have primarily focused on communications, with few direct health interventions provided by the nurse.

Challela[5] delineated four major responsibilities for the nurse member of an interdisciplinary team serving handicapped children. She cites the promotion and maintenance of health as the major, primary responsibility of the nurse. Tudor[6] addressed primary goals of nursing care in early intervention services; family support and a high level of health, development, and independence are suggested as goals for effective nursing practice. Una Haynes, a nurse who pioneered early intervention services to handicapped infants and young children, also has contributed significantly to a definition of a health/nursing role with this population. She advocated a pragmatic approach for the nurse and designed care plans for handicapped infants that stressed nutrition and feeding management, proper body alignment to facilitate sensory-motor experience, and parental support.[7] Barnard and Erickson[8] and others have stressed a family-centered approach and the use of behavior modification techniques in designing and implementing care plans for handicapped or disabled children and their families.

A conference of nurses specializing in services for handicapped infants was held in Salt Lake City, Utah, in 1976. This conference produced a statement, later submitted to the American Nurses Association, which addressed the role for nursing in early intervention programs for handicapped children.

> Although there has been a decrease in the birth rate over the past several years, marked advances in health care have resulted in a significantly increased survival rate of infants at risk for normal development. Consequently, there is a demand for increased community services which promote optimal development for these infants and their families.
>
> Nurses have a significant role as independent practitioners and as members of interdisciplinary teams in Early Intervention Programs for developmentally disabled and high-risk infants and children.
>
> Nurses provide:
> 1. Primary health care (prevention, health maintenance, health monitoring, nurturing, care-comfort, and restoration services).
> 2. Coordination and facilitation of services to promote a holistic child/family-care approach to services.
> 3. Liaison with other health care providers.[9]

Physical integrity has long been recognized as the foundation of all human advancement and achievement. Physical integrity, or lack of it, determines the individual's ability to experience and regulate internal and external stimulation, to attain and maintain homeostasis, to deal effectively with the environment, and to develop and maintain human relationships. All other life experiences are colored by the physical health and well being of the person. Nursing contributes significantly to physical integrity by providing primary health care, including prevention, health maintenance and monitoring, nurturing, care-comfort, and restoration to health. Although the term physical integrity might be used by some as a synonym for health, it is important that nurses and other health professionals identify a framework that will facilitate a health approach to caring for the handicapped infant.

MODELS OF HEALTH SERVICES

THE WELL CHILD MODEL

A model developed and used by maternal child health and the infant development programs at the Utah State Department of Health in 1977[10] can serve as a framework for health assessment and services to all children, including young handicapped infants. This model was adapted from the American Academy of Pediatrics National Health Status Goals[11] and identifies indicators of health in children, such as:

Adequate nutrition;
Adequate patterns of physical and emotional health;
Achievement of milestones in motor, communication, social, and cognitive development;
Protection against preventable disease and injury;
Absence of illness;
Correction of correctable abnormality.

The above indicators of health can direct goals for preventive, maintenance, and restorative services by nurses functioning independently or in concert with other health team members. The only areas of child health generally shared with educational disciplines are the achievement of developmental milestones, and the correction of those correctable abnormalities that are in the nonbiologic domains. In order to attain and maintain maximum child health, the nurse has responsibility to assure physical and mental health of the infant and to coordinate the work of team members into a holistic, family-centered, health-related focus.

THE PATHOPHYSIOLOGIC/MEDICAL MODEL

Expansion and modification of the well child model is necessary in order to anticipate special health needs and to reduce problems caused by a handicap or disability. Pathophysiology is a determinant of specific health needs and problems and has been the basis for what I term the Medical Care model. Interventions by nurses, therapists, and other team members patterned after this model have targeted the following assessment and intervention needs:
1. Therapy and special care routines.
2. Medications.
3. Prevention of complications or secondary handicaps.
4. Special equipment.
5. Safety.

Therapy and Special Care Routines

Prescriptive physical or occupational therapy is indicated in those infants who have orthopedic problems or other conditions involving neuromotor dysfunction, including those infants with a diagnosis of myelomeningocele, congenital hip, cerebral palsy-type disorders, neuropathy, or myopathy, or children whose limbs are malformed or partially absent. A general goal for therapy routines with infants is habilitative, striving to advance a normal sequence of motor skills, movement, and self-care abilities. In these cases a secondary overall goal is to prevent additional unnecessary deformity and dysfunction, for example, contractures, abnormal spinal curvatures, and so on.

Special care routines also include care of the shunt in hydrocephalus, crede of the bladder and other methods of urinary tract and bowel management with myelomeningocele, special body positioning for the child with cardiac lesions or with cerebral palsy, respiratory assistance or postural drainage for the infant with cystic fibrosis or other respiratory malfunctions, management of seizures, and so forth.

Within this framework, a major nursing function has been to assist the mother or family carry out therapy and management routines successfully in the home. With special training, study, and experience, the nurse can help families institute these routines based on her knowledge of pathophysiology and child care practices.

Medication Routines

Medications given to handicapped infants cover a broad range of drugs, some well known because of successful, long-term use and others that are new and whose short-term use provides limited data as to beneficial or adverse effects of use in infants.

Many infants with early discernible handicaps have some degree of neurologic dysfunction and are subject to develop or already manifest varying types of seizure disorders. Anticonvulsant drugs are in regular use with a large number of severely handicapped infants. Nursing's responsibility includes observation and documentation of the drug's effect on the infant, teaching parents proper administration and how to observe for adverse or expected side effects, providing physical assessment if an adverse reaction is suspected, and initiating prompt referral or reporting irregular medication responses to the physician.

Handicapped infants whose basic pathology includes hypertonicity of moderate or severe degree might also have sedative or muscle relaxant drugs prescribed. Fluoride and vitamin-flouride mixtures are given when indicated for maintenance of nutrition and prevention of caries.

Home management of the handicapped infant by the nurse will involve validating the following with the mother and other caregivers:
1. Knowledge of the drug, including the purpose and indications for use.
2. Appropriate methods of administering the medication, including proper timing, dosage, frequency of use, and indica-

tions for withholding the drug or contacting the physician for approval to alter frequency or dosage, and so forth.

3. Proper storage of the infant's drugs and all medications in the home.

4. A list of all drugs that the infant receives should be kept by the family. The list should note the name and telephone number of the pharmacy that generally dispenses the medications and the number of each prescription. This information can be extremely important in times of emergency, especially in cases in which the child's care is being provided by persons outside the immediate family, or when other circumstances make immediate, direct contact with the pharmacist advisable.

Nurses are referred to current pharmaceutical information guides, textbooks, or a current *Physicians Desk Reference* for updated information about specific drugs. Common problems occur frequently in managing medications for this population.

1. Special care is advised to insure correct, constant dosage of liquid suspensions of anticonvulsant medications. These suspensions require careful storage and proper handling to prevent variations in the actual amount of drug given per dose.

2. These drugs are often inappropriately mixed with formula or solid food and given through a nipple. Since nutrition and loss of appetite present major care problems for this population, it is imperative that medication be given separate from food; with the caregiver's consistent firmness, most infants will learn to accept medication as it comes from the pharmacy, and infants usually respond favorably to a small drink of plain water as a chaser when necessary.

3. Use of a plastic syringe with the needle removed, or the new commercial, syringe-type medicine dispensers available in many pharmacies, simplifies the problem of measuring an exact amount of medication to be given. At the same time, an effective means of insuring complete ingestion by the infant is provided. The infant and young child will often suck the medication from the syringe. It is advisable that a separate syringe be used for each medication given; this precaution is a necessity when the caregiver's ability to correctly measure and administer the proper dosage is in question.

Preventing Complications and Secondary Handicaps

Preventing or reducing contractures, decubitus, spinal or limb deformity, and unnecessary mental deterioration or disturbances has been the focus for the medical model of care for handicapped infants. This area of health care is fully addressed in the section of this chapter entitled "The Effects of Health Problems in Handicapped Infants."

Special Equipment Needs

The kinds and numbers of devices for use by the handicapped person multiply each year. Sophisticated learning devices and adaptive equipment are products of advanced technology and assist greatly in normalizing life for the handicapped and easing the burdens of caregivers.

During infancy special equipment includes braces of many varieties, body jackets and other limb or postural supports, colostomy and ileostomy devices, cardiac and respiratory monitors, and ventilators, and the adaptation of infant carriers, household furniture, or sitting and standing devices to promote motor abilities.

Safety Needs

As the infant becomes mobile his safety needs increase. One element of safety will involve proper use and storage of special equipment or devices used in the home. Safety measures applicable to all infants include protection from (1) extreme temperatures, (2) falling, (3) mouthing of contaminated toys, foods, and floor surfaces, (4) toys with sharp or broken edges or pieces small enough to swallow, and (5) unsafe cribs and high chairs.

Handicapped and disabled infants require a long time to develop sitting balance and upper trunk control. This fact makes it necessary to be aware of the need for proper sized and stable sitting chairs and devices in order to prevent falls.

Use of automobile restraints is a relevant preventive measure often overlooked with nondisabled infants, and the need for this protection is critical for a longer period with handicapped infants. A safety-approved car seat should be purchased and used for the handicapped infant who often undergoes more automobile travel than his normal peers as he is driven to clinics, the hospital, early intervention programs, and so on. Of special note is a recent report from the Society of Automotive Engineers[12] which evaluated restraint systems used in transportation of handicapped children. The report points out that neither traditional nor specially constructed wheelchairs have been designed to provide impact protection. Padded seat belts keep the child in the wheelchair during an accident but do not prevent the two most common head and spinal injuries associated with impact. Upper torso restraints are required in order to prevent excessive head excursion and torso flexion.

Parents of handicapped infants should be counseled about the need for the use of an approved car seat at the time of first contact by the nurse. If an infant is later referred to a preschool service, parents and education personnel will need additional guidance in order to safely transport the young child to such programs and other essential services.

EFFECTS OF HEALTH PROBLEMS IN HANDICAPPED INFANTS: A MODEL FOR PREVENTION AND HEALTH MAINTENANCE

High rates of postnursery illness, hospitalizations, and death during infancy have been reported in studies of preterm, low-birth-weight infants. I have noted many similarities in health problems between this group and infants with discernible handicaps. Most medical and nursing textbooks report as health problems in handicapped children only those secondary defects or abnormalities that are known to frequently occur in conjunction with specific diagnoses, for example, congenital heart disease and intestinal malformation in patients with Down syndrome, seizure disorders in patients with cerebral palsy, and hydrocephalus in patients with myelomeningocele.

Frequent re-occurring infections, failure to thrive, organically based behavior disturbances, and sensory disorders and impairment are common health problems of both high-risk and handicapped infants. Recognition of these real or potential health problems and the impact of health status on the developmental capacity of handicapped infants has been limited. Many early intervention services have been formulated within an educational framework and little attention has been given to the basic needs of daily care that enhance the immediate and ultimate health and development of the handicapped or high-risk infant.

An intense regimen of medical and health follow-up care is recommended for low-birth-weight infants by the Good Start Program, Meyer Developmental Center for Developmental Pediatrics, Texas Children's Hospital.[13] A multidisciplinary clinic acts as an adjunct service to the primary care physician to assist the family in managing the infant's health and developmental needs. Early identification of problems and the institution of appropriate health interventions assures optimal health for infants followed in the Good Start Program.

In a recent study, Littman and Parmalee[14] studied 126 preterm infants to examine outcome during the prenatal, intrapartum, and postnatal period as well as the state of health through later infancy. They found that fetal and neonatal complications are insults and not injuries and that the impact of the complications was transient. A high frequency of illness between the fourth and ninth month was found, and those infants with a greater number of medical problems beyond the neonatal period were performing less well on measures of development administered at two years of age. Late appearing health abnormalities and illness had an impact on the progress of the infants or at least were a reflection of developmental performance. These findings would indicate a need for close health surveillance for high-risk and vulnerable infants, as well as for infants with identifiable handicaps.

The model in Figure 1-1 presents the health problems manifested in most handicapped infants in the sequence of their appearance and suggests the cyclical nature of the health deviancies and their effects on the infant. For the most part, these problems are preventable when the health status of the infant is closely monitored, and they are at least partially remediable when recognized and treated early. The three steps of the cycle demonstrate the interrelationships of these health problems with one another and the additive and cumulative effects of these problems as major contributors to family and maternal (caregiver) stress.

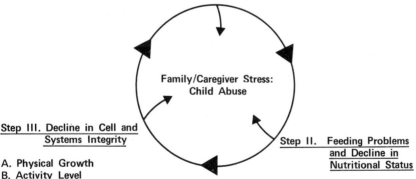

Step I. Pathology

    A. Initial — Structural, Functional, and/or Metabolic Abnormality

    B. Secondary — added handicaps, complications and/or chronic illness

Family/Caregiver Stress: Child Abuse

Step III. Decline in Cell and Systems Integrity

A. Physical Growth
B. Activity Level
C. Susceptibility to Infection/Illness
D. Elimination
E. Skin Care
F. Oral Health
G. Biorhythms, Response Levels
H. Vision Abnormalities
I. Reduced Appetite

Step II. Feeding Problems and Decline in Nutritional Status

FIGURE 1-1. The effects of health problems in handicapped infants.

The first behavioral deviation identified with handicapped and high-risk infants is difficulty in feeding. Reduced or altered intake of nutrients and fluids produces a decline in nutritional status which, in turn, results in loss of integrity at the systems and cellular level. A number of health problems are produced at least in part by loss of physiologic integrity. Decreased mental and motor activity, increased susceptibility to infections, elimination problems, decreased oral health, and loss of appetite are factors that singly or in combination further reduce cellular and systems integrity. These problems have an additive effect and tend to worsen aspects of the initial handicapping condition by producing secondary defects and acute or chronic complications or by reducing the benefits of treatment and intervention regimens. Each step in the cycle stimulates and aggravates the stress for the family (mostly for the mother or primary caregiver) as they cope with the ongoing care needs of the infant.

A detailed discussion of the model for the Effects of Health Problems in Handicapped Infants follows. Information regarding assessment and intervention is discussed from a nursing perspective as the nurse has major responsibility for preventive and maintenance health care in community based services for handicapped infants and preschool children. The discussion follows the sequence of health problems as they appear in the model.

STEP I: PATHOLOGY

The pathophysiology of handicapping conditions discernible and diagnosed during infancy results in (1) neurophysiologic dysfunction as evidenced by abnormality of muscle tone, cranial nerve dysfunction, and other neuromotor problems, and (2) metabolic dysfunction, and (3) structural deformity (soft tissue or skeletal), or a combination. These abnormalities constitute the basis for diagnosis of a handicapping condition as well as the driving force of the Effects of Health Problems of Handicapped Infants model (Figure 1-1). The basic pathophysiology sets into motion a series of physiologic, functional, and psychologic responses that have an impact on the health and developmental status and well being of the handicapped infant and his family.

STEP II: FEEDING PROBLEMS AND DECLINE IN NUTRITIONAL STATUS

The first major effect of any one or combination of these pathophysiologic factors is seen in abnormal feeding patterns. If damage has been extensive, the handicapped infant exhibits poor suck, and poor or absent coordination of suck and swallow, and the infant is difficult to feed. Feedings require long, strenuous efforts that tire both the infant and his caregiver. Abnormal exaggeration of gag, bite, and postural reflexes complicate the introduction of solid foods and spoon feeding. These and other specific feeding problems and recommended interventions are discussed in Chapter 4. Both hypotonic and hypertonic infants show early decline in nutritional status as a result of problems with feeding.

Decline in Nutritional Status

In a series of monographs focused on clinical application of principles of infant nutrition, Filer[15] defined terms commonly interchanged and misused by health professionals—feeding and nutrition. Feeding is the mechanical action by which food reaches the mouth and is transferred into the gut of the infant. Nutrition refers to the nature and nurturing properties of the ingested materials being assimilated as food. A major emphasis for child health care professionals is knowledgable counseling of the mother about decisions that ultimately control her infant's nutrition and also limit or enhance his feeding ability.

Foman,[16] the American Academy of Pediatrics,[17] the World Health Organization,[18] and other people and institutions influential in establishing health standards for infants promote breast feeding for all infants. Human milk is both adequate in volume and composition for human infants and promotes an optimal growth rate. In the past, breast feeding has been discouraged or only half-heartedly supported when the newborn exhibited an obvious defect, such as Down syndrome, myelomeningocele, cleft lip and palate, microcephaly, or required specialized long-term care because of immaturity (preterm, low birth weight) or physical irregularities, such as multiple births, hyperbilirubinemia, cardiac or respiratory insufficiency. The rationale for discouraging breast feeding was based in part on the premise that breast feeding would heighten the mother's psychologic involvement with the atypical infant, which has been viewed as undesirable by some professionals. Physical separation resulting from prolonged periods of hospitalization has been another realistic prohibiting factor in preventing the development of normal lactation in mothers who otherwise would have pumped their breasts in order to maintain lactation and provide breast milk for their baby.

Advantages of breast feeding a handicapped or atypical infant include:

1. Added time for physical closeness, bringing with it the numerous tactile, visual, olfactory, and social experiences thought to benefit both the infant and his mother;

2. Development of a natural suckling pattern as opposed to the suck pattern necessitated by most artificial nipples. The optimal development of oral-facial musculature is facilitated by the act of sucking milk from the breast;
3. Provides the handicapped infant with the immunologic benefits available from human milk;
4. Prevents the adverse effects of deficiencies and excesses noted with artificial feeding that are known to stress the developing systems of the infant as well as affect his future nutritional status.

Teaching and assisting a mother to breast feed her handicapped infant is no more time- and energy-consuming than attaining nutrition with formula and bottle feedings. A single circumstance that could necessitate choosing formula feeding initially or as the infant grows is the mother's ability to assume total responsibility for feeding the infant. If family pressures and responsibilities are heightened or a mother's emotional response to the handicapped infant is initially negative, bottle feedings might be preferred. Because of the need for mothers to occasionally leave their infants or home for brief periods, an occasional feeding (every two or three days) of breast milk from a bottle is encouraged. Nipple confusion is a common frustration for mother and infant if the bottle nipple is never offered at all during the first several months.

Instruction about proper selection of appropriate nipples for bottle feedings is important in order to insure adequate volume intake for the handicapped infant. Difficulty in coordinating suck and swallow is exaggerated when the infant is required to suck as opposed to the natural process of suckling as is required when he draws milk from the breast. Several commercial nipples are especially difficult for the handicapped infant to manage; the nipples with a short shaft do not allow the infant to pull the nipple far enough into his mouth and compress it slightly between the tongue and palate. The too short nipple causes the infant to produce a clicking sound as the vacuum he attempts to create in order to suck properly is broken. A high-arched palate increases the need for a longer nipple shaft. Use of the NUK nipple is purported to simulate the suckle action of drawing milk from the breast,[19] and also stimulate development of the oral musculature in a manner similar to breast feeding. Hospital and public health nurses working with infants who have poor suck or oral-facial disorders involving cleft palate report success in maintaining and increasing volume intake by use of the Ross Laboratory Volu-Feed Disposable Nurser with a premie nipple. The use of cross-cut nipples for handicapped infants must be avoided, as this increases the likelihood of aspiration when suck, swallow, and breathing are not well coordinated. Plunger type nippled feeders for solid foods can also contribute to this same problem and should never be used with the handicapped infant.

A number of factors have prompted mothers and health care advisers to offer solid foods before age four to six months, which is the recommended age to begin feeding solid foods to normal infants.[20,21]
1. Poor weight gain.
2. Fussiness or extreme irritability, both of which are common manifestations in infants with neuromotor immaturity or dysfunction.
3. Feelings of inadequacy in the mother that are exaggerated by inability to comfort the infant as well as difficulty in feeding the infant. These feelings are enhanced by pressure from other family members and friends to offer solid foods as a means of calming or comforting the infant.
4. Unfortunately, offering solid feedings during the first several months of life remains a practice in hospital care settings. Parents have observed other infants or their own young infant being fed solid foods during hospitalization and assumed that this was the right thing to do. Nurses need to carefully explain all feeding and other caregiving actions to parents in busy hospital settings.

When solid foods are introduced, feeding the handicapped infant presents a new set of frustrations and problems that are related to both the mechanical aspects of feeding and the infant's nutritional status. Immature or erratic tongue movements, abnormal head and body postures, a hyperactive gag or bite reflex, and other physical phenomena make the feeding of solid foods stressful for the infant and his caregiver. A more detailed description of abnormal patterns and habilitative approaches is found in Chapter 4.

Lack of activity, increased periods of abnormal muscle tone, frequent hospitalizations, or illnesses of the upper respiratory system all contribute to an irregular appetite pattern for the young handicapped child. Preferences for certain foods are reinforced by harried caregivers. In order to insure that the baby gets something or enough to eat, whatever foods the baby will eat or drink well are offered more frequently and given in larger quantities as long as poor appetite persists. Unless offered regularly during the first weeks of life and thereafter, infants tend to refuse plain water and consequently may suffer marginal hydration during periods of acute illness or rapid growth. Hospital practices have erroneously influenced some parents of sick infants to believe that Jell-o-water or glucose solutions are preferred to plain water for their baby's nonformula fluid offerings.

By the end of the first year or earlier, the diets of many severely handicapped infants are deficient in protein, iron, bulk, and fluids. Even though use of iron fortified formulas has reduced the incidence of iron deficiency during the first year, iron deficiency anemia remains a common nutrition problem throughout childhood for many handicapped children. Resistance to the texture of commercially or home-prepared strained meats is a problem manifested by gagging or choking, which can frighten the caregiver enough to limit offering meats to the handicapped infant. Minimal ingestion of solids during the first year becomes an even greater problem later in life and contributes to other areas of health concern, including dental hygiene, lowered resistance to disease, and elimination problems.

Nutrition assessment is needed to ascertain levels of vitamins, minerals, basic nutrients (CHO, fats, and protein), and the volume of fluid intake. If lack of bulk is contributing to constipation, care must be given in advising the use of wheat products and other high bulk foods in the diet before 12 months of age. Consultation with a nutritionist is helpful in controlling severe constipation seen in infants under one year of age who have multiple, severe handicaps. In older toddlers and preschool children, use of grain products (graham crackers, wheat, barley, and other cooked grain cereals, bran products, or wheat germ) can help reduce constipation and provides excellent sources of vitamins and incomplete proteins in the diet. Increasing fluid intake is effective in keeping the stool soft enough to promote defecation with minimal straining.

Infants with congenital heart disease, various neuromuscular disorders, and other chronic diseases find it difficult to consume a sufficient volume of food to promote adequate growth. In these circumstances it is customary to use concentrated feedings, such as high caloric formulas and beikost. Not properly diluting commercial formulas or evaporated milk, and the addition of eggs or extra powdered milk to regular milk, formula, or other milk-based foods have been practices used to promote weight gain for severely emaciated handicapped infants and young children. If greater quantities of foods are consumed from a spoon in cases in which the infant cannot suck enough to attain needed calories from formula or breast milk, the solid foods must be selected with careful attention to caloric density. When the infant receives overconcentrated formulas or foods, hyperosmolality of the body fluids occurs. A high solute load is imposed on a functionally immature kidney, jeopardizing the infant's water balance and rendering the infant vulnerable to dehydration and renal failure.[22]

Renal solute load is composed of nonmetabolizable dietary components, especially electrolytes, in excess of cellular needs, and the end products of protein metabolism. When the solute load is increased, fluid must be drawn from the body tissues to provide adequate excretion of metabolic wastes from the body. Hypertonic dehydration can occur and is compounded even more when water volume intake has also been limited by difficulty in consuming food. Several foods should be given with caution to young children and infants, especially when water volume intake has been limited by difficulty in consuming food. These foods—skim milk, whole cow's milk, cereals, and most commercially prepared baby foods—yield a high solute load. When extrarenal fluid losses are high as in diarrhea, febrile disorders, and conditions causing an increased rate of respirations, these foods should be limited or not given at all.[23] Most nutritionists now counsel against use of skim milk and whole cow's milk during infancy, and use of cereals should be limited during the first year to commercially prepared baby cereals that are also iron fortified.

Consideration of the renal solute load in infant feeding is also extremely important in the following circumstances:[24]

1. low fluid intake, including feeding of calorically highly concentrated diets;
2. abnormally high extrarenal water losses, as in fever, elevated environmental temperatures, hyperventilation, and gastrointestinal upsets causing diarrhea; and
3. impaired renal concentrating ability due to pathology such as renal disease, protein-caloric malnutrition, and diabetes insidipus, or due to immaturity of the renal system as seen in otherwise normal newborns.

Dietary modification for handicapped or high-risk infants should be made by a nutritionist, nurse, or physician following a complete, in-depth nutrition assessment.

Caution and a complete nutrition assessment are warranted before feeding techniques are altered by physical therapists, occupational therapists, and other interventionists. When an infant's nutritional status is marginal or the infant is highly vulnerable to nutrition deficit or excess, advancing feeding skills must be considered less important than maintenance of optimal nutrition. The infant's nutritional needs supercede all other prescriptive, therapeutic, or developmental interventions. An example is illustrated from a case record:

Eric was a six-month-old infant with microcephaly, grand mal seizures, and spastic quadriplegia. An occupational therapist had seen the baby in consultation with the public health nurse who was providing an early intervention program for Eric. Eric had made no attempts to place his hands on his bottle during feedings. The therapist advised the mother to place both of the baby's hands around the bottle each time she fed him and to immediately remove the nipple from the mouth whenever the baby moved his hands away from the bottle.

When the nurse learned of the therapist's recommendations she requested that the mother delay instituting the recommended changes until a nutrition assessment was completed. The nurse used guidelines for infant nutrition assessment as provided through the local health department's WIC program. Eric's height and weight were found to be more than two standard deviations below the mean for his age, and the nutrition assessment showed deficits in both fluid volume and caloric intake. The nurse discussed her findings with the therapist, and it was mutually agreed that the infant's nutritional needs outweighed the need for him to maintain his hands on the bottle during part or all of his feedings.

Basic principles guide the nutritional management of the handicapped infant:

1. Nutrition assessment is based on physiologic and anthropometric data correlated with chronologic age. In contrast, feeding skills are assessed and programmed according to the level of neurologic development and functional motor abilities of the infant.

2. Because of difficulty in sustaining adequate volume of food and fluid intake, calories ingested by the handicapped infant must be efficient. There is no rationale for offering these infants empty calories and nonessential, inappropriate foods.

   During the first year the infant's major source of nutrients should be human milk or an iron fortified infant formula; no cow's milk or other animal milk should be used unless prescribed by a pediatrician or nutritionist. When beikost is added, only single foods should be used; combination vegetable and meat dinners or cereal and fruit mixtures are to be avoided. Iron fortified infant cereals, and meats, vegetables, and fruits are the only solid food additions necessary to maintain good nutritional status. Contrary to advertising claims of commercial baby food companies, desserts are not needed after essential foods are eaten. Exposure to starchy, sweet desserts is unnecessary and might stimulate a preference or expectation of something sweet at the end of a meal, a habit that handicapped infants can ill afford.

3. Plain water, sterilized as necessary during the early months, should be offered daily. In conditions in which renal damage or malfunction is a real or potential complication, it is essential that water intake be promoted early and maintained throughout life. This need is urgent in cases of myelomeningocele, sacral agenesis, and other degenerative neuropathies or myopathies that affect renal and bladder function, as well as in infants with urinary tract anomalies or dysfunction.

4. Care must be exercised when manipulating or redirecting feeding patterns or skills. Quality nutrition is always a primary goal and must be maintained at the cost of delaying advancement of feeding skills.

5. Food rewards for shaping or modifying behavior should be avoided with handicapped infants. Special foods should not be

given to reward desired responses, nor should food be withdrawn or withheld in order to shape behavior. Use of food in shaping behavior should be attempted *only* if all other alternatives have been tried and have proven unsuccessful. Concepts of behavior shaping are useful in advancing feeding skills and modifying diet.

6. Supplemental vitamins should be used only upon recommendation by a physician or nutritionist. Nurses should inquire about the use of nonprescription vitamin preparations when recording the infant's health history. Many parents do not realize that many commercial infant formulas are fortified with the vitamins needed by infants and usually supply total daily needs. Some families believe that extra vitamins will help promote growth or prevent illness in their handicapped infant; use of megadoses or single or combination vitamins can present special hazards to the sick or severely handicapped, debilitated infant. The American Academy of Pediatrics has warned against the administration of megavitamins to children with mental retardation.[25]

   Recommendations for use of a fluoride supplement will depend on the fluoride content of the family's drinking water and the type of formula given to the infant if he is not breast fed. Fluorosis is an unnecessary and potentially damaging complication for all infants that can be avoided by careful history taking during health assessment.

7. Certain populations of handicapped infants are prone to under- or marginal nutrition. Children with central nervous system (CNS) disorders, especially those conditions resulting in spasticity or hypertonicity, require high caloric intake in order to sustain growth. Infants with disorders that manifest a predominance of hypotonicity (Down syndrome, floppy infants, hydrocephalus, or neuropathy or myopathy such as that seen in spina bifida, or myotonic disorders), require fewer calories as their activity levels do not increase with advanced age at the same rate as normally developing infants. When cardiac defects, gastrointestinal abnormalities or disorders, or metabolic malfunctions exist, there are additional problems in maintaining adequate nutrition. In these cases ongoing nutrition consultation for the mother, the nurse, and the medical care provider is recommended. Special adjustments of caloric density or the proportions of carbohydrate, fat, or protein content of formulas and foods must be monitored by specialists knowledgable in management of nutrition during infancy.

8. Instructions pertaining to the proper preparation of baby foods at home should be discussed and supported by written materi-

als for those families desiring to avoid use of commercially prepared infant foods.

STEP III: DECLINE IN CELL AND SYSTEM INTEGRITY

Physical Growth

Several factors are known to influence physical growth including heredity, neural and hormonal controls, nutrition, disease, and environmental factors such as socioeconomic class, emotional stress, season, and climate. Reduced rates of growth in all parameters have been noted as a common finding in studies of handicapped populations.

Many studies have investigated the various factors thought to affect the common findings of short stature, underweight, delayed bone development, and frequent microcephaly associated with severely mentally retarded, multiply handicapped children. The influence of hormones, nutrition, and socioeconomic and cultural factors are relevant, but data do not support any single factor as the cause of a high incidence of undergrowth in this population.[26] Castells and associates[27] suggested that defects in the hypothalamus disturb the regulation of growth hormone secretion, resulting in stunted growth for children suffering CNS abnormality.

Studies by de Groot and Stutterheim[28] on 72 institutionalized severely mentally retarded children examined linear growth over a three-year period. The relationship among weight, bone-age, skinfold thickness, nutritional state, intercurrent illness, and antiepileptic drugs was determined. Elevation of chloride and sodium levels in the blood of these children suggested a slight dehydration and constituted the only frank biochemical deviations from normal levels. De Groot found no consistent relationship between length and any of the studied items that would support that other factors such as acquired or genetic growth disturbances, state of mind and emotional stability influenced linear growth. A differentiation between dwarfism caused by perinatal damage and the primordial dwarfism in cases of chromosomal disorders was made by Dooren.[29] Early or primordial dwarfism usually occurs without marked bone-age retardation, whereas dwarfism occurring later in pregnancy shows retarded skeletal maturation.

Growth of infants and young children with Down syndrome was investigated by Cronk.[30] A sample of 90 children with Down syndrome was followed for 36 months and measurements of recumbent length and weight studied. Rate of growth for both length and weight was most deficient during the first two years. About 30 percent demonstrated excess weight for length by 36 months; of this group, excess weight became manifest in 50 percent during the second year of life.

Failure to thrive is diagnosed when infants fall below the third percentile in height and weight for age. Organic disease, including central nervous system disorders or malformation, is a known cause of the failure-to-thrive syndrome.[31] Although the dwarfism described by earlier studies cited can be attributed to the etiology of a handicapping condition, improper dietary management, especially during the first months of life, can have an added detriment. Improper diet causes further limitation of structure, cell numbers, and functions of multiple body systems—the central nervous system, and skeletal, cardiovascular, gastrointestinal, and endocrine systems. The well-nourished infant with possibly greater intellectual potential is also thought to be less vulnerable to a congenital virologic insult than his less well-nourished counterpart.[32]

Maximum total development can only be attained with early recognition of the handicapped infant's extreme vulnerability to additional insults to physical growth and maturation, and with subsequent appropriate interventions to prevent illness and to assure dietary adequacy. Proper health management can minimize the deficits in physical growth caused by improper nutrition, repeated frequent illness, and inadequate hygiene.

Proper assessment of growth is necessary for identification of nutritional adequacy and the general well being of the handicapped infant. Growth assessment is primarily concerned with stature; other aspects of growth involve changes in weight, body composition, and maturity. Roche[33] found that in handicapped children factors such as feeding skills and unusual growth patterns may have more of an effect on dietary intake than they do on other children. As growth patterns change, nutrient intakes must be adjusted.

Anthropometric measurements, including length, weight, and head circumference, should be obtained at frequent intervals. Recumbent length is required on all children under two years. If nutritional status of the handicapped child is good, two complete measures per year are recommended.[34] High-risk children on special diets and infants with severe handicaps and questionable nutritional status might well require measurements once or twice per month.

Measurements should be recorded and charted serially. It is good to remember that most growth charts, including the National Center for Health Statistics (NCHS) forms, provide reference to percentiles of growth for normal infants and children. Horton, Rotter, and Rimoin[35] constructed standard growth curves for achondroplasia based on measurements of height, growth velocity, upper and lower segments, and head circumference. These authors suggest that similar growth curves for each of the skeletal dysplasias would be useful.

All tools used for anthropometric measurements should be in good working order: tapes should not be smudged nor torn (metal tapes are required for accurate occipital frontal circumference (OFC) determinations); scales must be balanced; and sliding headboards or footboards (of the Infantometer) should fit snugly and maintain right angles. Steps in measurement are given for both normal and handicapped infants.

    A. Measurement of the Infant's Length/Height (Birth to 2 years)
        1. Mount a yard or metric stick on a wall with a corner, alongside table or bench, or use the Infantometer (infant length measuring device).
        2. Place the infant in a supine position on the bench or Infantometer with the top of the infant's head against the top or wall.
        3. Straighten the infant out; take measurement at eye level, with the right heel flexed.
        4. Record measurement.
    B. Steps to Weigh an Infant
        1. Make certain the scale is accurately balanced.
        2. Have the infant nude or in a dry diaper only.
        3. Place the infant on beam balance scales and balance; read measurement.
        4. Record measurement.
    C. Measurement of the Infant's OFC (Occipital Frontal Circumference)
        1. Place the metal tape so that it covers the occipital protuberance and the ends come together midforehead, above the supraorbital ridges.
        2. After making certain the tape covers the actual circumference, pull the ends together, read, and then record the measurement (in cm).
        3. To ascertain an exact correct measurement, allow the tape to loosen, then reposition it and take a second (or sometimes even a third) reading.
        4. Remember, a single recording of the OFC can be meaningless. It is helpful to have the initial (newborn) measurement; a series of additional measurements are needed to determine a normal or abnormal rate of head growth.
        5. Measurements of head growth should be obtained periodically for the first two years of life on all children.

Activity Levels

Marginal or undernutrition results in changes of quantity, structure, and function in nerve and muscle cells that limit (1) the strength of neuronal stimulus, (2) the timing and strength of muscle response, and

(3) the recovery period for both neuronal and muscle structures. The overt behavioral manifestations of these impairments include limited weakened response to stimulus, reduction of self-initiated movement, loss of tone, and changes in skin color and temperature.

Sequelae of limited movement and reduced activity include the following:

1. Demineralization of bone tissue.
2. Predominance of prone and supine positions prevent the beneficial effects of gravity in elongating the thorax, which subsequently results in downward expansion of the rib cage and lungs, and produces mature breathing patterns.
3. Lack of muscle use in the limbs reduces the blood and lymph circulation to these areas, causing lowered skin temperatures in the limbs and limited metabolic exchange.
4. Limited movement of the trunk and limbs also reduces normal function of the gastrointestinal and respiratory systems.
5. Reduction in rich sensory motor experiences which themselves can stimulate additional activity and movement in the infant.

Mental alertness and response, already altered from age-expected norms because of pathophysiology, can suffer additional decrement, resulting in reduced response to sensory stimuli. This decrement of mental functions manifests as apathy, lethargy, and loss of affect with either pleasant or aversive stimuli. A study relating the varied performance of eight-month-old infants before and after treatment for nutritional anemia was reported by Honig and Oski.[36] Significant changes in scores for mental development as measured by the Bayley Scales for Infant Development were demonstrated in an experimental group whose hemoglobin levels were brought back into normal range, demonstrating that a single biochemical deviation in otherwise healthy infants resulted in demonstrable change of cognitive function. This same biochemical deviation is much more detrimental when the infant is already dealing with multiple chemical or structural deviations resulting from pathophysiologic change. Prevention or amelioration of biochemical deviations in handicapped infants can likewise enhance their cognitive, social, affective, and motor performance. A high level of alertness and responsiveness enhances the impact of specific environmental changes and developmental experiences and facilitates advancement in multiple areas of development.

Bax[37] reported results of a five-year study of an experimental health-care program for preschool children, which showed a close relationship between health problems and developmental and behavioral disorders during the early years. The children studied who had frequent infections were most likely to have developmental and behavioral problems. Handicapped infants are even more vulnerable to these unfavorable sequelae of frequent, repeated infections. Whenever there is alteration of the infant's mental or motor performance not explainable by environmental factors, an assessment of health status is warranted.

Careful assessment of motor function and body postures should lead not only to motor programming and correct body alignment but should also address the health implications of limited body movement. Monitoring the respiratory status, the presence of constipation, careful handling of fragile long bones, and preservation of body warmth are special interventions related to either the hypertonic or hypotonic infant who is essentially immobile.

Special attention should be given to assess nutritional adequacy and presence of undetected illness or injury. The latter assessment will include an interim health history including possible exposure to illness or incidence of possible injury, as well as a physical examination by the nurse or physician. Continued behavioral changes and evidence of illness or injury are indications for referral to a physician who can conduct a more indepth diagnostic evaluation of the infant. Fujimoto and associates[38] have reported significant health benefits in conducting a special clinic to manage health needs of young children with Down syndrome.

Parents, therapists, and other early intervention team members need to be instructed about the importance of ruling out an organic basis for behavioral change before assuming (1) that the infant is deliberately resisting care or special treatment regimens, or (2) that the infant is deteriorating or regressing in cognitive or motor ability.

Example: Allison was a three-year-old child who was totally blind and moderately mentally retarded. The team who worked with her in a facility-based service for handicapped preschoolers was perplexed by Allison's sudden vigorous resistance to placement of solid chunks of food in her mouth. She fought and kicked when staff tried to place small bits of cracker and cereal between her cheek and gum to stimulate tongue motion and chewing. Her level of compliance in other activities changed, and she appeared to be more socially withdrawn.

The situation worsened, and the team requested consultation from the preschool coordinator of the State School for the Deaf and Blind. A strict behavior modification regimen had been instituted with no success, and the team felt that the behavior was evidence of more severe retardation or autism, as the child now resisted all physical contact by the staff.

The consultant from the School for the Deaf and Blind had both a nursing and special education background, and she decided from the history that there might be an organic basis for the child's behavioral changes. With help from the staff, she used a flashlight to examine inside

Allison's mouth. Extensive decay in one tooth and redness and swelling along the gum tissue surrounding the tooth was observed. A dental examination was suggested. The dentist found active periodontal infection and several rotted teeth. After these problems were treated with medication and dental surgery, Allison returned to the classroom, where she continued a similar rate of progress as had been recorded prior to her behavioral change several months earlier.

Susceptibility to Infection or Illness

Owing to immaturity of immune response systems, all infants are susceptible to a number of infections, especially those involving the respiratory and gastrointestinal tract; this problem is of great significance to the handicapped infant. Factors such as diminished respiratory exchange due to lowered activity levels, the tendency to choke and aspirate fluids during feedings because of irregular suck, swallow or breathing patterns, or a combination, and the reduced integrity of mucous membranes of the respiratory systems due to marginal or under nutrition and subsequent dehydration make the handicapped infant vulnerable to increased upper and lower respiratory disorders and otologic infections.

Otologic Problems

In Down syndrome and other chromosomal aberrations, the oral-facial structure deviates from normal and the risk of oral-pharyngeal and ear infections is increased. Even though pneumonia is no longer the cause of death for many persons with severe handicaps as it was before the use of antibiotics, respiratory illness is still a common cause of repeated hospitalizations and illness for many young handicapped infants and children.

Frequent repeated bouts of otitis media with or without accompanying upper respiratory symptoms are prevalent in Down syndrome population. Otitis media affects many children during the first two years of life, and chronic infection results in conductive hearing loss, accounts for delays in speech and language development, and causes auditory processing deficits and disturbances in auditory and visual integration. Later on these children may also experience learning deficits, such as reading and spelling disorders.[39]

Several recent studies report a high incidence of hearing loss and middle ear pathology in persons with Down syndrome. Schwartz and Schwartz[40] studied 38 preschool-aged Down syndrome children and found that 60 percent of the children demonstrated otoscopic and acoustic impedance, evidence of middle ear effusion. Krajicek[41] examined 107 persons with Down syndrome and found a 60 percent prevalence of middle ear pathology in one or both ears. In addition, 41 percent of this series were judged to suffer from middle ear anomalies resulting in permanent congenital hearing loss. This group concluded that these anomalies had been masked by the presence of otitis media.

Sanger[42] used an extensive review of the literature to relate the influence of trisomy 21 on the embryogenesis of the human face to the high incidence of structural deviation that affects auditory function in this population. Factors that contribute to the high incidence of middle ear disease and other upper respiratory disorders in children with Down syndrome include absent or malformed nasal bones, which account for the flattening of the nasal bridge;[43] missing or smaller than normal sinus structure;[44] underdevelopment of the maxillary complex and deficiency in the palatal vault;[45] hyperplasia of the adenoids, and laryngeal and pharyngeal tonsils;[46] and brachycephaly, which is associated with abnormal muscle tension that contributes to the dysfunction of the eustachian tube and increased middle ear effusion.[47]

Early use of amplification has been suggested as one approach to minimizing the language delay and other learning disorders that may have mistakenly been attributed solely to the mental retardation of Down syndrome and not in part to early uncorrected hearing deficit.[48,49] Early identification and prompt treatment of otitis media and acute upper respiratory disease are necessary to reduce the compounding effects of disease and congenital hearing loss. In addition, adequate audiologic evaluation at periodic intervals is needed so that linguistic, social, and cognitive skills can be maximized by specific intervention actions.

Emphasis on the auditory evaluation is important, as there has been a tendency for young handicapped children to be subjected to multiple fragmented screening procedures, but less frequently have they enjoyed the advantages of regular, complete auditory evaluations. The best method available to diagnose middle ear anomalies is a combination of air conduction audiometry and tympanometry together with a pneumatic otoscopy. Cooperation between education and health professionals is required to plan, implement, and evaluate a complete audiologic evaluation. Cooperative effort thus assures immediate confirmation of conditions requiring medical care or other therapy and referral to appropriate services.

In all phases of service—prevention, early identification, and proper treatment of middle ear disorders—the nurse's role is paramount. Middle ear disease must be considered when ruling out causes for extreme fussiness or other behavioral changes in a handicapped infant; in some instances these behavior changes are mistakenly attributed to the infant's neurologic deficits or disability. The presence of infection, especially otitis media, pharyngitis, and other respiratory infections as a cause of extreme fretfulness should be investigated routinely.

Respiratory Dysfunction

The nurse is advised to monitor carefully breath and chest sounds of severely disabled infants on a routine basis. Even without overt symptoms of cough, fever, and so forth, these infants often have evidence of chronic respiratory infection as manifested by harsh productive or nonproductive cough, or by fluid sounds with inspiration or expiration. Breath sounds in infants are evaluated by auscultation with stethoscope, or in severely debilitated infants by simply placing an ear to the infant's chest or back.

Increased respiratory exchange occurs normally with crying, laughing, or as a result of limb or body movement. Bicycling the legs very slowly and firmly with deliberate effort to compress the knees against the abdomen assists expiration and can be helpful in attaining the goal of increasing respiratory exchange. (Note: This activity would be contraindicated in infants with known or suspected cardiac or respiratory problems or hip deformities.) Often therapeutic motor activity alone offers the postural changes and limb and trunk movement that will stimulate respiration. If not, the daily regimen should be modified to include postural drainage and the use of percussion techniques to promote drainage of excess mucus from the respiratory tract.

Other interventions for preventing or reducing respiratory congestion include liquification of mucus in the respiratory tract, which is promoted by insuring adequate fluid intake and adding moisture to the room air of the home by use of a humidifier during naps or at night-time. Keeping mucous secretions moist facilitates movement of thickened secretions by the infant.

When the infant does suffer otitis media or respiratory infections, either an acute or chronic illness, the parents' knowledge of the need for prompt assessment and treatment must be determined. Proper administration of medications, plus assuring proper use and care of humidifiers, croup tents, and thermometers, and maintaining nutrition and hydration during illness are important goals for teaching and intervention by the nurse.

Elimination

In etiologies producing renal dysfunction, parents must learn aspects of care that prevent or ameliorate acute and chronic infections of the renal tract, such as maintaining adequate fluid intake, measuring and recording urinary output, crede maneuvers, and so on. The family also needs to recognize signs and symptoms of bladder and urinary tract infection or malfunction. Abnormal vaginal secretions may signal vaginitis and are also seen as sequelae to prolonged dehydration or bladder and urinary tract problems.

Besides the problems associated with renal function and vaginitis, most handicapped infants whose pathology involves central nervous system dysfunction have some degree of constipation. Constipation may be manifested by infrequent bowel movements, extreme effort required to defecate, and passage of hard, dry pellets of stool. Infants with Down syndrome who have constipation related to megacolon may also exhibit occasional bouts of explosive type diarrhea and ribbonlike stool.

Constipation is generally managed through changes in diet that will increase the fluid content, carbohydrate content, and bulk in the diet, or combinations of the above. Use of nonmedicated glycerine suppositories may produce partial, temporary relief by stimulating a bowel movement, but this method should never be considered a permanent solution for constipation in infants. An increase in body or leg movements or more frequent position changes often helps. Prescriptive and nonprescriptive drugs such as stool softeners or laxatives may be used for temporary relief of constipation. The possibilities of fecal impaction or parasitic infestation should be investigated when the bowel or stool patterns become erratic or show sudden, marked changes.

> *Example:* A two-year-old girl with Down syndrome had been both bowel and bladder trained but suddenly became encopretic. Teachers in her preschool used behavioral modification techniques, but the child continued with loose, frequent stools both at home and at school. The mother reported no dietary changes or illness that would account for the uncontrolled, diarrhea-type stools. The nurse referred the child to the pediatrician for examination to rule out an organic basis for the problem. A stool culture proved positive; the child had a parasitic infection and was treated with medication. Within a week her bowel movements were normal and the child was once again toilet trained.

In myelomeningocele and other paralytic disorders, sphincter control is absent or variable in function. Innervation of the abdominal and perineal muscles that normally complement the peristaltic action of the bowel to produce defecation is also absent or less than normal. Bowel management routines are fairly successful in these children and ideally should begin during the latter half of the first year. During the first months of life, the mother may be instructed in use of the crede maneuver as a method of emptying the bladder more completely. Later on, bladder management for these infants may be accomplished by various techniques, such as periodic clean catheterization, crede following voluntary urination, or in some cases, surgical control through ureteroileostomy.

Management of ostomys, ostomy appliances, and skin care, and the need to provide psychologic support for the parents and the infant are similar in cases of colostomy and ureteroileostomy. Placement of the stoma and choice of a size-appropriate appliance are crucial considerations for infants requiring ostomies. Nurses can play a key role prior to surgery by helping the surgeon to determine optimal placement of the stoma through consideration of abdominal contour, areas of stress naturally created by trunk and limb movement, and diaper and clothing needs. Techniques for management of ostomies have improved through the past years, but adhesives and attachment straps or buckles are still difficult to manage with infants. Assistance from a local ostomy group or consultation with a stomal therapist is recommended for the family and the nurse who are unfamiliar with the new appliances and techniques of care.

Skin Care

Good skin care must be stressed early to the infant's caregivers. At best, toilet training is likely to be delayed a year or more with the majority of these babies; the severely, multiply handicapped infant will possibly be incontinent for three years or longer. Excoriation, skin breakdown with subsequent infection, or a chronic diaper rash are caused by concentrated urine; and because these children are comparatively immobile, they are unable to shift body weight and relieve pressure in order to maintain good circulation to the sacral and perineal areas. A preventive and restorative approach to care of diaper rash challenges the mother and nurse during the first year (and longer for the severely multiply handicapped child).

Three degrees of diaper rash have been identified, and the handicapped infant will likely suffer from one or more. Mild rash is similar to chafing and presents erythematous, raised areas on the genitals and buttocks. Ammonia rash is more severe, with bright red weeping papules which might ulcerate on both genital and buttocks areas. An infected diaper rash is the most severe form; the entire diaper area may become reddened, endurated, and painful owing to invasion by *Candida albicans*, staphyloccocci, *Escherichia coli*, or other intestinal bacteria.

Treatment involves care of both the baby and his diapers, and according to Alexander and Brown[50] has four goals:
1. To remove the source of irritation,
2. To reduce the immediate skin reaction,

3. To relieve discomfort of the area,
4. To prevent secondary infection.

Prevention of diaper rash begins with proper instructions to the mother regarding (1) care of the baby's diapers, (2) frequent diaper change, and (3) complete cleansing and drying of the genital and buttocks areas following urination and defecation. The use of disposable diapers may be a convenience for the mother, but many infants wearing disposable diapers have a high incidence of infections, including pyoderma, and monilial and miliaria rashes.[51] Proper washing of cloth diapers with soap products, thorough rinsing, and periodic vinegar soaks or rinses can prevent accumulations of ammoniates and soap residue in diapers. Special diaper care is critical for infants who are likely to be diapered for many years. As the child grows older and larger, his urine volume increases, and the long-term accumulation of ammonia in the diaper aggravates skin breakdown or ulcerations.

Ointments, creams, lotions, and other solutions have been advocated for use in protecting the infant's diaper area by providing a barrier that prevents urine and moisture from reaching the skin or for use in healing infected lesions or excoriated areas. Use of any protective or healing substance should be alternated with periods of exposure of the diaper area to the air, or exposure to short periods of direct sunlight. Caution is indicated in limiting the exposure of young infants to direct sunlight as the infant's skin burns quickly. A medicated, water-soluble ointment or cream is often prescribed for stubborn or infected lesions. With some etiologies, such as spina bifida and spinal cord lesions, circulation to the diaper area is impaired, further increasing the chances of skin breakdown. Gentle massage of the diaper area during bath time and at diaper change can stimulate circulation and hasten the healing process. NOTE: When the nonambulatory infant or child is able to sit, his caregivers must make certain that he is moved so that his weight is shifted at least every 15 to 20 minutes. Otherwise, the constant weight and pressure will contribute to diaper rash and more serious dermal lesions, including decubiti in the sacral area.

The skin of infants is far more susceptible to superficial bacterial infections, and reactions to primary irritants is a common occurrence. Infants are also more prone to develop erythema as a result of drug reactions or skin eruptions. Extremely debilitated or moderately inactive handicapped infants and those whose nutrition or hydration status is compromised are extremely susceptible to dry and flaking skin, excoriation, and skin breakdown. Caregivers should receive instruction in the observation, prevention, and management of skin disorders in handicapped infants. Preventive measures include frequent position changes, gentle massage during bath time, and the judicious use and choice of soaps for bathing the infant and washing the infant's clothing and blankets. Reddened areas, rashes, or evidence of maceration and breakdown should be reported early to the primary health care manager for examination and treatment as indicated. The use of a lamb's wool or sheepskin mattress may alleviate breakdown of skin over bony prominences and promote healing of excoriated or decubitus lesions.

Oral Health

Craniofacial malformations are characteristic of certain congenital disorders, including Treacher-Collins syndrome, Apert syndrome, Crouzon syndrome, dwarfism, gigantism, and many chromosomal aberrations. Along with cranial pathology there are various facial deformities that occur in developmentally disabling conditions such as maxillary hypoplasia, hypertelorism, micrognathia, and exorbitism. Cleft lip or cleft palate also occurs singly or in conjunction with other structural deformities peculiar to syndromes resulting in severe handicaps or mental retardation. Infants born with these disorders are usually identified at or soon after birth and generally are referred to multidisciplinary diagnostic care centers. Need for dental care and eventual orthodontic care has been well recognized in these cases.

A larger group of handicapped infants who have a need for close attention to dental development and hygiene consists of those infants with neuromotor dysfunction of the head and neck (cerebral palsy type disorders). Similar factors have an impact on the dental health of many handicapped infants:

1. Feeding problems that result in nutritional deficits or excesses;
2. Medication (primarily anticonvulsants) that causes gingival hypertrophy and hypoplasia;
3. Neuromotor dysfunction that produces (a) abnormal postural responses, (b) heightened sensitivity to intrusion into the oral cavity, (c) difficulty swallowing, (d) sporadic tongue thrusting, (e) retarded jaw movements,[52] and (f) hypersensitive, prolonged gag and bite reflexes—all of which affect eating ability and complicate oral hygiene;
4. Increased incidence of systemic illness, nutrition deficits or excess, and malocclusion all may affect the formation of the teeth, making the tooth structure vulnerable to decay or damage.

Normal dentition occurs between the seventh month and two years. General health counseling relative to dental care begins with instructions for prenatal use of fluoride compounds. The incidence of dental caries is significantly reduced by the addition of a ppm sodium fluoride to the drinking water, especially during times of tooth formation.[53] An appropriate level of fluoride is thought to deactivate the proteolytic enzymes before they can ingest the protein matrix of the enamel, and its role in prevention of caries is well accepted.[54]

When primary teeth erupt in infants with congenital defects known to be associated with oral-facial malformations or in infants with neuromuscular involvement of the head and neck, careful frequent oral examinations should be made by health professionals. Extra teeth, congenitally missing teeth, caries, malpositioned teeth, displaced and malformed alveolar segments, fractured incisors, unusual eruption patterns, infected periodontal or gingival tissues, or functional malocclusion are all indicators for early dental or orthodontic referral, regardless of the infant's age or diagnosis.[55]

Children with Down syndrome have a unique set of oral health problems. Periodontal disease has a high incidence in this disorder and is generally severe in nature. Alveolar bone degeneration is also common[56] and, in combination with periodontal disease, causes early loss of teeth. Dentition is often abnormal, and delayed tooth eruption, congenital absence of both primary and deciduous teeth, and anomalies of form and structure are commonly seen.[57]

Paradoxically, the incidence of caries is lower in Down syndrome than that for the general population. While studies have found the saliva in Down syndrome to have elevated pH, sodium, calcium, and bicarbonation concentrations, the causative factor for low incidence of caries and the high incidence of periodontal disease remains unknown. The need for early attention to dental hygiene is clear. Often measures of good dental care contribute to advancing oral control and feeding skills. Oral desensitization, brushing, and facilitating tongue and lip control can simultaneously (1) promote oral and dental hygiene, (2) advance control of oral and tongue musculature, and (3) consequently serve as prespeech therapy.

The effects of anticonvulsant medication on oral health include alterations in normal physical findings. Anticonvulsants cause thickening of the calvarium, coarseness of facial features, root abnormalities, stomatitis, and gingival hyperplasia.[58] In patients given phenytoin the gingival tissues become hyperplastic leading to (1) malalignment and rotation of teeth, (2) retention of food, debris, and plaque in the mouth, (3) unpleasant cosmetic appearance, and (4) production of malodor. Braham and associates[59] recommend that a comprehensive preventive and restorative dental program be initiated at the time that drug therapy is instituted and be mandatory for all diagnosed patients with epilepsy.

Ideally, intervention should be preventive in nature and involve educating the mother about fluoride, nutritional needs of the infant, and appropriate cleansing techniques after dentition begins. Special techniques that promote good oral hygiene serve a dual purpose, as these same techniques are useful in promoting oral control and prespeech oral competence.

Nutrition counseling should emphasize the importance of maintaining the integrity of host and tooth cells by insuring protein, vitamin, and mineral intake adequate to maintenance and growth needs. Preventing prolonged exposure of tooth surfaces to fermentable carbohydrates will reduce the incidence of dental caries associated with bottle mouth syndrome in young children.[60] Handicapped infants are vulnerable to this problem, as the period of dependence on the bottle for nutrition and hydration can be prolonged by physiologic and psychologic factors:

1. Physiologic factors include prolongation of abnormal oral and body postures and reflex patterns, and the inability to attain or sustain motor control of muscles controlling ingestion, mastication, and swallowing of both liquid and solid substances.
2. Psychologic factors include parental fears of reducing the quantity and quality of diet; difficulty and frustration associated with attempts to advance the infant to a spoon or cup use; and overuse of the bottle to quiet and comfort an irritable infant.

Both factors can be minimized by early assessment and intervention to remediate nutrition and feeding irregularities. As early as six months of age most handicapped or developmentally delayed infants who are nippling well can be started on the cup. Very gradual increased exposure to the cup daily can accomplish weaning from bottle to the cup for total fluid and nutrient needs by 12 to 18 months of age. When teaching parents, the need to avoid propped bottles, numerous frequent small bottle feedings, and the regular use of sweetened juices and sugar or Jell-o-water solutions by bottle should be related both to maintenance of nutritional status and promotion of oral health.

Dental care should begin as soon as the first tooth erupts. A 2 × 2 inch gauze or a clean washcloth can be used to wipe off teeth, ridges, and gums and the rest of the infant's mouth. By the middle of the second year many toddlers will begin to imitate tooth brushing. Caregivers should finish the brushing job, using a small, soft-bristled brush (no dentifrice is needed). The handicapped infant or child will probably require special positioning for this task. Water-piks are no substitute for brushing, as they only wash out debris and may choke and frighten an infant.

An early visit to the dentist, ideally by the end of the first year, is recommended for all handicapped infants. Instructions for use of flossing materials, disclosing solutions, and special care techniques should be demonstrated and given in writing. Dietary instructions should reflect nutrition principles applied to control of caries:

1. Follow a sound diet plan.
2. Limit the frequency of eating sweets.
3. Decrease the intake of sticky sweets; use detersive foods or brush teeth after eating sweets.

4. Use of detersive foods as appropriate for age and nutritional needs.
5. Use fluoride supplement as directed by a dentist or physician.

Biorhythms

Physical growth—change in body size, proportion, and composition—is a rapid and dramatic phenomenon during infancy, and maturation of all body systems during these early months produces physiologic regulation. A first major adaptive task of the infant is to establish regulation of physiologic cycles, that is, respiration, cardiac rhythm, renal function, sleep-wake cycles, and feeding patterns.[61] During the first six months of life, the infant's physiologic and behavioral responses stabilize and become somewhat predictable.

Bassler[62] has summarized the contributions of researchers into a timetable of physiologic rhythms in infancy.

1. A single circadian rhythm, the periodicity of electric skin resistance, which is an indicator of automatic systems activity, exists in the first weeks of life.
2. During the second and third weeks of life the rate of urine flow becomes rhythmic with heavier urine flow occurring during the day and lesser flow at night.
3. Body temperature does not show variations in a rhythmic pattern until between five and nine months.
4. At about five to nine months circadian periodicity in blood glucose level and in the constituents of urine and in urine flow can be demonstrated.
5. Between 4 and 20 weeks signs of a circadian rhythm in heart rate are evident.
6. Before 18 months there is rhythmic excretion of potassium, sodium, and phosphate; from 18 to 24 months a circadian variation in creatinine and chloride excretion appears.

Rhythmic variations in hormone levels occur in infants and are relevant to assessment and interventions for health management. About five weeks after birth, infants show a high level of growth hormone during REM sleep states.[63] Adrenal tides do not begin to develop until around three years. Since the rise in secretion of corticosteroids is inversely related to eosinophil levels, Bassler[64] speculates that the young child, lacking the rhythm of adrenal tides that produces a drop in eosinophils between midnight and 3 A.M., is at a disadvantage to ward off illness and noxious agents.

SLEEP AND SLEEP-WAKE CYCLES. Sleep serves several purposes. A restorative effect is suggested by evidence of increased secretion of growth hormone during stages 3 and 4 of non-REM (NREM) sleep.[65] Many neurotransmitters have been studied extensively in the search for support of a biochemical theory of sleep function and linked to sleep-stage production. Sleep is thought to be a time of information (sensory) sorting, processing, and storage, linking its function to psychologic status. Studies of sleep deprivation in adults found disorientation and disruption of mental processes and emotional disequilibrium to be outcomes of unnatural or limited sleep experiences.[66,67,68]

Numerous research studies have confirmed a sequential change in sleep patterns that begins during fetal life and continues into adult life. Polygraphic records at all age levels have documented two major sleep states, active or REM (rapid eye movement state) and quiet, or NREM (nonrapid eye movement) state. A transitional state is an intermediate or immature state of poorly organized sleep, which is typical of preterm infants, newborns, and some abnormal infants.[69]

The functions of REM and NREM sleep are not fully understood. One study on the effects of sleep deprivation in the neonate caused some investigators to conclude that active (REM) sleep might serve to facilitate development of selected central nervous pathways, and that quiet (NREM) sleep might reflect the level of brain maturation.[70] A positive correlation exists between REM and quiet wakefulness in that the EEG is extremely active during both periods. High levels of mental processing activities are also occurring during both periods. During NREM or quiet sleep, alpha waves are more depressed.

As the infant advances in age, the amount of REM decreases, and by two years of age the child's REM-NREM sleep pattern resembles that of an adult. This period of alteration in sleep pattern correlates with the period of most rapid brain growth for the infant or child. The length of an infant's sleep cycle also changes; at birth, normal term infants display a 40- to 50-minute cycle, but by eight months the infant has a 90-minute, adultlike sleep cycle.[71]

One investigator has proposed a basic rest activity cycle (BRAC) continuous throughout the 24-hour day that is expressed both as active and quiet sleep states and as waxing and waning of attention during wake periods.[72] BRAC is described as being a function of the central nervous system, and the known relationship of neurophysiology in controlling sleep and wake states supports this position.

For sleep to be of maximum benefit it must be synchronized with the biologic clock, that is, when body temperature oscillations are not synchronous with imposed sleep-wake cycles, sleep is poorest in quality.[73] Investigations have shown that resynchronization can occur and is accomplished in three to five days time, and the resynchronization process is associated with chronic feelings of fatigue and restlessness.[74,75] A morning nap has been shown to be largely REM sleep, while the afternoon nap is dominated by NREM activity. This difference could affect efforts to resynchronize or stabilize erratic sleep patterns, and suggests that a child or infant who is unable to sleep at night should avoid afternoon naps. Scheduling naps during the morning might assist in restorative functions needed because of stress or illness.

Information relating to the evolution of diurnal sleep patterns is relevant and useful to parents and nurses. Research of sleep-wake cycles during infancy by Parmalee[76] indicates that a diurnal cycle emerges in many infants by about five to six weeks of age. By age 12 to 16 weeks, this diurnal pattern is well defined and daytime sleep occurs during definable nap periods. An important maturational level is achieved by about thre~ months, when half the sleep is REM and half is NREM.

Early manifestations of neurologic function have been studied through investigations of sleep patterning. Sleep disturbances are common sequelae in premature infants and infants with central nervous system insult or injury. Feinberg,[77] and Goldie and associates[78] found less REM sleep in mentally retarded persons. Other studies suggest that the infant's inability to develop a normal sleep cycle and a normal sleep pattern are signs of neurologic dysfunction.

Barnard[79] cites criteria defining a sleep problem:
1. A child who has not been able to maintain an eight-hour sleep duration after three months of age;
2. Any case in which parents feel there is a sleep problem;
3. Cases of recurring problems (more than three times per week) in getting to sleep for naps or night sleep.

Use of these criteria categorize a large majority of handicapped infants as problem sleepers. Parents report common concerns; the handicapped infant is resistant to night sleep or fails to sleep through the night; his daytime naps are erratic in length and frequency; he goes to sleep at night very late and wakens early; and he wakens and fusses many times each night.

Assessment of sleep patterns can be partially achieved by use of the Sleep Activity Record produced by the Nursing Child Assessment Satellite Training Project.[80] This assessment process elicits information regarding (1) the infant's environment and physical arrangements for sleep; (2) determination of the exact nature of sleeping problems as perceived by the parents; (3) the outcome of the infant's nonsleep or irregular sleep behavior; (4) expectations of the parents for sleep behavior; (5) other sources of stress to either the infant or the mother or family; (6) the results of previously attempted interventions; and (7) the presence of acute or chronic illness.

Only frustrations associated with a difficult feeding process are more stressful to the mother and family than stress engendered by problems related to sleep, or more precisely, to problems related to irregular sleep patterns of the handicapped infant. It is usually the mother who struggles to keep up her own physical and mental energy as she tests new ways to make the infant's sleep times more consistent with family routines. She is most often the family member who gets up at night with the fussy, nonsleeping infant in order to protect the sleep of the father, siblings, or others. A common outcome of these problems has been for the mother, out of desperation, to move herself and the handicapped infant into separate sleeping quarters as a means of maintaining order in the home at night. Besides creating unnatural stress on the mother, this solution adds undue stress to the marital relationship. I have had mothers confess somewhat guiltily that this practice also served to avoid the possibility of another pregnancy, an issue which for many couples can be an additional source of controversy and marital stress.

Nurses can intervene to help parents induce more normal sleep patterns for all infants.

First, the environment can be adapted to foster the development of normal sleep patterns and rhythms by use of the following measures:
1. Promoting quiet and darkening rooms for nap and night sleep.
2. Synchronizing sleep times by establishing a fairly strict care routine for feedings, bathtime, naps, outings, and bedtime.
3. Using special relaxation techniques such as rocking or stroking. Many parents will need assurance that these activities will not lead to spoiling the infant.
4. Producing relaxation in the spastic or hypersensitive infant whose primary postural response is one of extension by use of special hammocks to force a flexed body posture.
5. Swaddling is an ancient yet effective means of quieting or comforting an anxious irritable infant.[81]
6. Providing adequate covering is necessary to ensure a constant body temperature during sleep. The handicapped infant often lacks body fat, the tissue integrity, and normal movement patterns that facilitate normal peripheral circulation required to maintain constant body temperature. If his extremities become cool, he might suffer enough bodily discomfort to bring him from a quiet to a restless state of sleep, or it might even cause him to waken and fuss.

    The use of stockings under trousers or pajamas with feet attached is recommended. For many severely debilitated babies, the use of heavy blanket sleepers does not negate the need for several additional layers of blanket over the feet and body, and this is almost always necessary for the infant whose movements are severely limited.

7. Using the bed as a place for the infant to play should be discouraged. Hanging toys or mobiles should be used in the areas of the home that will place the infant in the center of family activity during his waking times. In other words, he should learn to associate his bed with sleep. A certain blanket, toy, or fuzzy animal that accompanies the bed routine (both nap and night sleep) can reinforce the sameness of these experiences and help establish routine. A small, semifirm stuffed animal or toy placed at the infant's head or placed along the back for support gives the very young or small infant something to lean into and can provide the security of object contact that seems to facilitate sleep and comfort.
8. Establishing a pattern for sleep-rest cycles is facilitated by ensuring consistency of the sleeping area and sleep surface. Naps in usual play- or awake-time areas, for example, the infant seat, floor, or playpen, should be discouraged.

An important step in counseling parents and finding solutions to a handicapped infant's extreme sleep problems is helping parents to realize and accept the following:

1. Some crying or nonsleep that does not respond to any maneuvers or interventions will lessen as maturation occurs;
2. The behavior, that is, irregular sleep patterns, may be a result of the pathophysiology and is unrelated to the quality or quantity of care that is given.

Professionals attempting to provide early intervention services or to develop therapeutic regimens or in any way to intervene with an infant must remember the infant's basic needs. The intervener must insure that the intensity, timing, and organization of interventions support physiologic growth and biorhythm patterns—naptimes, feeding times, fussy periods, and alert-quiet periods.

Response Patterns

TEMPERAMENT. Studies of infant temperament are relevant to handicapped infants, especially those with CNS dysfunction. Three primary categories of behavioral response or temperament have been described by Thomas and Chess:[82] the easy going child, the slow-to-warm-up child, and the difficult child. In general terms, the difficult child evidences (a) high activity levels; (b) unpredictable and arhythmic functions, including sleep-wake cycles, feeding patterns, and elimination schedules; (c) intense reactions to stimuli and a low threshold of responsiveness; (d) a generally unfriendly mood, which makes him less adaptable to new or altered situations; and (e) high distractability, with a shortened attention span and persistent responses. These characteristics tax the patience and understanding of the most adequate parents and caregivers. It is important to recognize the similarity of the above behaviors to those seen in children with suspect or known neurologic dysfunction or dysmaturity. The infant who suffers from organic insult or injury and who also brings a genetic repertoire of behaviors characterizing him as a difficult child in the framework of the Thomas and Chess studies is at double risk for behavioral-interaction disorders and difficulty in social adjustments.

In 1977, Chess investigated temperament and the handicapped child.[83] The first investigation was a longitudinal study involving 68 premature children with congenital rubella. The later study found that sensory impaired, that is, deaf-blind or hearing impaired children, exhibited behaviors suggestive of a difficult temperament. Chess suggested that management and educational plans for multihandicapped children should determine the basic temperamental patterns before intervention, and that assessment of temperament should take an equal place in the list of factors to be studied in arranging to meet the needs of the individual child.

The infant with multiple severe handicaps who evidences generalized CNS damage or dysfunction is often extremely irritable and difficult to comfort and nurture. The high-pitched cry, so commonly considered to be a sign of CNS damage during the newborn period, might not alter or lessen during the first weeks and months to a more discriminative response as is seen in normally developing infants. The changes in response that occur with normal development allow the infant to give increasingly clear signals and cues indicating his need for food or comfort to his caregiver. Neuromotor deficit or dysfunction prevents or delays the emergence of clear signals and cues by many handicapped infants.

Following care (feeding, diaper change, or other comforting measures), the same intense, piercing high-pitched cry often persists unrelentlessly in the severely damaged baby, which heightens the mother's frustration and prevents her from experiencing the satisfaction of meeting her infant's needs. Consequently, as discussed previously, difficulty in feeding alters the nutrient or volume intake significantly for these same infants, further compounding the infant's inability to be soothed and comforted by satiation with food and a successful feeding experience.

Supportive counseling can help parents understand that the infant's behavior is caused by organic damage or malfunction. Meanwhile, the nurse must work with the family to test out the effect of various, active comfort or quieting measures.

1. Preventing random flailing motions of the arms and legs can help calm some hypersensitive infants. This is accomplished

by gently yet firmly securing the baby's arms and hands close to his body with hands or by use of a swaddling technique.

2. Encouraging the infant to suck or chew on his fist or fingers has a calming effect and can assist some infants to gain self-control. This is preferable to the introduction of a pacifier as a means of promoting nonnutritive, comforting suck, as finger sucking or chewing actions can be initiated or discontinued as the *infant* perceives the need for and the reward of this comforting maneuver.

3. Rocking motions, especially in concert with swaddling, may comfort the infant. A hammock device can assist by maintaining a posture of flexion and even body support.

4. Although seemingly impossible in some situations, promoting a calm approach in manner and voice helps some infants gain and sustain control.

5. Controlling sudden, intense auditory, visual, or kinesthetic stimuli is indicated for the irritable, hypersensitive infant.

6. Adhering to a strict daily routine may help stabilize responses as the handicapped infant achieves neurologic maturation.

7. Allowing and encouraging parents to express the intense feelings triggered by an irritable, nonconsolable infant can be helpful. To know that feelings of anger, frustration, guilt, and helplessness are expected and normal in these situations is comforting to some degree.

A more tangible help might be to provide respite care for the infant, through assistance of family, friends, neighbors, or respite care services in the community. All too often, referral for respite care or support from professionals is given only after a crisis situation is identified. Prevention of a care crisis should be part of the total family care plan whenever staff identify stresses and problems created from coping with a difficult or impossible-to-console infant. A preventive approach should actively support and assist families to find and use respite care services on a regular, planned basis. Where community respite services are unavailable or limited, nurses can help facilitate the development and expansion of respite care systems.

Use of respite care facilities and support systems are hampered by a mother's inability to separate from her handicapped infant. Difficulty in allowing others to participate in infant care is a natural response of any mother, which is complicated by the multiple, complex care needs of a handicapped infant. These situations can be alleviated by careful observations of the mother's readiness to begin separation, and by support and deliberate programming with both parents and the total family, which is designed to achieve separation over a period of time through a systematic approach which gradually increases participation in care of the infant by others.

Coyner[84] reported a sequence of maternal behaviors that signals readiness and ability of a mother to separate from her infant; this sequence of observable behaviors also demonstrates the level of confidence achieved by a mother in her own care-giving skills. The sequence described is recommended as a guide to observations, counseling, and family interventions that can reduce separation anxiety for the mother during the early periods of infancy, and promote the child's ability to separate from his mother at a later age.

Maternal-Infant Separation Process

Ability of the mother to separate from her infant is indicated when the mother voluntarily shares the care of the infant with others, including the father, siblings, grandparents, close friends, or babysitters.

First Phase: During this phase the mother is present or immediately available during periods of shared caregiving. The sharing of caregiving activities is listed in the sequence of occurrence. It is imperative to note that those activities shared first require a small amount of sharing or caregiving time from the new caregiver, offer limited periods of new caregiver-infant interactions, and also require little infant care knowledge or skill from the new caregiver.

First Shared Activity: Holding and playing (looking, smiling, reciprocal verbalizations, and so forth) during waking, alert periods.

Second Shared Activity: Changing the diaper or other clothing.

Third Shared Activity: Bathing. This activity is generally first shared with the father, grandmother, or other adult persons and is seldom shared with siblings or less experienced caregivers.

Fourth Shared Activity: Feeding. This is the caregiving action most difficult for the mother or primary caregiver to share, especially when the infant is atypical or is a difficult-to-feed infant. When the primary caregiver is confident about sharing this activity with at least one other significant person, she is usually ready to try out brief periods of care by others when she is not present, which moves her into the Second Phase of the Maternal-Infant Separation Process.

Second Phase: Now the mother is able to remove herself physically from the infant so that one or more of the above Phase One activities are carried out by someone else during her absence.

First subphase action: Short periods of partial care by others, excluding feeding. If at all possible, the mother will arrange the period of absence to coincide with periods of sleep or minimal care needs by the infant.

Second subphase action: Short periods of total care by others, including feeding. The others involved in giving the infant care will be one or two select, trusted adults, often the father, grandmother, an aunt of the infant, or a trusted friend or neighbor of the mother.

Third subphase action: Longer, infrequent total care by close family members. Now the mother is able to leave the infant in the care of others overnight, or throughout the daytime periods.

Fourth subphase action: Longer, or infrequent total care by persons outside the immediate or extended family. The mother of a handicapped infant might not reach this phase until the child is beyond infancy.

Fifth subphase action: Regular periods of total care by persons outside the regular family. The young child and his mother can now enter into classrooms, daycare settings, regular babysitting experiences, and so on, with minimal separation anxiety exhibited by either member of the dyad.

Ideally, the possible need for respite care should be suggested to the mother before the need is indicated. Reality often dictates that respite care is indicated because of a family crisis; any movement along the two phases and the opportunity for the mother to share the infant's caregiving *before* a crisis should make a forced separation or respite experience less traumatic for the mother and her infant.

Vision Abnormalities

Handicapped infants have a high incidence of eye and visual disorders. Neuromotor dysfunction produces eye muscle imbalance in infants with generalized hypertonic or hypotonic function, resulting in strabismus, esotropia, exotropia, or nystagmus. Congenital cataracts and glaucoma, palpebral colobomas, blepharophimosis, dermoid cysts, and ptosis are abnormalities peculiar to selected congenital defects. In infants and children with cerebral palsy, athetoids have a higher incidence of hyperopia.[85] Early recognition of congenital cataracts and glaucoma and other diseases of the eye structure (keratitis, optic neuritis, iritis, and choroidoretinitis) is important as techniques of treatment are effective.

Cortical blindness is a diagnosis given severely handicapped infants when functional tests and diagnostic examinations fail to confirm visual response. Many infants termed cortically blind during the neonatal period have shown gradual increased (though limited) visual responses within the first 4 to 6 months.

The presence of a visual disorder by itself constitutes a handicap; combined with other multiple complex disorders, loss of vision can reduce the infant's capacity for social, emotional, motor, and intellectual development. It is imperative that problems relating to vision be identified and treated early and that ongoing monitoring of all aspects of vision be provided.

Whenever central nervous system disease is suspected, a diagnostic evaluation should include an ophthalmologic examination. Reports of visual function should be shared with the ophthalmologist by early intervention staff and parents at the time of initial diagnosis and in follow-up visits. Routine health examinations by the nurse or physician should include careful inspection of the eye structure as well as detailed functional assessments of vision.

Screening tests for the older infant, toddler, and preschooler should ascertain visual acuity, hyperopia, myopia, color blindness, muscle imbalance, and depth perception.[86] Empirical observations of visual function by parents and professional staff are often accurate in determining the visual abilities of handicapped infants; however, these observations are not substitutes for periodic ophthalmologic evaluation when problems of vision or visual structures are suspected or confirmed.

Use of low vision tools and techniques for visually impaired infants can aid in optimal developmental learning and experiences. If refraction is recommended, parents and staff should be aware of the need to maintain proper position of the infant's glasses. Only a small portion in the center of the lens is exactly correct for the infant's prescription. If the glasses are not positioned so the infant looks though this area, his view is distorted and lack of proper correction results; this situation usually causes the infant or child to actively reject glasses. Rejection is also triggered when an elastic strap that is attached to the ear piece of the glasses and around the back of the head to hold the glasses in place is too tight, thus causing the ear pieces to press into the side of the infant's head above each ear. The area above the ear should be examined frequently for evidence of excess pressure from the glasses, including redness or open sores.

Besides evaluating proper position of glasses and observing functional vision, the health professional should be prepared to instruct parents and staff about the following:

1. Etiology and prognosis of visual disorders or abnormalities.
2. Special therapeutic needs, including medication, patching, surgical interventions, and follow-up examinations.
3. Appropriate screening and diagnostic techniques.
4. Referral sources.

Reduced Appetite

Reduction of appetite is promulgated by a combination of previously discussed factors—inadequate nutrient intake, repeated or chronic illness, decreased activity levels, and general neuromotor dysfunction. Anorexia compounds the problem of dietary management by further increasing nutrient deficits which serve to refuel the cycle of additional health problems for the handicapped infant. When the cycle continues with minimal or inadequate interventions, the rate of secondary complications and additional pathology is greatly increased. Additional systems break down in growth or functional ability; secondary skeletal deviations are seen; there is additional loss of neuromotor control; numerous infections occur more frequently and become chronic; and the child is locked into a chain of health problems that become less remedial as he advances in age.

A SPECIAL CHALLENGE FOR HEALTH MANAGEMENT: THE INFANT WITH SPINA BIFIDA (MYELOMENINGOCELE)

It has not been the purpose of this chapter to discuss specific diagnoses or categories of handicapping conditions that affect infants. I have found that the infant born with a significant neural tube defect, especially spina bifida cystica (myelomeningocele) presents an array of structural and functional deficits that challenge the expertise and skills of health care specialists in many disciplines. For this reason, a brief discussion of the pertinent health needs of these infants is presented.

Spina bifida cystica, or myelomeningocele, is a severe handicapping condition, which is identifiable at birth and causes multiple handicaps from birth that require intensive health care throughout life. Infants with this disorder suffer total or partial loss of limb function, contractures of the lower limbs, bowel and bladder dysfunction, and other sensory impairments; up to 80 percent also develop some degree of hydrocephalus. Figure 1-2 is a model that illustrates problems of management of spina bifida and pinpoints the results of inadequate management interventions by health professionals.[87] In addition to the health needs shown in the Health Problems Model, there are significant health management needs peculiar to this disorder.

Approximately 80 percent of babies with myelomeningocele have hydrocephalus. Shunt systems are installed early to promote drainage of excess cerebrospinal fluid from the ventricular system into the circulatory system and with excretion via renal function. The nurse should know the type of shunt used, the drainage site and mode of entry of excess cerebrospinal fluid into the circulatory system, signs of stoppage or other malfunctions of the shunt system, and techniques of routine or special care, such as recommendations about pumping of the shunt reservoir or observation of both the pump site and other incision areas.

If medical management of the hydrocephalus is used (use of Di-

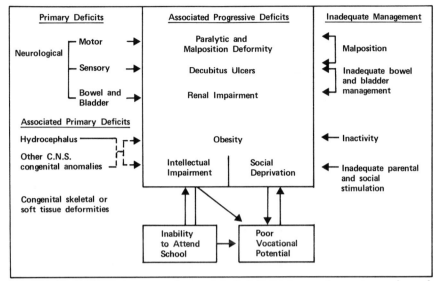

FIGURE 1-2. The primary and associated deficits in myelomeningocele and their relationship to the problems of management. (From: SWINYARD, C (ED): *Comprehensive Care of the Child with Spina Bifida: Rehabilitation Monograph XXXI.* New York University Press, New York, 1966, p 198, with permission.)

amox or other diuretic drugs), nurses, other staff members, and parents must understand proper techniques of administration, adverse side effects, and signs of drug toxicity. Regardless of treatment modality, the nurse must instruct the family about observations of the fontanels, correct measurements of cranial growth, and signs and symptoms of increased intracranial pressure.

Bowel management routines can be instituted from about six months of age, if mothers are willing and ready to commit the necessary time and effort. Glycerine suppositories or saline enemas can be used to establish a regular time to stimulate a bowel movement. Nutrition consultations regarding the appropriate additions of fiber to the diet are helpful.

Children with myelomeningocele often respond favorably to an early urine management routine. Intermittent clean catheterization has been proven effective as a means of routinely draining the bladder completely and thus reducing or preventing ureteral reflux and other renal tract infections and disorders. This procedure is taught early in life, and teaching and establishing a successful catheterization routine are responsibilities of the clinic nurse and community health nurses that are shared with the parents. Surgical intervention, ileoureterostomy, has been used to provide a means of urinary diversion and preserve functions of the lower and upper renal systems. Procedures to prevent diaper rash, excoriated buttocks, and decubiti as discussed earlier in this chapter are important for these infants during the many months prior to the accomplishment of any bowel or bladder management regimen. During the early months, urine and feces may continuously cover the perineal and buttocks areas, giving rise to excoriation, infection, and decubiti.

Special dietary instruction and nutrition consultation is begun at birth and continued on a routine basis in order to maintain hydration, assure adequate urine volume, and prevent constipation and fecal impactions.

Preparation for Diagnostic Procedures

Much effort is required to help parents understand the many ongoing diagnostic procedures experienced by the infant with myelomeningocele or hydrocephalus. Electroencephalograms (EEG), x-rays, computerized axial tomography (CAT) scans, intravenous pyelograms (I.V.P.), cystoscopy, and frequent blood and urine testing are some of the more common procedures that will begin early and continue throughout the life of the child with myelomeningocele.

Written guides that explain the tests and their use in comprehensive care of the child need to be written in simple terms and used by all members of the health team. Besides participating in the preparation of such materials, parents should be encouraged to keep a written record or log of their child's experiences and his response to these diagnostic procedures, medications, and hospitalizations. This information can be of great value to diagnostic technicians and physicians ordering care, especially if the family moves or there is a change in physicians or other health care providers.

The nurse is often assigned to work with aspects of team care that involve counseling parents. A national organization for families of children with myelomeningocele has been organized;* this group develops written materials and pamphlets regarding special care needs and home management. The University Hospital School in Iowa City, Iowa, has produced an excellent guide for parents of infants with myelomeningocele,[88] as well as a larger (binder) publication for management of the child with myelomeningocele.[89]

FAMILY AND MATERNAL STRESS

Family or maternal stress is evident at each point of the cycle involving the effects of health problems in handicapped infants and is com-

---

* The Spina Bifida Association of America, 343 South Dearborn St., Chicago, Illinois 60604.

pounded by the cumulative and additive effects of constant concern about maintaining growth and a state of well being for the handicapped infant. While interventions must be psychologically supportive and sympathetic to the parents' emotional and mental stresses, at the same time interventions must be action-oriented. Only one possible outcome of these parental stresses—child abuse—will be discussed; readers are referred elsewhere for information about the psychologic impact of the birth of a handicapped infant on the family.

Child Abuse

One outcome of increased maternal or family stress is the potential for neglect or abuse of the handicapped, atypical infant. Evidence of child abuse among handicapped or developmentally disabled children is cause for great concern among health professionals. Currently, child abuse legislation and services throughout the nation are derived from a social-psychologic model. This model purports child abuse to be a result of stresses and strains placed on relatively ordinary people living in our complicated society; this explanation accounts for occurrence of child abuse at all socioeconomic and educational levels. The day-to-day care and management of the handicapped infant taxes the physical, financial, and emotional resources of even the most stable, secure family.[90] Little wonder that recent investigators found a high incidence of abuse cases to be infants or children with mental or motor delay.[91-93] The abused child is in double jeopardy; in a significant number of cases he is already handicapped, and insults of physical abuse can add to his initial pathophysiology. In other cases, his previously normal developmental course is altered when the abusive injuries cause a developmentally disabling, handicapping condition; in these cases, the potential for additional, continuing abuse is heightened, and intense, long-term intervention by multiple agencies or services is often indicated.

Solomons[94] discussed three main factors known to be involved in child abuse and related these to abuse of the handicapped child.

1. Stress and strain on the family.
2. Unrealistic parental expectations regarding the child.
3. Emotional and societal isolation of parents.

Families already at risk for neglect or abuse prior to the birth of a handicapped or otherwise atypical child require ongoing expert support and guidance to insure the health and safety of the handicapped child.

Kaminsky[95] has demonstrated the interrelationship of risk factors and specific assessment and intervention approaches to the infant, child, and his parents in a model depicting the relationships of child abuse and mental retardation throughout the developmental cycle, which is shown in Figure 1-3.

In the role of patient and family advocate, the nurse assumes responsibility for the health and well being of both the infant and his family. This holistic approach to assessment and intervention should alert the nurse to factors that will place the child or his family at high risk for abuse. Interventions that help stabilize the family and its individual members as they cope with the handicapped infant and his multifaceted care needs should be given priority. Prescriptive programs designed to facilitate developmental advancement for the infant must be carefully designed and considered in the context of total family-centered care. Polier[96] used the term professional abuse to describe the failure of professionals to use their knowledge and power with the family to effect the type, nature, and extent of services received.

Solomons[97] proposed areas of focus and introspection for those intervening with the handicapped child and his family which merit consideration by all health professionals.

1. Parental guilt may be compounded because the parents have had thoughts about injuring or have deliberately injured the handicapped child.
2. The therapeutic regimen that demands inflicting pain or discomfort on the child places the abuse-prone parent in an intolerable situation.
3. If the professional encourages unrealistic expectations of performance by the child, this can enhance the possibility of abuse.
4. When parents become the therapist and improvement or change is minimal or is not possible, the frustration engendered potentiates the possibility of abuse.
5. Not many professionals really consider the total burdens placed on the total family by the handicapped child—financial, time, physical, and emotional.

The professional nurse and other team members are prepared to monitor the total health needs and well being of the infant and his family. Assessment skills and counseling expertise of staff can assist in the identification and appropriate intervention with abuse-prone families. Total health management of the handicapped infant will require the services of many health professionals. Nutritionists, occupational and physical therapists, psychologists, and social workers all share important functions in the team, but the nurse and the physician share the responsibility to coordinate services in such a manner that the health and development of the family and its individual members are protected and promoted.

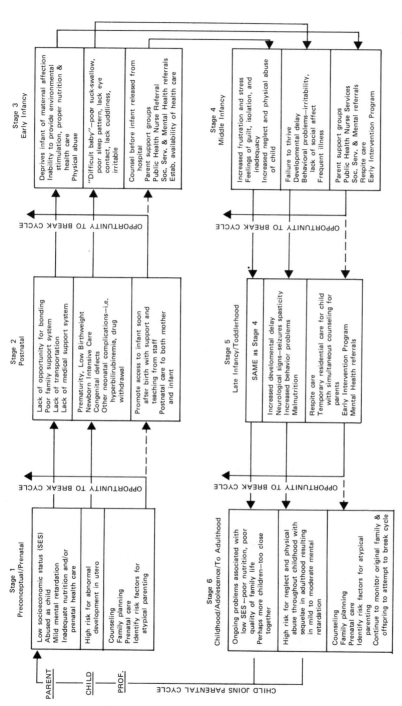

FIGURE 1-3. Relationship of child abuse and mental retardation throughout the developmental cycle. (From: KAMINSKY, C: Presentation, 3rd Annual Birth Defects, Mental Retardation, Medical Genetics Symposium. University of Utah, Salt Lake City. July, 1980, with permission.)

Other Health Interventions

Health professionals must be aware of all referral sources in the community that can bring health, education, and social services to the handicapped infant and his family in order to meet the goal of total family health and development. Medical care and diagnosis is available in most areas through state-operated Crippled Children's Services, Easter Seal Society Centers, Shriners' Hospitals, and Children's Hospitals and Medical Centers. Social service agencies can provide special assistance for indigent, migrant, and welfare families and protective and foster care services; in many areas social service agencies operate and oversee respite care centers and other community-based residential and sheltered work centers. Education agencies in some states provide infant and preschool programs in addition to school services for handicapped children. Other agencies that can be of help to the family include the following:

> Legal and advocacy agencies and groups.

> Public and private nonprofit organizations serving the retarded, handicapped, or disabled person, including local and state Association for Retarded Citizens groups, United Cerebral Palsy, Inc., Easter Seal Organizations, and the Spina Bifida Association.

Within their own professional organizations, health professionals can advocate for and support the rights and needs of handicapped persons of all ages through group action at the local, state, and national levels. Professionals who join and actively participate in the other special organizations for the handicapped can help parents, community leaders, and governmental units to collaborate in order to develop and offer services that benefit the handicapped child, his family, and his community.

A GUIDE FOR HEALTH ASSESSMENT AND PROMOTION: THE NURSE'S ROLE

Collaboration between health team members can be viewed from a framework that combines the traditional, pathology-oriented model with the holistic model of health promotion discussed in this chapter. The nurse functions in the following ways, based on documented assessments and the model of care and service goals of an early intervention program:

1. Carries out treatment needs based on the pathology of disability or dysfunction. In this role the nurse shares responsibility with the physician, therapist, and other nurses.

2. Prevents or reduces secondary handicaps and health complications. In this role the nurse works primarily within a nursing framework, sharing only limited responsibilities with physician, therapists, and other nurses.
3. Promotes the development and growth of the child and his family. This is a primary nursing function that will be shared with the psychologist, social worker, other nurses, therapists, and physician, depending on the setting of her practice.

ASSESSMENT

When a handicapped infant is admitted to a service it is recommended that the nurse obtain and document the following basic information:

1. A health history.
   Special emphasis will be needed to ascertain pertinent prenatal and postnatal events, including a general prenatal course, conditions of the infant during and following birth, and his physical and developmental status since birth. Special notation of any confirmed or suspected food or medication allergies will be helpful, as well as learning the number and length of hospitalizations and the infant's response to possible long, repeated periods of hospital care.
2. Physical assessment.
   Certain parts of the routine physical assessment are significant to a health and developmental assessment of high-risk and handicapped infants by the nurse:
   Assessment of muscle tone and skin turgor
   Assessment of height, weight, and head growth (the occipital frontal circumference or OFC)
   Assessment of sensory function—visual, auditory, tactile, gustatory, olfactory, and kinesthetic responses
   Assessment of dentition and oral integrity
   Assessment of primary and secondary reflex and postural patterns.
3. Nutritional status.
   Dietary intake, including an assessment of caloric and volume intake, is important, as well as documentation of the child's level of feeding skills.
4. Health care history.
   This information should identify all who have contributed to the infant's health care since birth, including the availability and use of routine pediatric supervision, specialist physicians, therapists, nurses, and other health professionals who have evaluated the child or made specific recommendations re-

garding health problems or developmental therapy needs. The nurse will need to obtain the necessary records that document these findings and recommendations.

5. Developmental assessment.

Some measure of developmental function should be attained and documented by the nurse. Use of a formal screening tool, such as the Denver Developmental Screening Test, or more sophisticated evaluations of function, such as those produced by the Milani Comparetti, Bayley Scales of Infant Development, Hunt-Uzgiris scale, or others, should be used by nurses who have received special instruction in their use.

6. Environmental assessment.

This portion of the assessment will examine the infant's inanimate and animate environment, according to Yarrow's model.[98] Subjective observations of the infant's physical surroundings are of value, or the nurse might choose to use the Caldwell HOME inventory to ascertain the quality of the home environment.[99] Use of the Barnard model of mother-infant interaction/characteristics can help the nurse document the mother-infant relationship.[100] Further assessments and observations will help the nurse evaluate other relationships in the family that ultimately have a significant impact on the infant and on the nurse's ability to assist both the family and infant meet their developmental and health needs.

The above areas should receive special attention from the nurse during her initial and subsequent periodic re-evaluations of the infant and his family. It is recommended that the health (nursing) appraisal be repeated and brought up to date at least every six months; all assessment data should be documented and recorded according to agency policy or professional standards of care. Health monitoring will be a vital part of continued nursing contacts with the family and might be done in cooperation with other team professional staff, if the nurse is employed as a team member in an early intervention program.

Use of a problem list is invaluable to the nurse and can provide other professionals with pertinent information to help them and the nurse formulate specific, relevant health goals for the infant. Each health problem that is identified needs to be noted on the list and resolution or remediation documented as a routine part of nursing care. Over a period of time this practice can help the nurse delineate her role and value to both the team, herself, and the family in the maintenance of the handicapped infant's health. Documentations of health education efforts with families and staff on a separate flow sheet will assist in planning and evaluating health teaching interventions.

INTERVENTION

Health guidance, as related to real problems encountered or the prevention and promotion of wellness and good health for the infant, requires careful planning and documentation in the health record. Health guidance should include, but is not limited to, the following activities:

1. Advising specific actions or offering anticipatory guidance regarding specific identifiable health problems.
2. Teaching or counseling directed towards the prevention of specific health problems, including complications of the handicapping condition or associated health irregularities.
3. Teaching or counseling related to maintenance of optimal physical and mental well-being of the infant and other family members.

Direct nursing intervention occurs when the nurse acts directly on, with, or in behalf of the handicapped infant or his family. Activities such as counseling, administration of a therapeutic technique, routine, or medication, adjustment of the physical environment, health education, assessments of physical integrity or function, referral to other health, social, or educational services, and communication with other care providers are within the realm of the professional nurse. Documentation of all efforts and of the outcome of nursing intervention—whether direct patient care or health guidance—is a necessary component of expert professional care.

Communication with other health care providers should be in both verbal and written form. It is recommended that the primary care nurse in an early intervention setting prepare a summary of her assessments and intervention plans to be shared every six months with other health care providers, especially specialist and primary care physicians. Howard[101] and other pediatricians closely associated with and supportive of early intervention services have articulated the need for a new definition of partnerships between the pediatrician and early intervention team members. My experience has shown that the submission of regular written health and care summaries to physicians by the nurse promotes significant on-going liaisons and has led to earlier diagnosis and treatment of primary and secondary health problems in handicapped infants, as well as better coordination of information and support to families of these children.

If the nurse is functioning as a developmental specialist and prescribing developmental therapy techniques, as well as providing health-related interventions, periodic reports should summarize both current health and developmental data. The summary should also note cooperative efforts with other members of the health-education team in those instances in which several agencies or professionals are involved with the infant and his family on an on-going basis.

REFERENCES

1. *Healthy People: The Surgeon General's Report on Health Promotion and Disease Prevention.* US Department of Health, Education and Welfare (PHS) Publication No 79-55071, 1979.

2. CROSSLAND, CL, DeFRIESE, GH, AND DURFEE, MF: *Child health care and "the new morbidity": Toward a model for the linkage of private medical practice and the public schools.* Commun Health 6:204, 1981.

3. GODFREY, AB: *A sensory motor approach for slow to develop children.* Am J Nurs 75:56, 1975.

4. BROWN, J AND HEPLER, R: *Stimulation—A corollary to physical care.* Am J Nurs 76:578, 1976.

5. CHALLELA, M: *The interdisciplinary team: A role definition for nursing.* Image 11:9, 1979.

6. TUDOR, M: *Nursing intervention with developmentally disabled children.* Matern Child Nurs J 3:25, 1978.

7. HAYNES, UH: *Nursing approaches in cerebral dysfunction.* Am J Nurs 68:2170, 1968.

8. BARNARD, KE AND ERICKSON, MP: *Teaching Children With Developmental Disabilities: A Family Care Approach.* CV Mosby, St Louis, 1976.

9. COYNER, AB: *Proceedings of Conference: Nursing Role in Early Intervention Programs for Developmentally Disabled Children.* University of Utah College of Nursing, Salt Lake City, 1976.

10. COYNER, AB AND HO, E: *POME, Fiscal Year 78: Child Health Conferences and Infant Development Program.* Bureau Maternal Child Health, Family Health Services, Utah Division of Health, 1977.

11. American Academy of Pediatrics: *National Health Status Goals.* June, 1976.

12. SCHNEIDER, LW, MELVIN JW, AND COONEY, CE: *Impact Sled Test Evaluation of Restraint Systems Used in Transportation of Handicapped Children.* Society of Automotive Engineers, Inc, Warrendale, Pa, ISBN 0148-7191, 1979.

13. DESMOND, MM, ET AL.: *The very low birth weight infant after discharge from intensive care: Anticipatory health care and developmental course.* Curr Probl Pediatr X(6), 1980.

14. LITTMAN, B AND PARMALEE, AH, JR. *Medical correlates of infant development.* Pediatrics 6:470, 1978.

15. FILER, LJ (ED): *Overview. In: Infant Nutrition: A Foundation for Lasting Health? The First Year of Life: Nutritional Needs, Current Feeding Practices.* Health Learning Systems, Inc., Bloomfield, NY, 1977.

16. FOMAN, SJ, ET AL.: *Recommendations for feeding normal infants.* Pediatrics 63:52, 1979.

17. Committee on Nutrition: *Pediatric Nutrition Handbook.* American Academy of Pediatrics, Evanston, Ill, 1979.

18. *Twenty-Seventh World Health Assembly, Part 1: Infant Nutrition and Breast Feeding.* Official Records of the World Health Organization, No 217:20, 1974.

19. *The Incredible, Insatiable Sucking Desire.* Reliance Products Corp, Woonsocket, RI, 1978.

20. FOMAN, *op. cit.*

21. ANDERSON, AS, PURVIS, GA, AND CHOPRA, JG: *The introduction of mixed feeding in infancy.* In Committee on Nutrition (EDS): *Pediatric Nutrition Handbook.* American Academy of Pediatrics, Evanston, Ill, 1979, p 139.

22. ABRAMS, CA, ET AL.: *Hazards of overconcentrated milk formula.* JAMA 232:1136, 1975.

23. ZIEGLER, EE AND FOMAN, SJ: *Fluid intake, renal solute load, and water balance in infancy.* J Pediatr 78:561, 1971.

24. BERGMAN, KE, ZIEGLER, EE AND FOMAN, SJ: *Water and renal solute load.* In FOMAN, SJ (ED): *Infant Nutrition.* WB Saunders, Philadelphia, 1974, p 245.

25. Committee on Nutrition: *Megavitamins and Mental Retardation: American Academy of Pediatrics Policy Statement.* American Academy of Pediatrics, Evanston, Ill, 1981.

26. DE GROOT, CJ AND STUTTERHEIM, A: *Aspects of physical growth and nutrition in severely mentally retarded children.* In MITTLER, P (ED): *Research to Practice in Mental Retardation, Vol III: Biomedical Aspects.* University Park Press, Baltimore, 1977, p 327.

27. CASTELLS, S, ET AL: *Cerebral dwarfism: Association of brain dysfunction with growth retardation.* J Pediatr 85:36, 1974.

28. DE GROOT, *op. cit.*

29. DOOREN, LJ: *Growth and Sexual Maturation in Cerebral Defects.* Unpublished thesis, Lieden, The Netherlands, 1974.

30. CRONK, CE: *Growth of children with Down's syndrome: Birth to three years.* Pediatrics 61:564, 1978.

31. BRASEL, JA: *The effects of feeding practices on normal growth, failure to thrive, and obesity.* In Infant Nutrition Foundation for Lasting Health? Health Consequences: Infant Health, Long Term Consequences, Part 2. Health Learning Systems, Bloomfield, NJ, 1977, p 10.

32. SCHEINER, AP, ET AL: *The study of children with congenital cytomegalovirus infection.* In MITTLER, P (ED): *Research to Practice in Mental Retardation, Vol III: Biomedical Aspects.* University Park Press, Baltimore, 1977, p 261.

33. ROCHE, AF: *Growth assessment of handicapped children.* Public Health Currents. Ross Laboratories, Columbus, Ohio, November/December, 1979.

34. *Ibid.*

35. HORTON, WA, ROTTER, JI, AND RIMOIN, DL: *Standard growth curves for achondroplasia.* J Pediatr 93:435, 1978.

36. HONIG, AJ AND OSKI, FA: *Developmental scores of iron deficient infants and the effects of therapy.* Paper presented at the Society for Research in Child Development, New Orleans, 1977.

37. BAX, M: *The intimate relationship of health, development, and behavior in the young child.* In BROWN, CC (ED): *Infants at Risk: Assessment and Intervention.* Johnson & Johnson Baby Products, Pediatrics Round Table Series, 1981, p 108.

38. FUJIMOTO, A, ET AL: *An evaluation of comprehensive health care in the management of Down's syndrome.* Am J Public Health 68:406, 1978.

39. ZINKUS, PW, GOTTLIEB, MI, AND SCHAPIRO, M: *Developmental and psychoeducational sequelae of chronic otitis media.* Am J Dis Child 132:1100, 1978.

40. SCHWARTZ, DM AND SCHWARTZ, RH: *Acoustic impedance and otoscopic findings in young children with Down's syndrome.* Arch Otolaryngol 104:652, 1978.

41. KRAJICEK, MJ: *The presence of congenital middle ear anomalies and otitis media in the Down's syndrome population.* Unpublished doctoral dissertation, University of Northern Colorado, Greely, Colorado, 1977.

42. SANGER, RG: *Facial and oral manifestations of Down's syndrome.* In KOCH, R AND DE LA DRUZ, FF (EDS): *Down's Syndrome (Mongolism): Research, Prevention and Management.* Brunner/Mazel, New York, 1975, p 32.

43. BENDA, CE: *The Child With Mongolism (Congenital Acromicria).* Grune & Stratton, New York, 1960.

44. GASMAN, SD: *Facial development in mongolism.* Am J Orthodont 37:332, 1951.

45. SHAPIRO, BL, ET AL: *The palate and Down's syndrome.* N Engl J Med 276:1460, 1967.

46. ARDAN, GM, HARKER, P, AND KEMP, FH: *Tongue size in Down's syndrome.* J Ment Defic Res 16:160, 1972.

47. COLEMAN, M, SCHWARTZ, RH, AND SCHWARTZ, DM: *Otologic manifestations in Down's syndrome.* In *Down's Syndrome: Papers and Abstracts for Professionals* 2:1, 1979, p 1.

48. BROOKS, DN, WOOLEY, H, AND KANJILAL, GC: *Hearing loss and middle ear disorders in patient's with Down's syndrome (mongolism).* J Ment Defic Res 16:21, 1972.

49. KRAJICEK, op. cit.

50. ALEXANDER, MM AND BROWN, MS: *Pediatric Physical Diagnosis for Nurses.* McGraw-Hill, New York, 1974.

51. WIENER, F: *The relationships of diapers to diaper rashes in the one-month-old infant.* J Pediatr 95:422, 1979.

52. KOSTER, S: *Orthodontic treatment of handicapped persons.* In WEI, SHY AND CASKO, J (EDS): *Orthodontic Care for Handicapped Persons.* University of Iowa, Iowa City, 1977, p 28.

53. NIZEL, AE: *Nutrition in Preventive Dentistry: Science and Practice.* WB Saunders, Philadelphia, 1972.

54. *Ibid.*

55. REGER, RH: *A model program of implementing orthodontic care for the handicapped.* In WEI, SHY AND CASKO, J (EDS): *Orthodontic Care for Handicapped Persons.* University of Iowa, Iowa City, 1977, p 18.

56. BROWN, RH AND CUNNINGHAM, WM: *Some dental manifestations of mongolism.* Oral Surgery 14:664, 1971.

57. SANGER, *op. cit.*

58. BRAHAM, RL, ET AL: *The Dental Implications of Epilepsy.* US Department of Health, Education and Welfare Publication No (HSA) 79-5217, 1979.

59. *Ibid.*

60. NIZEL, AE: *Nursing bottle syndrome: Rampant dental caries in young children.* Nutrition News 38:1, 1975.

61. STROUFE, LA: *Socioemotional development.* In OSOFSKY, JD (ED): *Handbook of Infant Development.* John Wiley & Sons, New York, 1979, p 462.

62. BASSLER, SF: *The origin and development of biological rhythms.* Nurs Clin North Am 11:575, 1976.

63. LUCE, GG: *Biological Rhythms in Psychiatry and Medicine.* NIMH, Public Health Services Pub No 2088, US Government Printing Office, Washington, DC, 1970.

64. BASSLER, *op. cit.*

65. SANFORD, S: *Sleep in the critical care setting.* In *Current Practice in Critical Care, Vol 1.* CV Mosby, St Louis, 1979, p 239.

66. KAY, D, ET AL: *Human pharmacology of sleep.* In WILLIAMS, R AND KARACAN, I (EDS): *Pharmacology of Sleep.* John Wiley & Sons, New York, 1976, p 83.

67. MOSES, J, ET AL: *Sleep stage deprivation and total sleep loss: Effects on sleep behavior.* Psychophysiol 12:141, 1975.

68. VOGEL, G: *REM deprivation III: Dreaming and psychosis.* Arch Gen Psychiatry 18:3112, 1968.

69. PRECHTL, HF, WEINMAN, H, AND ADKIYAMA, Y: *Organization of parameter in normal and neurologically abnormal infants.* Neuropediatr 1:101, 1969.

70. ANDERS, FF AND WEINSTEIN, MS: *Sleep and its disorders in infants and children: A review.* Pediatrics 50:312, 1972.

71. Bassler, *op. cit.*

72. KLEITMAN, N: *Basic rest-activity cycle in relation to sleep and wakefulness.* In KALES, A (ED): *Sleep: Physiology and Pathology: A Symposium.* JB Lippincott, Philadelphia, 1969, p 33.

73. Sanford, *op. cit.*

74. TAUB, J AND BERGER, R: *Acute shifts in the sleep-wakefulness: Effects on performance and mood.* Psychosomatic Med 36:164, 1974.

75. TAUB, J AND BERGER, R: *The effects of changing phase and duration of sleep.* J Exp Psychol 2:30, 1976.

76. PARMALEE, AH, WENNER, WH, AND SCHULZ, HR: *Infant sleep patterns: From birth to sixteen weeks of age.* J Pediatr 65:576, 1964.

77. FEINBERG, L, BRAUN, M, AND SCHULMAN, E: *EEG sleep patterns in mental retardation.* Clin Neurophysiol 27:128, 1969.

78. GOLDIE, L, ET AL: *Abnormal sleep rhythms in mongol babies.* Lancet 1: 229, 1968.

79. BARNARD, KE, AND DOUGLAS, HB (ED): *Child Health Assessment Part I: A Literature Review.* US Department of Health, Education and Welfare, Bethesda, Maryland, 1974.

80. BARNARD, KE, AND ERIKS, J: *Nursing child assessment sleep activity record.* In *Nursing Child Assessment Satellite Training Project Learning Resource Manual.* University of Washington School of Nursing, Seattle, 1978, p 44.

81. CHISHOLM, JS AND RICHARDS, M: *Swaddling, cradleboards and the development of children.* Human Development 2:255, 1978.

82. THOMAS, A AND CHESS, S: *Temperament and Development.* Brunner/Mazel, New York, 1977.

83. CHESS, S: *Temperament and the handicapped child.* In FRANKENBURG, WK (ED): *Proceedings: Second International Conference on Developmental Screening.* JFK Child Development Center, Denver, 1978, p 309.

84. COYNER, AB: *Meeting the psychosocial needs of handicapped infants and toddlers.* Presentation given at Utah Chapter American Assoc Mental Deficiency Annual Meeting, Salt Lake City, 1979.

85. DONLON, ET: *Visual Disorders.* In CRUICKSHANK, WM (ED): *Cerebral Palsy: A Developmental Disability.* Syracuse University Press, New York, 1976, p 287.

86. THERO, C: *Vision screening.* In KRAJICEK, MJ AND TEARNEY, AI (EDS): *Detection of Developmental Problems in Children: A Reference Guide for Community Nurses and Other Health Care Professionals.* University Park Press, Baltimore, 1977.

87. SWINYARD, C (ED): *Comprehensive Care of The Child With Spina Bifida: Rehabilitation Monograph XXXI.* New York University, New York, 1966.

88. HENDERSON, M AND SYNHORST, D: *Care of the Infant with Myelomeningocele (Spina Bifida) and Hydrocephalus.* University of Iowa, Iowa City, 1975.

89. WOLRAICH, ML AND HENDERSON, M: *What You Should Know About Your Child with Spina Bifida.* Iowa University Affiliated Program Publication, Iowa City, 1979.

90. SOLOMONS, G: *Developmental disabilities and child abuse.* Newsletter of the American Academy for Cerebral Palsy and Developmental Medicine 30:12, 1978.

91. ELMER, E AND GREGG, G: *Developmental characteristics of abused children.* Pediatrics 40:569, 1967.

92. SANDGRUND, A, GAINES, R, AND GREEN, A: *Child abuse and mental retardation: A problem of cause and effect.* Am J Ment Defic 79:327, 1974.

93. NELSON, K AND ELLENBERG, J: *Epidemiology of cerebral palsy.* In SCHOENBERG, R (ED): *Advances in Neurology: Neurological Epidemiology.* Raven Press, New York, 1978, p 419.

94. Solomons, *op. cit.*

95. KAMINSKY, C: *Child abuse and mental retardation.* Presentation, Third Annual Birth Defects, Mental Retardation, Medical Genetics Symposium, Salt Lake City, 1980.

96. POLIER, J: *Professional abuse of children: Responsibility for the delivery of care.* Am J Orthopsych 45:357, 1975.

97. Solomons, *op. cit.*

98. YARROW, L, RUBENSTEIN, J, AND PEDERSON, F: *Infant and Environment.* Hemisphere Publishing, Washington, DC, 1975.

99. BRADLEY, R AND CALDWELL, B: *Home observation for measurement of the environment: A validation study of screening efficiency.* Am J Ment Defic 81:417, 1977.

100. BARNARD, K AND EYRES, S: *Overview of the nursing child assessment project.* In *Nursing Child Assessment Satellite Training Project: Learning Resource Manual.* University of Washington, Seattle, 1977, p 24.

101. HOWARD, J: *The role of the pediatrician with young exceptional children and their families.* Exceptional Children 48:316, 1982.

Chapter 2

MEETING DEVELOPMENTAL AND HABILITATIVE NEEDS OF INFANTS AND TODDLERS

Raeone S. Zelle

In the first chapter a framework was presented for appraising the infant's level of wellness and meeting his health needs. It is very apparent why the subject matter rated priority. A healthy state is the underpinning of the infant's functional adaptability. In this chapter a framework is presented for assessing normal patterns of development and elements in a growth-fostering environment. This framework provides the background for assessing patterns that deviate from the norm, interpreting their functional significance, and planning intervention that supports the inner resources of the infant or child and his family.

The framework is an outgrowth of my study of neurophysiologic, neurodevelopmental, and sociologic theory and constructs and my professional relationship with colleagues in nursing and other disciplines. The framework is also an outgrowth of my interaction with developmentally disabled infants and children and their families. I have observed and descriptively recorded the evolvement of the development of these children on a longitudinal basis, including over a ten-year span with some of the children.

Over the years it has become more and more apparent that a developmental milestone is meaningless in isolation. The behavior only has significance in relationship to other behaviors in a dynamic context. When the focus changes from the end point to the process of development, one realizes that functional adaptations emerge from behavioral patterns that both complement and facilitate one another. Thus, development is an indivisible whole; no aspect can be singled out. It is mind-boggling to try to envision the complex interplay of microsystems within the infant or child reflected by the intertwined behavioral patterns. These behaviors both influence and are influenced by another intertwined set of microsystems within the family unit. The infant's behavioral patterns also have an impact on a broader interplay of macrosystems in his neighborhood, community, and culture, both directly and as a member of the family unit. There is a reciprocal impact on his behavior by this broader environmental milieu. This entangled web of relationships has been greatly simplified in a model (Fig. 2-1).

In recent years researchers have focused on the process of development. I have drawn from these studies and from my own longitudinal observations of a selected number of normal infants in order to describe patterns of development that evolve at different ages. The descriptions are provisional because there is much yet to learn. To prevent utter chaos, the patterns were unwoven. However, I have attempted to reweave them within the limitation of static words by describing how motor, oral and language, cognitive, and affective patterns are interrelated both within a stage of development and from stage to stage.

Researchers have reported phases in the developmental process, which will be discussed throughout the stages. Some of these phases are progressive and others are repetitive in nature; developmental patterns are, therefore, pictured in a spiral on the model. There is expansive movement upward as the infant organizes environmental experiences in a progressively higher order internal framework. There can also be movement downward to repeat components in the evolvement of an earlier pattern. Rood[1] identified three repetitive phases in the evolvement of a motor skill, which I have adapted somewhat. First, the infant develops enough stability to cocontract muscles in a teamwork fashion and maintain a position. For example, he assumes a quadruped position. In the second phase, the infant superimposes proximal mobility on distal stability; the hands and knees remain fixated on the surface, and the infant rocks back and forth with a movement of the shoulder and hip joints. In the third phase, distal mobility is superimposed on proximal stability. The distal parts move, while the proximal parts are dynamically holding; the infant alternately lifts his hands and knees to creep in a reciprocal pattern. As will be seen throughout the stages, the infant repeats this process over and over again. He moves through patterns of stability, flexibility, and integration. The same holds true for manipulative skills of a more cognitive nature. The infant stabilizes his banging schema (bangs better and better); he then flexibly modifies the schema (bangs two objects together), and integrates the schema with another schema (bangs a peg to displace it through a hole).

There is a directional dimension in some of the patterns, which is illustrated in Figure 2-2. Although the dimensions appear to be dis-

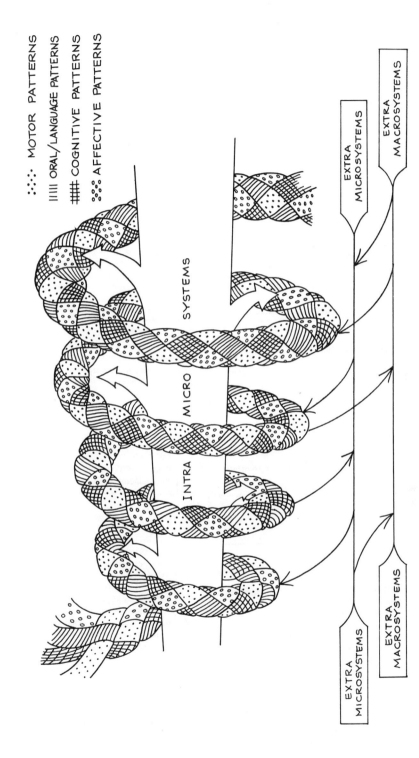

FIGURE 2-1. Intertwined developmental process.

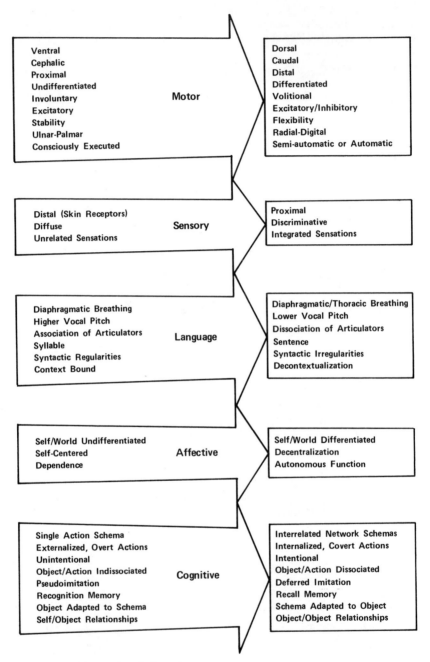

Ventral Cephalic Proximal Undifferentiated Involuntary Excitatory Stability Ulnar-Palmar Consciously Executed	**Motor**	Dorsal Caudal Distal Differentiated Volitional Excitatory/Inhibitory Flexibility Radial-Digital Semi-automatic or Automatic
Distal (Skin Receptors) Diffuse Unrelated Sensations	**Sensory**	Proximal Discriminative Integrated Sensations
Diaphragmatic Breathing Higher Vocal Pitch Association of Articulators Syllable Syntactic Regularities Context Bound	**Language**	Diaphragmatic/Thoracic Breathing Lower Vocal Pitch Dissociation of Articulators Sentence Syntactic Irregularities Decontextualization
Self/World Undifferentiated Self-Centered Dependence	**Affective**	Self/World Differentiated Decentralization Autonomous Function
Single Action Schema Externalized, Overt Actions Unintentional Object/Action Indissociated Pseudoimitation Recognition Memory Object Adapted to Schema Self/Object Relationships	**Cognitive**	Interrelated Network Schemas Internalized, Covert Actions Intentional Object/Action Dissociated Deferred Imitation Recall Memory Schema Adapted to Object Object/Object Relationships

FIGURE 2-2. Maturational direction.

crete, they coalesce in an expression of developmental maturation. For example, motor patterns evolve in a cephalocaudal progression from head to foot at the same time that they progress outward from proximal to distal and obliquely in a rotational direction—ulnar-palmar to radial-digital orientation of the hand. There can be a reversal in the direction as a response to injury and stress, for example, excitatory forces again dominate over inhibitory forces. The maturational direction can be opposite in two different systems. Whereas there is a proximal-distal progression of motor development, a parameter of sensory maturation (sensitivity to skin receptors) proceeds in a distal-proximal direction. However, a relationship was not found between proximal and distal motor functions with one an antecedent of the other in a recent study.[2] The developmental process is complex. No wonder confusion and controversy abound.

There is also confusion and controversy over which environmental elements nourish development. Investigators are beginning to look at parameters that are general in scope and that consistently relate to development across different stages, sexes, and developmental areas. They are also identifying parameters that are highly specific in scope relating to development in a particular stage, age range, or developmental area. Even more important from a practical standpoint, researchers are beginning to focus on individual differences. In the second section of each stage, I have described an environment that I feel is growth fostering in a general way. The notions are based on my experiences and available research information. It is hoped that a more solid and predictive framework is forthcoming from the collaborative effort of researchers and professional persons practicing in the different settings. The payoff in terms of the health and development of infants and children will be considerable, especially from a preventive standpoint.

We know even less about the developmental process of the infant who has a disability. Studies that have begun to look at this process reveal the infant's strong desire to use what he has to organize his world and his inner sense of self. Because the infant's pathway may be altered by substitutions, circuitous routes, and a different timetable, the professional intervener and parent cannot become bound by a notion of developmental fixity and rigid necessities. They must attempt to see reality as the infant or child sees it by sensitively observing his behavioral patterns and interpreting them within a functional framework. They will thus recognize dysfunctional aspects of patterns that are interfering with his adaptability. For example, the infant tries to move toward his caregiver, but abnormal muscle tone involuntarily moves him away. However, the intervener and caregiver have to monitor any tendency to separate out a dysfunctional pattern in an earnest attempt to strengthen it. They then sever its relationship with other behavioral patterns and isolate the infant's or child's vulnerability. Instead, the focus should be on supporting the resources that the child has within himself to reweave the patterns in a way that exploits strengths and minimizes interfering forces. How can the child, through his own actions with minimal passive assistance, control the effect that the environment has on him and at the same time increase his adaptability so that he can expand his interaction with the environment?

In the third section of each stage, I have provided a framework for assessing possible ways that impairments can alter the infant's or child's interaction with both humans and inanimate objects in the environment. This is again a humble attempt; there is so much more to learn. Also, dysfunctions can be expressed in as many different ways as there are individual infants and children. To further illustrate the complexity: An infant may have abnormally low muscle tone (hypotonia) during the first one or two years. The impairment may then change to abnormally high muscle tone (hypertonia) or fluctuation of muscle tone in extreme ranges, and the infant has to reshuffle his patterns of adaptation.

I will discuss the multifaceted ways that abnormal muscle tone can be expressed and related precautions in Chapter 3. I also describe aberrant regulatory mechanisms that affect the state behavior, especially of the younger infant, and the threshold to sensory input. Thus, the content in Chapter 3 further defines and complements some of the content in the third and fourth sections of each stage.

In the fourth section I move from assessing the functional implications of impairments to providing a framework for integrating habilitative approaches in the daily care routine. This is also a humble attempt because the rationale for habilitative approaches is still in an exploratory stage. The infant is presently the only expert, and the suggested approaches cannot be used in a cookbook fashion with generalized applicability. The suggestions from this book and other sources must be adapted and modified on the spot with the infant or child at the helm, and a very different approach may be the outcome. At times, the infant or child will feel frustrated in the role of director if his signals are vague or confusing, and thus misleading.

The family will no doubt enlist the help and support of a number of interveners. It is important that the interveners share a core framework and understand each other's language. The members of the different disciplines should also feel comfortable handling and interacting with infants and children who have different types of disabilities. The interveners can then more flexibly intertwine their roles and expertise. Each discipline is not attempting to tug unevenly on a pattern in the weave or declare possession of a pattern and pull it out from the rest. This serves as a counterforce to the child's and family's inner efforts to remain whole. The individual style and expertise of each team member will place one or the other in the forefront at different points in time as the one who can be the most helpful.

In keeping with this philosophy, I have drawn upon the specialized expertise of a person in another discipline, A. Joy Huss, M.S., OTR, RPT, to help me translate sensory-motor patterns and habilitative approaches to the framework presented in this chapter. Of course, the expertise of Ms. Huss relative to habilitative approaches and therapy modalities extends far beyond the scope of this book.

For ease of reading, the author has used the word caregiver in singular form throughout the sections. In the real-life situation, a number of persons may assume the role of caregiver at different points in time, for example, mother, father, sibling, grandparent, or babysitter. The infant may also be forming a close, intimate relationship with more than one person. I have translated habilitative activities directly to the caregiver/infant dyad. Again, in the actual situation the caregiver in the dyad will no doubt be a number of different persons as the role is interchanged throughout the day. More than one member of the family or the whole family will be involved in some of the activities. Also, it can be assumed that an intervener or interveners collaborate with the caregiver to flexibly adapt approaches to an individual infant or child. To further enhance the flow of words, I ascribe the female gender to the caregiver and intervener and the male gender to the infant or child.

As was mentioned earlier, habilitative approaches are integrated in the daily routine and intertwined with spontaneous interaction between the infant or child and the caregiver. Thus, there is a flow of activities with a multidimensional emphasis in certain sections. An outline of expected habilitative outcomes is placed at the beginning of the section to orient the reader to the focus and scope of the approaches. Subheadings would be antithetical to the intertwined model because of the inference that one of the developmental parameters is more important than another.

FIRST STAGE: BIRTH THROUGH FOUR MONTHS

FRAMEWORK FOR ASSESSING
NORMAL DEVELOPMENTAL PATTERNS

Description of Normal Motor Patterns

Referring to Figure 2-2, the ventral (flexor) muscles are initially more active than the dorsal (extensor) muscles, and the neonate assumes a cuddly, flexed posture. He is at the mercy of gravity and is therefore dependent on full postural support either on a horizontal surface or in the caregiver's arms. Gravity stimulates the tonic labyrinthine reflexive response characterized by a more exaggerated flexor posture in prone position. The infant hugs the surface with the arms adducted in close to the body. The shoulders are also adducted, the elbows are flexed, the forearms are internally rotated, the hands are fisted, and the thumbs are adducted with the ulnar fingers more active. The hips are flexed, and the pelvis is posteriorly tilted, which pushes the buttocks up in the air. The legs are flexed and abducted, and the feet are dorsiflexed. The head is retracted (pulled into the shoulders), and there is a fatty pad on the dorsal surface of the neck because of the lack of extension. In contrast, the tonic labyrinthine reflex stimulates extensors more in the supine position, which decreases the exaggerated flexor posture. The force of gravity pulls the flexed arms in a more abducted position and pulls the head asymmetrically to one side. The hips and knees are still flexed and abducted but to a lesser degree. The feet are still dorsiflexed.

As illustrated in the above description, the neonate's posture and movements are governed by gravity and what has been termed primitive reflexes. Comparetti[1] postulated that these responses are not true reflexes because they are variable and modifiable. He defined the primitive responses as residual fetal patterns to present oneself in the proper position for birth and for propulsion through the birth canal. Comparetti contended that the primitive responses are functionally meaningful even before birth, with functional correlates along the continuum of development. Gilfoyle and Grady[2] described the primitive responses as the neuromechanisms for stability and mobility patterns. There are a number of good resources that describe the reflexes and the age of evolvement and integration.[3,4] Equally important is an understanding of the functional significance of the so-called reflexes both in terms of the infant's present pattern of movement and adaptations and later patterns.

The phasic reflexes mediated at the spinal level are primitive mobility patterns. There is a burst of activity in response to a brief, intermittent stimulus, which immediately abates or changes unless the stimulus is repeated. The movement involves a quick alternation from one extreme of the range to the other because of the lack of stabilizing elements. For example, the infant pulls his legs up in extreme flexion in response to a tactual stimulus to the foot. The flexor withdrawal response and other phasic reflexes, primary walking, crawling, crossed extension, Moro, and avoidance response of the hands, collectively involve movements through the physiologic range of flexion, extension, adduction, and abduction. The primary walking and crawling responses also provide the earliest reciprocal experience. The placement reaction involves a flexion-extension sequence of the foot, and this response continues throughout life to prevent tripping over obstacles.

The gross phasic movements are primarily protective in nature. The infant moves his limbs away from a tactile stimulus, and he shields himself from an approaching object by pulling his head back and interposing his hands between his face and the object. He also extends and turns his head on face contact to avoid suffocation. However, not all of the infant's responses to tactile stimuli are in the nature of avoidance, again for survival reasons. He turns in a rooting response and orients to the nipple. Both the avoiding and orienting lateral head movements are primitive precursors of later rotation patterns.

The phasic responses are nonspecific, unlocalized, and excitatory or emotionally charged in nature. The phylogenetically older pathways are more thinly myelinated, and there is a spread of input to other neurons. Also, there is a lack of inhibition mediated by higher centers to isolate and control responses because of the immature development of neuronal networks.[5] The burst of movement requires a great deal of energy with the sympathetic component of the autonomic nervous system dominating. However, the neurologically intact infant has internal regulatory mechanisms that restore him to a lower energy state. He has the capacity to shut out or habituate to a repeated, unpleasant stimulus.[6]

In contrast, the tonic reflexes mediated at the brain stem are primitive stability patterns. There is a change in the distribution of muscle tone throughout the body as a result of a change in the position of the head or body in space and related proprioceptive input. The infant maintains contact or a posture until a new stimulus intervenes. Background stability serves to maintain a position and prevent overreaction all along the continuum of development, and this regulatory effect has its rudimentary beginning in the early tonic responses.[7]

The tonic reflexes are also precursors to other functional patterns. The tonic labyrinthine response (TLR), which was discussed earlier, is a postural accommodation to space when the infant is very dependent on a support. He molds to the surface in a prone position with exaggerated flexor tone and increases body surface contact in a supine position with less flexor tone. The force of gravity serves as a resistance to strengthen later, more functional, antigravity flexion and extension responses. The asymmetric tonic neck reflex (ATNR) is initiated by proprioceptive input from turning the head to one side. The midline is the reference point with extension on one side of the body and flexion on the other side. This asymmetric pattern is used in later functional skills—writing or walking. In early infancy, it is felt that the ATNR reflex initiates hand watching by placing the hand of the extended arm within the visual field. With the symmetric tonic neck reflex (STNR), the waistline is the reference point. When the head is raised, the upper extremities are extended and the lower extremities are flexed and vice versa when the head is lowered. This pattern is involved in later skills, such as pulling up to a standing posture with stability of the upper extremities and mobility of the lower extremities. In infancy, this response is observable in the chainlike reaction of increased extension of the arms with head raising. The primary standing reflex involves extension of the lower extremities in relationship to gravity and momentary, stabilized weight bearing with the whole foot on the surface. This is a precursor to normal extension in bipedal patterns. The traction response involves a tonic reaction of the finger flexors to maintain contact with an object. There is also synergistic flexion of the wrist, elbow, and shoulder. This total flexor response is inhibited with the evolvement of postural extension, and only flexion of the fingers and adduction of the thumb remain in a grasp reflex.[8] The contrasting mobility and stability elements of phasic and tonic reflexes are illustrated in Figure 2-3.

Since development moves along a cephalocaudal continuum, the focus of the first four months is the development of head control and stability in the shoulder girdle. In prone position, the infant has two opposing forces that he moves against to develop neck extensors—the more developed neck flexors (ventral muscles) and gravity. Propensity for vertical righting also facilitates extension of the head toward a position it will assume when the infant sits and walks—nose and face

PRIMITIVE REFLEXIVE RESPONSES

Phasic Reflexes

Primitive mobility patterns

Tonic Reflexes

Primitive stability patterns

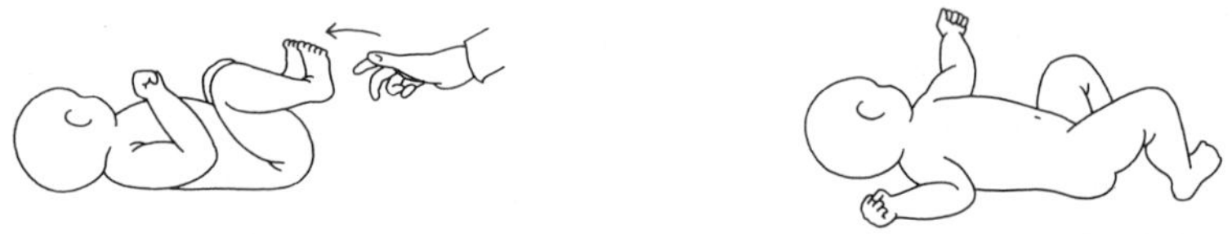

Burst of activity with quick alteration from one extreme of ROM to another, immediately abates or changes unless stimulus is repeated. Primarily protective, excitatory effect.

Moro
Avoidance response of hands
Flexor withdrawal
Crossed extension
Primary walking
Placement reaction
Crawling
Rooting

Maintains contact or posture elicited by a change in the position of the head or body in space until new stimulus intervenes. Rudimentary inhibitory, regulatory effect.

Tonic labyrinthine reflex
Asymmetrical tonic neck reflex
Symmetrical tonic neck reflex
Primary standing
Traction response

FIGURE 2-3. Primitive reflexive responses.

DEVELOPMENTALLY DISABLED INFANTS AND TODDLERS

vertical and mouth horizontal in relation to the force of gravity. Head righting is weak at first but improves with practice and elicits a change in the position of the arms. The arms gradually move forward away from the infant's body and provide a stabilized base of support to maintain the prone position when the infant raises his head. The arm support compensates for the lack of equilibrium (balance) reactions. When the flexor pattern is still dominant, the arms are flexed; and the propped weight is on the forearms and pronated, fisted hands. As the infant practices raising his head higher to achieve vertical righting, the arms become more extended in a chainlike reaction. However, they remain in a slanted position with the elbows forward in relation to the shoulders because of minimal extension in the trunk area and lack of proximal stability in the shoulder girdle. The focus is on neck extension at this point. The lower extremities remain in the primitive pattern of hip flexion, knee flexion, and foot dorsiflexion.

The infant experiences a difference in flexor and extensor tone from the STNR chainlike reaction related to the position of the head. There is more extension of the arms when the infant raises his head higher to orient to the environment and more flexion of the arms when he lowers his head to orient to the surface or to rest. With repeated practice of these movements, the neck and shoulder girdle muscles become stronger. Also, antigravity extension of the head begins to integrate the tonic labyrinthine reflex, decreasing the prone, flexor posture. Another contributing movement is the reciprocal kick, which lengthens the hip flexor muscles. The buttocks gradually come down, which decreases the posterior pelvic tilt in the prone position. As one end comes down, the other end (head) can simultaneously be raised higher, ultimately to a 90-degree angle and vertically righted position.

These background components lead to a more adaptive support position of the arms and hands. They are freed from the total support role and move to a forearm support position that involves a more complex combination of flexion and extension. The weight is on flexed elbows, which are in line with the shoulders because of increased proximal stability and increased extension in the neck and upper trunk area. This is the first stabilizing pattern involving cocontraction of the muscles in the neck and shoulder girdle.[9] The weight is also distributed differently on the forearms. They are more externally rotated, and the radial side of the hand is now free, which enhances the support function of the ulnar side of the hand. This pattern is later involved in higher manipulative skills such as writing. All the weight-bearing experiences provide proprioceptive and tactile feedback, which the infant organizes in a beginning, albeit vague, internalized sensory-motor schema of his arms. Prone weight bearing is therefore a precursor to prehension. The infant's head is also maintained in a functional midline orienting position, and the chest is lifted higher off the surface.

Because movement patterns are dependent on a balance between flexion and extension, the infant exercises the ventral muscles when in the supine position. He has the same propensity to right his head to the vertical position. The very young infant tilts his head forward to orient to his caregiver when she holds him facing her. He keeps practicing head flexion; and at the end of this stage, he can right his head vertically or almost vertically to orient to his caregiver when she approaches the end of the crib. As the neck muscles strengthen, he can also maintain his head in a midline position in supine with the chin more tucked in. The gap between the surface and the back of the neck is decreasing as the neck muscles elongate. With increased stability in the shoulders and waning of the ATNR, the infant begins to overcome gravity with arm movements. He adducts the arms in close to the body, which places the hands in a more functional midline position. He clasps his hands and then begins to explore other areas of his body, bringing his knees and then his feet in contact with the hands as he develops some control of abdominal and hip flexor muscles. The knees are flexed and the hips remain on the surface when he explores his feet. At the end of this stage, the infant maintains his head in alignment with his body when pulled to sit after a slight initial lag, again because of the influence of the head righting reflex and the increased strength of the neck flexor muscles. He helps pull with the arms, and the legs come up in flexion also. The infant uses the flexor muscles to roll from supine to sidelying position but still in one unit.

A similar process is thus occurring in both the supine and prone positions. The progravity tonic labyrinthine reflex is being integrated. The infant practices antigravity flexion in supine and antigravity extension in prone position as illustrated in Figure 2-4 and summarized in Table 2-1. He is less at the mercy of gravity.

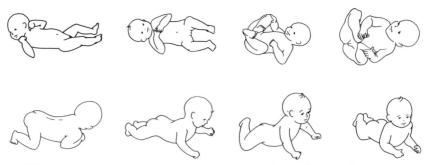

FIGURE 2-4. Antigravity responses progressively evolve in the prone and supine positions.

TABLE 2-1 Progressive evolvement of antigravity responses (First Stage)

POSITION	*ORDER	ANTIGRAVITY MOVEMENT
Prone	1	Turns head laterally to clear nose from surface
E	2	Raises head 45 degrees, flexed arms in
X		support position, weight on internally
T		rotated forearms and pronated, fisted
E		hands
N	2	Raises head 90 degrees, extended arms in
S		slanted, support position, weight on
I		pronated, semi-fisted hands
O	3	Raises and maintains head in midline
N		position, weight on flexed elbows, externally rotated forearms, and ulnar side of hand
Supine	1	Tilts head forward to orient when held in en face position
F	2	Maintains head in midline position with chin more tucked in
L		
E	2	Brings hands to midline in contact with each other
X		
I	2	Flexes knee up in contact with hand
O	3	Flexes knees and brings feet up in contact with hands
N		
	3	Maintains head in line with body when pulled to sit after slight initial lag
	3	Rolls from supine to sidelying with arms and legs flexed

* 1—Beginning of stage; 2—Midway in stage; 3—End of stage

When the infant can maintain his head in the midline orientation in both the prone and supine positions, this is the beginning of axial stability and a reference point to determine where the head is in space and whether he or the world is moving. There is an interrelationship between the vestibular system (with end organs sensitive to head movements and forces of gravity) and neck and extraocular muscles.[10] The two-month-old infant uses his eyes to orient to stationary peripheral objects. The head does not turn also because of immature neural circuitry and the lack of effective communication between the visual and vestibular systems. At three months, eye movements are readily followed by a rotation of the head toward an object in the periphery. The eyes maintain fixation on the object while the head is moving because of visual communication with the vestibular system via the cerebellum.[11] With the precocious development of the visual system, the three-month-old infant has ocular control almost equal to that of an adult, which will be discussed in more detail in the following paragraph and the section on Cognitive Patterns.

EVOLVEMENT OF PREHENSION SCHEMAS. The rudimentary elements of prehension skills also evolve in this stage. Even the newborn is capable of a primitive form of reach; he moves his arm toward his caregiver or a bright object at 7 to 10 days of age or younger.[12] The newborn also responds to a stimulus in the palm of the hand with a traction response, which has been described. By two or three months, the infant can converge his eyes on an object as near as five inches, and the blink response evolves. He is therefore able to focus on his hand which is especially in view when he is in the ATNR posture. He also fixates on a suspended object and reaches out in a circuitous, swiping action.[13] The effort elicits the traction response with increased flexor tone and fisting of the hand.[14] By three or three-and-one-half months, the infant can oppose gravity and engage in bilateral activity more frequently. He clasps his hands in midline and may assume and maintain this response when an object is suspended in midline. Or, he may reach out with one or both hands toward the object, alternately glancing between the object and the hand nearest the object. It is as if there is an eye-object, eye-hand comparison. There is unnecessary movement during the reaching action because of the lack of proximal stabilization.

By the end of this stage, the infant has had more experience weight bearing in prone position which has increased proximal stability. He reaches with both hands or with one hand, leaving the other one in midline. There are also fewer unnecessary movements. The flexor traction response has subsided with increased extensor tone, and the hands are no longer fisted, which paves the way for the reach and grasp schema. The infant alternately glances from the object to one or both raised hands until there is fumbled contact.[15] The object is crudely grasped with an ulnar orientation because of internally rotated forearms and the lack of differentiation between the arm and hand. He cannot adapt his hand to the object. The ulnar grasp facilitates stability of the wrist and palm area of the hand as a background component for the later radial-palmar grasp and individual finger use.[16] The avoidance response is also diminishing toward the end of this stage in response to all the tactile stimulation to the hands, and the infant maintains the reflexive grasp longer and may bring the object to his mouth. The progressive evolvement of prehension schemas is summarized in Table 2-2.

TABLE 2-2 Evolvement of prehension schemas (First Stage)

FUNCTIONAL ADAPTATION	QUALITATIVE DESCRIPTION
Automatic, reflexive orientation to an object	Grasps object placed in hand, spread of flexor tone to wrist, elbows, and shoulders Primitively moves arm toward a stimulus
Rudimentary coordination of eye and hand movements	Focuses on hand when in ATNR position Visually follows hand movements Reaches with circuitous, swiping motion; effort elicits increased flexor tone
Beginning accommodation of reflexive reach and grasp to object	Reaches and bats object with one or both hands, alternately glancing between object and nearest hand Reaches with one or both hands, alternately glancing between object and hand(s), crudely grasps object with ulnar orientation

Description of Normal Oral and Language Patterns

As explained in the previous section, the neonate has no neck to speak of and no separation between the head and shoulder girdle because of the undifferentiated flexor posture. The larynx is high, with the upper border opposite the second or third cervical vertebra. When the infant sucks, the larynx moves almost in the nasopharynx, and milk goes down on either side of the larynx, bypassing the air. With this defense against penetration of oral contents, the infant can breathe while sucking and comfortably swallow in a reclined position. The vertical mobility of the larynx is restricted because of the high position, and there is an anterior-posterior movement during swallowing.[17,18] Since the raised larynx is in close proximity to both the nasal and oral cavities, the infant's vocalization has a hypernasal quality.

The tongue literally fills the small oral cavity and pressure against the palate at rest helps widen the arch. The vertebral wall is forward, which in turn places the tongue in a more forward position, and mobility is restricted by both the forward position and crowded quarters.[19] The reflexive sucking movement involves a downward and forward displacement of the tongue and mandible followed by an upward and backward movement of the tongue and mandible, which results in a stripping or milking action. Large vascular loops in the lips of the newborn have an adhesive effect which helps maintain an oral seal.[20] Fat pads in the cheek also provide stabilization to achieve intraoral pressure and keep the nipple in place while the mandible is still loose and lax. The infant has his own suck-swallow-pause pattern which demonstrates the temporal organization imbedded in the brain stem.[21] The pattern serves as a background for communication, eliciting interaction with the caregiver during the pause phase. It is as if the intermittent pauses were designed to perpetuate this very important input. The nonnutritive sucking pattern is adaptively different with a shorter burst, longer pause, faster sucking rate, and less swallowing.[22,23] The infant is already demonstrating an ability to alter patterns to accommodate to different sensory input.

The configuration of the infant's rib cage is also different, which affects his breathing pattern. The thorax is somewhat cone shaped, and the ribs are in a horizontal plane at about right angles to the spinal column; they later angle downward. The spine and sternum are cartilaginous and thus soft and flexible, which provides an unstable base for the ribs, and the intercostal muscles are weak.[24] Chest mobility is therefore limited; lung expansion is primarily accomplished by lowering the diaphragm. Because of the angle of insertion, the efficiency of the diaphragmatic contraction is decreased. The diaphragm descends to a lesser degree, which limits the increase in the abdominal pressure and expansion of the rib cage. The contraction of the diaphragm tends to suck the compliant lower rib cage inward (posteriorly) in the supine position because of the horizontal insertion which also decreases the expansion of the rib cage.[25] Breathing is shallow and rapid to provide adequate ventilation.[26]

The work of breathing is even greater during active (REM) sleep. There is direct inhibition of motor neurons and a loss of tone in intercostal muscles, which further decreases the stability and stiffness of the rib cage. Some of the force of the diaphragmatic contraction is dissipated, sucking in the compliant upper ribs as well as inspiring air. Thus, the strength of the diaphragmatic contraction must be increased to maintain the same air volume, and more effort is exerted during active sleep than during quiet sleep or the awake state.[27] The breathing is referred to as paradoxical, because the thoracic and abdominal movements are approximately 180 degrees out of phase or counterdirectional, characterized by an inward movement of the rib cage as the abdomen moves outward. During most of the quiet (NREM) sleep periods, the thoracic and abdominal movements are in phase or codirectional.[28]

Because the very young infant spends a considerable amount of time in the active (REM) sleep state, and because he has a lower proportion of high oxidative, Type I fibers in the intercostal and diaphragmatic muscles,[29] he is more prone to respiratory fatigue. Signs of fatigue often precede apneic episodes, which occur more frequently during active sleep.[30]

As is evident, the infant's breathing pattern is very variable with fluctuations in the rate and type of respirations within certain states and from one state to another. This is further discussed in Chapter 3. In view of conflicting findings in the literature, it may be impossible to establish a norm in terms of even the respiratory rate for infants as a whole or an individual infant in this stage.

Because breathing and oral movement patterns are still very immature, the neonate's vocalization is limited. He makes vegetative sounds (grunt, hiccup) and cries in an audibly different range to express hunger and pain, which elicits protection, provision for physical needs, and social attention from a sensitive caregiver. He also has other ways to communicate with his caregiver, because innervation of the oral and facial muscles begins remarkably early even before birth. Barnard and associates[31] outlined an impressive number of subtle and potent engagement and disengagement cues that the infant communicates with facial and bodily movements. Most of the behaviors have evolved by one month of age. The infant can also integrate a number of behaviors into an organized action: he expresses his dislike of a disturbing stimulus by breaking his visual gaze, turning his face to the side, frowning, grimacing, and emitting a fussy sound.[32]

The infant's responsiveness to sound begins in the third trimester and has evolved to rather sophisticated levels by birth.[33] He orients to speech over noise and selectively prefers the female voice, discriminating his mother's vocalization at less than three days of age.[34] The very small infant also demonstrates an imbedded temporal rhythm by moving in synchrony with the spoken word.[35] The physiologic uterine sounds and possibly audible human voices provided a base for sensitivity to the rhythm, intonation, frequency, variation, and phonetic components of speech.[36]

As the stage progresses there are developmental changes in the breathing pattern related to a number of factors. Wilder[37] found a relationship between an increase in the duration of the respiratory cycle during crying and the development of motor patterns that require stabilization of the neck and shoulder girdle, such as the prone propped position. She reasoned that the positional fixation involves impoundment of air within the thorax, which requires coordination of respiratory and laryngeal muscles, and the infant must be able to coordinate these same muscles to prolong the expiratory phase during crying. The I-fraction during a crying respiration decreases each month, reflected by a shorter inspiratory phase and a more prolonged expiratory phase. The I-fraction approaches the value in mature speech at three months of age.

The respiration rate and variability decreases in all states, and there is a diminution of the out-of-phase paradoxical breathing during active sleep.[38,39] There is also a sharp decline in the apneic episodes in the active sleep state during the first three months.[40] These changes are no doubt related to maturation of respiratory control mechanisms, a less compliant rib cage and spine, some development of thoracic muscles, and increased resistance to fatigue. There is an increase in the proportion of Type I oxidative fibers in the ventilatory muscles, which is felt to reflect, in part, an adaptation to the functional demands of extrauterine breathing. The adult value in terms of the percentage of Type I fibers in the internal and external intercostal muscles is achieved at two months of age,[41] and the percentage of Type I fibers in the diaphragm increases from 25 to 40 percent.[42]

Even though there are progressive changes in the breathing pattern, respirations are still predominantly abdominal. Wilder measured consistent, albeit relatively minor, participation of the thoracic muscles in crying and noncrying vocalization, whereas thoracic participation occurred in only 35 percent of the observed cycles of vegetative breathing at four months.

Wilder also observed physiologic asynchrony in the abdominal and thoracic movements during both crying and noncrying vocalization in some infants as early as two months of age. The chest wall continues to rise and expand, which maintains the thorax in an inspiratory position after the expiration begins with an inward movement of the abdomen. This is a holding maneuver to provide some opposition to the elastic recoil forces of the lungs and slow down the expulsion of air. Because of the immature motor development, overshooting occurs during the infant's budding attempts to exert active control over passive expiratory movements. The overshooting results in subcycles or mini-respirations—momentary expansion and contraction of the abdominal and/or thoracic circumference during the course of a continuously voiced expiration. This same overshooting is evident in the development of other motor skills, such as reaching and grasping.

More pronounced physiologic asynchrony was observed during noncrying than crying vocalization, which implies a difference in the expiratory control during these two types of vocalization in infancy that is not fully understood at this time. During noncrying vocalization, there is a longer lag time, with the thorax holding in an inspiratory position for a longer interval after the expiration has begun. This is a rudimentary beginning of the adaptation in mature speech. More braking is applied to maintain the subglottal air pressure in a relatively limited range, which is lower than the pressure for crying. However, the respiratory adaptations during noncrying vocalization are unstable during the first eight months, and there is no unique waveform as there is for crying. At times the waveform resembles vegetative breathing with an almost equal inspiratory and expiratory phase. Also, there is an inherent limitation in the volume of air to control and the length of the utterance because the lung capacity is still relatively small, even though there have been rapid changes in the development and enlargement of aveoli during the first three months.[43]

The developmental changes in the breathing pattern intermesh with structural changes in the oral and pharyngeal cavities and continuing maturation of the neuromuscular system to facilitate increased control during feeding and vocalization. With increased stabilization in the neck and shoulder girdle, the posterior third of the tongue and larynx begin to descend in the neck to initiate the formation of the supralaryngeal cavity, which will continue to expand in subsequent stages. A related shift from a one-tube to a two-tube system also begins to occur. When the shift is complete, sometime around the ninth month,[44] the oral cavity lies between the lips and velum, and the pharyngeal cavity is at a right angle to the oral cavity between the velum and larynx. The palate also opens up transversely toward the end of this stage, and the tongue becomes more mobile owing to the beginning elongation from its base and the increase in the size of the oral cavity.[45] There is less protrusion of the tongue because the vertebral wall is in a less forward position. There is also increased elevation of the tongue toward the gum ridge during swallowing, and the infant is developing more control of the lips during the sucking movement. Thus, oral movements are less obligatory and stereotyped, and the primitive sucking and biting reflexes are becoming inhibited. Another important factor in the modification of oral functions is the feeding and mouthing activities in the early months that provide the infant with copious sensations that challenge his capacities for accommodation.

Nonvegetative vocalizations begin to evolve with the production of cooing sounds around eight weeks. There is disagreement concerning when the different vowel sounds first appear, because it is more difficult to differentiate these sounds in young infants. The vocal tract is still plastic, with overlapping of the frequency range among the vowels versus the later demarcated quality.[46,47] The front vowels, e, ee, i, may appear first, involving a forward position of the main body of the tongue and manipulation of the jaw position. Another front vowel, ae, and two middle vowels, uh and ʌ, evolved by 16 weeks in a recent study.[48] The main body of the tongue moves toward the center of the mouth when forming a middle vowel. Consonants produced at the periphery of the vocal mechanism involving either a back velar adjustment (g, ng) or a front labial movement (p, b, m) may also evolve by the end of this stage accompanied by concomitant bodily movement.[49,50] These sounds do not require as much air expenditure as consonants that evolve later. It is evident that the tongue now has enough room and a certain degree of longitudinal flexibility to impede the air flow in a particular way necessary to form some vowels and vowel and consonant combinations. The lips become involved in the constriction of the air flow if labial consonants are produced. The infant also develops enough respiratory control to laugh in response to movement and auditory and tactile stimulation.

The frequency (pitch) of the vocalization decreases during the first 21 days after birth and then increases until about four months of age, stabilizing toward the end of the first year.[51] The reason for this developmental trend is not fully understood.[52] The vocalization becomes somewhat less hypernasal with the beginning descension of the larynx in the neck a little farther away from the nasal cavity.

All the above maturational parameters are coupled with a pleasurable social relationship to expand the infant's communicative repertoire. He can combine behaviors into more complex units to express engagement and disengagement, such as reaching toward the caregiver, rhythmically opening and closing his hands, smiling, gurgling, and cooing.[53] Likewise, a certain word may receptively begin to be connected with a set combination of events. The four-month-old infant may recognize the peek-a-boo game if the same vocalization, action routine, time, place, and person are involved.[54]

In summary, the oral-facial muscles are situated in a privileged structural position in view of the maturational directions described in the introduction. They are cephalic, rostral, and ventral.This phylogenetic advantage explains the rather precocious maturity of the orofacial neuromusculature, which has both survival and social significance, and is further outlined in Table 2-3.

Description of Normal Cognitive Patterns

The infant's responsiveness to environmental stimuli is dependent on his level of consciousness. He is most receptive to his environment when there is an optimal level of internal inhibition and minimal motor activity—the awake, alert inactive state. As described in Chapter 3, these periods are relatively brief in duration during very early infancy because of an immature regulatory mechanism, competing physiologic demands, and an immature ability to process sensory input. Environmental stimuli can be mediated to affect state changes, the duration of time in a particular state, and the level of arousal. Again, this is nature's

TABLE 2-3 Evolvement of oral and language patterns (First Stage)

Functions with predominantly stereotyped, relatively undifferentiated patterns in neonatal period

    Breathes with a shallow, rapid, predominantly abdominal movement

    Responds to tactual stimulation with an obligatory rooting, suck-swallow, and bite response

    Vocalizes with a limited repertoire—vegetative sounds and crying

Demonstrates some ability to alter stereotyped responses in neonatal and early infancy period

    Selectively orients to speech over noise

    Alters sucking, swallowing, and breathing to accommodate to nutritive and nonnutritive sources of sensory input

    Modifies crying to differentially express hunger and pain

    Coordinates facial and bodily movements to express engagement and disengagement

Further modifies breathing and oral patterns concurrent with beginning structural changes

    Produces hypernasal cooing sounds around eight weeks

    Responds to tactual input with a progressively less obligatory suck-swallow, rooting and bite response

    Moves lips somewhat more actively during sucking

    Moves tongue more flexibly with increased elevation to gum ridge during swallowing

    Produces front vowels—e, ee, I, and ae; and possibly middle vowels—uh, ʌ, by end of stage

    Produces back consonant sounds—g, ng; and possibly front labial consonant sounds—p, b, m, concurrent bodily movement

    Vocalizes with a progressively higher pitch, beginning diminution of hypernasality

Develops increased ability to coordinate and associate behaviors both expressively and receptively

    Combines vocalization and movements in more complex units to express engagement and disengagement

    Receptively associates a certain word (peek-a-boo) with a set combination of events

---

way of facilitating attachment. The caregiver orchestrates her repertoire of behaviors to elicit observable changes in the infant's behavior, which provides refueling feedback.

There has been an increased awareness of the infant's competence during periods of alertness. He can adapt his reflexive patterns to turn his head and orient to a soft rattle or human sound. The infant can control interfering motor activity and fixate on his mother's face or a bright object and selectively move his eyes in a horizontal and even a vertical excursion to follow his mother's face or the object.

There is controversy over whether the infant has a fixed focus at 7 or 8 inches or if he sees equally unclearly across a wider and yet still limited range of 15 to 29 inches.[55] If he has a fixed focus, it is as if nature designed a protective bubble that adaptively includes the distance of his mother's face during breast feeding. The neonate shows a preference for stimuli that occur in human social interactions. He is attracted to elements of angularity, contrast, and curvilinearity present in the human face[56] and to higher pitched sounds in the female voice as mentioned earlier. The infant prefers milk smells above water or sugar water and identifies the breast pad of his mother six days after birth. He responds differently to the taste of human milk and a special cow's milk formula designed to simulate human milk.[57]

Piaget[58] postulated that sensory input remains in separate spaces —visual space, auditory space, and buccal space. The infant can relate to input via only one sensory modality at a time. He can suck or look, but he cannot simultaneously suck and look. The findings of one study[59] suggest that the infant can relate only to one or another of the smaller units of a pattern rather than the whole pattern. There is controversy whether he has a rudimentary short-term memory at this very early age manifested by a response decrement to one stimulus and a revived interest to a new stimulus.[60,61,62,63] He may view the world as if he were looking through a train window. Sensations appear, disappear, and reappear in separate frames.

Because of his immature processing capacity, the infant is born with mechanisms to select which stimulation he will attend to. He uses ocular and head movements and state changes to regulate his arousal and attention level and maintain homeostatic control. He moves through rest/activity cycles alternately orienting and turning away. He also alternates between alert and drowsy or sleep states. The infant has the ability to reflexively withdraw from stimuli as described in a preceding section, and he can also shut out repetitious or unpleasant stimuli with a response decrement. Thus, he has the ability to both protect and nourish his rapidly developing nervous system.

The nourishment comes from his ability to search for, find, and respond to another person and also from primitive, repetitive actions, such as scratching, nutritive and nonnutritive sucking, or movement of the limbs. The reflexive actions become modified as a function of experience and what Piaget termed primary circular reactions which center on the infant's own body. He repeats a movement over and over in a rather rhythmic cycle to recapture an unexpected sensory response that he stumbled upon. For example, the infant sucks his hand which has accidentally come to his mouth. With repeated practice the chance adaptation becomes strengthened and consolidated into a firmly established schema. The hand movement comes under the control of the sucking schema, and the infant can place the fist or fingers in and out of his mouth with increased economy and control. He can also maintain the hand in his mouth for longer periods. The same process applies to the visual sense. When the infant's extremities assume the ATNR posture, his one hand moves in and out of his visual field as he moves in and out of the posture as discussed earlier. The hand ceases to exist when it disappears from view, and he cannot voluntarily bring the hand back into view. He attempts to control something of interest, and his looking holds the hand in place for progressively longer periods of time. By two months of age, the infant can focus on and examine objects directly in front of the eyes as well as out in the periphery. His eyes gain increasing control over the hand, and he moves it at different distances and angles, which maintains the display that the eyes contemplated. The hand-watching schema thus evolves with coordination of the visual sense and somatosensory input from the body. Hand clasping also evolves as a spectacle that the infant can produce for himself. Initially, he occasionally glances at his hands as they approach each other or during the mutual tactual exploration. The infant then progresses to visually monitoring the approach of his hands and subsequent clasping activity. His eyes see what his hands feel, and there is a coordination of the visual and tactual sense.[64] Other circular reactions adaptively evolve to entertain the infant, for example, dribbling and retraction of saliva, head bobbing-pause rhythm.

The very young infant can also yoke his movements to grossly imitate some of the facial and body gestures of an adult—open and close his mouth, protrude his lips or tongue, and move his fingers. This is a precursor to true imitation, because the infant assimilates the adult's action in his primary circular reactions as though it were a repetition he himself had just made. There is a lack of differentiation between the infant and other humans.[65]

The infant begins ordering reality around body modes. Experience with the sucking schema becomes the basis for forming rudimentary classes of nonnourishing suckable objects and nourishing suckable objects when hungry. The infant also relates the nursing position with nutritive sucking, which involves a coordination of tactual and kinesthetic signals. The hand becomes inserted in different actions or schemas: something to look at, something to suck, something to clasp. However, the hand the infant sucks, the hand he looks at, and the hand he grasps are three different hands. His perceptual integration is still very primitive. The infant cannot relate his hand to more than one schema at a certain point in time.

Periods of alertness gradually increase as competing physiologic demands decrease. By three months of age, the infant sleeps longer at night with more periods of deep sleep; and other physiologic functions are becoming better organized. His inner regulatory mechanism and processing capacity have matured to the point that he can remain alert and attentive to external stimuli for up to 15 minutes or longer. Increased ocular and head control allows him to prehend the world with his eyes. The infant generalizes the visual schema to new and different objects, truly looking for the sake of seeing. He visually scans the environment, moving his head and eyes laterally, upward, and downward when in a supine, prone, or well-supported sitting position. He can accommodate his eyes to bring an object into focus and either hold the fixation or pursue an object, matching eye and head velocity to object velocity to maintain a stationary image on the retina. His eyes now work better as a team and binocular vision is enhanced.[66] The infant can scan contours and boundaries of his caregiver's face and objects. He can also control three gaze directions relative to his mother's face—central position with form perception; peripheral position with only motion, speed, and direction retained; and total loss of visual contact. Each position provides a different sensory-motor experience.

A sufficiently predictable stimulus world and the coordination of sensations through the reciprocal action of schemas provide the basis for the formation of primitive internal referents. Sensations are no longer isolated in separate spaces. The infant begins to develop expectations of how a recurring stimulus should look, smell, sound, feel, and/or move. He relates a stimulus event to an organized template of past experiences and perceives a match or mismatch. In this way, he expands his ordering of reality. He becomes more consistent in discriminating his mother's face from a stranger's face[67] and thus forms a rudimentary class of mother and not mother. He develops expectations that certain things go together; and if the violation of his expectation is too severe, he becomes disturbed. In one study,[68] three-month-old infants became upset when their mothers' voices were projected away from the mothers' faces. If there is too much discrepancy between a stimulus and his expectation, the infant cannot process the event and loses interest. On the other hand, if there is just the right degree of discrepancy, the stimulus event elicits alertness and interest. There is no question among researchers that the three-month-old infant has short-term memory and habituates—becomes bored with the repeated presentation of a stimulus.[69,70,71] It is as if he says, "Oh, that again!" His interest is revived by a new and yet not too dissimilar stimulus.

Although the infant is acquiring what Piaget termed recognition memory, everything external to him remains undifferentiated during this stage. The infant does not perceive that objects are independent entities that move from place to place in space. His tracking of movements from point A to B and then back to A toward the end of this stage is a precursor to this understanding. He also stares at the place where a disappearing object was last seen.

The elaboration of primitive schemas is also an important precursor to the later differentiation of objects and actions. As described in the section on motor patterns, an interesting stimulus elicits a rudimentary reaching action in the very young infant. With increased maturation, he is able to reach out and swipe an object. The infant then smiles and coos to express his joy at creating a spectacle. By the end of this stage, he coordinates eye-hand and hand-mouth movements in more complex ways. The infant can crudely reach and grasp an object that the eye sees, if the hand and object are both in view. The infant even brings the object to his mouth, with the mouth moving down to meet his hands. Thus, there is further accommodation of reflexive responses to the stimulus, which has come about through a process of repetition, generalization, and differentiation; this is outlined in Table 2-4. Interaction with the environment is also moving in an outward direction, and the awkward contacts with objects herald the beginning of secondary circular reactions described more fully in the next stage.

Description of Normal Affective Patterns

The infant draws no boundary lines between himself and another person or between himself and the actions of another person or object. He has the illusion that the touch, voice, and body of his mother is his own—a sense of oneness and quasi-unity with her. Mahler, Pine, and Bergman[72] refer to this period as the symbiotic phase of the separation/individuation process. The authors also point out that the infant senses small degrees of difference in temperature, texture, smell, and turgor as he molds into the contours of his mother's body and then uncurls the mold. This is the beginning of the boundary formation process. Thus, the beginning of separation is simultaneous with the beginning of attachment to a significant person.

The infant is born with appealing characteristics which Stern labels babyness—a large head, protruding forehead, large eyes, and fat cheeks.[73] He is also born with an innate preference for the stimulus world that his caregiver provides. The mother's eyes are within the range of his visual bubble when he nurses, and the mutual gaze is an early potent form of communication. The caregiver and infant can remain locked in this interaction much longer than two adults with the possible exception of two adults deeply in love. The infant uses other proximity seeking behaviors to interact with the caregiver—forward movement of the head, upward tilt of the face, and a primitive effort to reach toward the caregiver. He nestles his soft, fuzzy scalp in the corner of her neck and nuzzles against her breast. The infant also emits cues to regulate the level and duration of stimulation from his caregiver in accordance with homeostatic needs—averting his gaze or turning his eyes and

TABLE 2-4 Evolvement of cognitive patterns exemplified by visual schema (First Stage)

Nourishes his system with reflexlike, single action schemas in newborn period
    Centers schemas on and around his own body
    Registers sensations from different spheres of activity in separate spaces
Slightly modifies reflexive response to accommodate to a stimulus
    Fixates and follows face or object in horizontal and vertical excursion
    Yokes movements to grossly imitate some facial and bodily gestures of
        another person—pseudoimitation
Adapts reflexive response to orient to stimuli in more active ways
    Follows a moving object in a horizontal, vertical, and circular orientation
    Attempts to prolong or recapture a new sensation by re-enacting the move-
        ment in a rhythmic cycle (primary circular reaction)
Consolidates reflexive responses in a well-established schema through repeti-
    tious primary circular reactions
    Keeps hand in view once it enters visual field by chance (visual control of
        hand movements)
    Moves hand at different distances and angles (reciprocal coordination of
        visual and manual schemas)
    Simply repeats action schema to satisfy need to look, lack of intentionality
Generalizes schema to an increasing number of objects in a more directive way
    Scans environment, moving head and eyes in all directions
    Scans contours and boundaries of caregiver's face and objects
Generalizes and elaborates schema
    Begins to direct schema outward to objects in external environment
    Reaches and bats object, alternately glancing between object and nearest
        hand
    Crudely grasps object when both object and hand are in view (coordination
        of vision and grasping schemas)
Forms primitive internal referent from experiences—recognition memory
    Loses interest in repeated stimulus, renewed interest in new stimulus
    Begins to recognize mismatch between mother's and stranger's face
    Becomes disturbed if stimulus is too discrepant
Primitively germinates the concept of an object
    Tries to prolong or recapture sensations through primary circular reactions
    Stares at place object was last seen to disappear
    Self, action schema, and objects still undifferentiated
Rudimentarily orders reality around body modes
    Forms rudimentary class of nonnourishable suckable objects and nourish-
        able suckable objects
    Places object in a separate action schema or category—something to suck
    Progresses to placing object in two action schemas or categories—some-
        thing to grasp and suck

head away for a recovery period. The infant's babyness, helplessness, and brightened response to his caregiver's face and voice elicit a repertoire of behaviors from his caregiver that are adapted to the infant's immature processing capacity. Thus, if the infant's cues are clear and the caregiver is sensitive to his homeostatic needs and involvement/ recovery cycles, intricate dyadic patterns evolve.[74] A mutual dialogue develops in a specifically human way, which provides the foundation for interpersonal relationships and all psychic functions according to Spitz.[75] The infant associates satisfaction and wholeness with his caregiver, and he senses that his communicative signals successfully restructure the external world to meet his needs.

The infant responds to his mother with a smooth, cyclic curve of involvement and recovery and smooth and cyclic motor movements. The mother cycles also in a "kind of swan's mating dance."[76] The infant very early on senses when he has a different dance partner. His father may use a rhythmic but more playful jazzing-up approach, which elicits a heightened response from the infant as early as two or three weeks. The infant responds with a more "wide-eyed, playful and bright face,"[77] and the play period may be shorter if the infant becomes overloaded. It is more difficult for a stranger to adapt to the infant's cyclical rhythms, and a clear response difference has been observed by Brazelton as early as four weeks. The infant responds to the stranger with a jagged, homeostatic curve of attention and an abrupt break for a recovery period before he returns for another period of orientation. This is a more expensive, demanding response pattern. The infant also responds to inanimate objects with the same jagged, more demanding response; and when his caregiver and objects are both in view, the infant preferentially focuses on his caregiver.[78]

The smile is a very potent interactive signal and progresses through maturational changes during this stage. The response is initially reflexive and a way of discharging inner tension, occurring primarily during drowsy or light sleep states. By three weeks, the infant smiles responsively to the human voice. At five or six weeks, the human face supercedes the voice as an elicitor of the smile. At two to two-and-a-half months, the human face elicits an automatic smile with a high degree of regularity, and the infant's mother elicits a more intense response than an unfamiliar person. By the third or fourth month, the smile becomes an instrument to elicit social responses.[79]

Toward the end of this stage, the periods of wakeful alertness have expanded as discussed in an earlier section. The infant and mother spend more time in focused interaction, getting to know each other. The infant develops a primitive inner sense of how his mother moves, smells, looks, and sounds. He moves into what Bowlby[80] terms Phase II, attachment-in-the making, which is characterized by fairly consistent visual discrimination of his mother.

More recent research broadens the scope of social and personality development beyond a simplistic dyadic model. The findings suggest that the infant forms an attachment to both parents, which is imbedded in a complex network of relationships between the infant and his parents and between the two parents.[81] Chibucos and Kail[82] found a relationship between the quality of the father-infant interaction at two months and the security of the infant-father attachment at seven-and-a-half months. This finding implies that quality is more important than quantity.

Experiences also enable the infant to form a very primitive, vague, internal sensory-motor representation of his own body. He senses vague differences as he alternately molds and distances from his caregiver's body. The infant also derives sensations from his movements and self exploration beginning with the hands and progressing to the knees and feet.

If his environment has been contingent, the infant has experienced contrastable inner sensations of discomfort and pleasure, dissatisfaction and satisfaction. His emotions as well as his perceptual system begin to be differentiated by these experiences. The infant expresses these beginning differentiations with his expanding repertoire of behaviors and vocal sounds, and his cues become even more clear. This differentiation and elaboration of affective patterns is outlined in Table 2-5.

GROWTH-FOSTERING ENVIRONMENT

The infant within himself is a world of microsystems and regulatory mechanisms that strive to maintain homeostasis. This very young evolving system needs a predictable, consistent outer world to support inner homeostatic control. The infant is also dependent on environmental stimulation to acquaint him with the social world and facilitate the wiring-in of neural structures that are very incomplete at birth. With the right blend of environmental stability and variety, the infant begins the long process of organizing incoming messages into invariant sets as the backdrop for introducing order to the mobile changing world as well as the infant's own mobility.

The caregiver is the most qualified in the role of master chef to combine just the right blend of background staples and novel additions of flavor, texture, and color to optimally nourish the rapidly developing nervous system. The recipes cannot be found in a prescriptive cookbook, they must be dynamic and ever changing with on-the-spot im-

**TABLE 2-5 Evolvement of affective patterns
(First Stage)**

Perceives self and others as an undifferentiated whole
    Makes no differentiation between sensations and source of stimulation
    Senses an existence of oneness and quasi-unity with his caregiver
Modifies reflexive responses to seek proximity
    Moves his head forward and tilts the face upward
    Primitively reaches toward the caregiver
    Molds into the caregiver's body
Emits cues to regulate the level and duration of interaction
    Averts his gaze or turns head and eyes away
    Alternates between alert and drowsy or sleep states
Begins to coalesce behaviors with caregiver's behaviors in interactive fit of human relatedness
    Responds to caregiver with a smooth, cyclic interactive rhythm
    Responds to stranger with a more jagged, energy-consuming curve of attention
Begins to form an attachment to a significant person
    Organizes affective experiences into a very primitive inner referent of the caregiver
    Smiles more intently in response to the caregiver's face
Relates to his caregiver in more socially active ways
    Remains awake, alert, and more outer directed for longer intervals
    Expresses emotions more differentially (pleasure, displeasure)
    Uses the smile as an instrument to elicit a social response
Senses his own body in a vague, primitive way
    Feels small degree of difference as he molds to the caregiver's body and uncurls the mold
    Simultaneously experiences touching and being touched as he explores his own body

provisation. The recipes are the outgrowth of the chef's background and style and the unique palatal preference of the small infant within the broader framework of the family.

There is a very intimate relationship between the master chef or caregiver and the infant, which is imbedded in a matrix of reciprocity. This is vividly demonstrated in spontaneous play that springs forth during brief alert periods in the course of handling and care. The caregiver uses exaggerated facial expressions and changes in the pitch and loudness of her voice together with touch and movement to maintain the alert state within an optimal range. There is a vocal burst-pause pattern as if the infant were making a verbal response that exposes him to the time frame of a dialogue.[83] The high-pitched, rhythmic sing-song quality of the caregiver's voice, the slow rate of change of stimulus variations, and the slow, rhythmic handling movements provide a temporal pattern adjusted to the infant's perceptual and processing capacities which in turn facilitates these capacities.[84] The caregiver also uses a pattern to soothe the infant. She increases and then gradually decreases the tempo of her speech and movements, which acts as a pacemaker.

The infant fuels the interaction with alert facial expressions, and he also signals a need for a rest period by averting his gaze. The caregiver is sensitive to his signals and intuitively pulls back to respect self-regulatory mechanisms and competing physiologic demands. She remains available to resume the play period if the infant signals readiness, which adapts the stimulation to his optimal span of attention.

No interaction can always be perfectly timed; overshooting or undershooting is bound to occur, which calls for a revision in the recipe. The optimal range is sometimes exceeded, which has functional significance; exposure to a certain amount of stress helps expand the infant's adaptability. The difference in the interactive style of the mother and father also expands the infant's adaptability. The sociability of the infant has been related to the amount of interaction with the father.[85]

Contingency is a potent element in a predictable, consistent environment. The sensitive caregiver responds to the infant's signals of discomfort, hunger, and other needs. This contingency facilitates polarized sensations of hunger and satiety, discomfort and comfort, a low level of arousal and an alert sensorium, and other contrasts, whereas noncontingency can result in ongoing intermediate states (half-full) or a preponderance of one sensation (hunger). If the environment is predictable, sensory cues will be more predictable.

In the course of meeting the infant's care needs, he receives tactile, vestibular, and proprioceptive input from position changes, cuddling, nuzzling, kissing, and rocking. Handling also elicits his own bodily movements and sensory feedback. In some cultures, the infant receives a great deal of input by being attached to his mother's body during most of the day. In the American culture, he has been placed in a horizontal, more static position during sleep periods, which dominate in the 24-hour interval. There has been a renewed emphasis on the proximal receptors, and studies have related vestibular and tactile input to increased ocular control, heightened visual alertness, and improved motor skills.[86,87] More and more caregivers are now carrying their infants in a commercial support that holds him next to their body. However, there is a controversy regarding the comfort of these carriers. The rocking chair, suspended cradle, and the pram are also experiencing a comeback in the nursery.

With increased internal control and contingent caregiving, the infant is gradually able to sustain longer periods of attention during the day. Play periods are elaborated because of a higher threshold for stimulation. The caregiver creatively modifies and adapts behavioral sequences to maintain optimum control over the infant's attention, excitement, and affect, which have been termed the energizing forces of cognitive development.[88] She maintains a regular tempo with repetitive runs in the modality or modalities she is using to create expectation. The caregiver then superimposes variation to facilitate the evaluative process in keeping with the infant's focus on mismatches during the latter part of this stage. For example, she says, "I'm gonna getcha." and then changes the tempo—"I'mm gooonna getcha . . . I'mmm gooooonnnaaa getcha."[89] The caregiver encourages and supports the variation provided by the different playful styles of the siblings, now that the infant is more adaptable. She helps them observe for signs of an impending sensory overload which signals a need for a rest period.

As the infant's ocular control increases, he is positioned where there is a flow of activity but not too high a sound or activity level or chaos. The infant can then scan his environment and focus on interesting events during part of an awake, alert interval. He tracks his caregiver and other family members as they approach, move away, and move about in the room. Suspended objects will capture his interest for a while, including the increased feedback when he accidentally bats them. However, the infant should not have a barrage of objects around him with no way to turn away for a recovery and processing period. There is the danger of overloading because of the more jagged and energy-consuming curve of attention that may be elicited by objects. Also, each infant has his own individual style and preferences. Suspended objects that interest one infant may not be the right combination of stimulus dimensions for another infant. There can be no cookbook guide.

As the infant becomes less sensitive to temperature changes, he will enjoy being uncovered with more freedom to move. He is placed on the floor or other solid surface in both the prone and supine positions to practice movement patterns involving antigravity extension and flexion and beginning bodily exploration. More varied vestibular and tactual input can also be incorporated in spontaneous play because of his increased tolerance for stimulation. The caregiver and other family members can sway the infant up in the air while well supported in the trunk area, tilt him to each side while suspended vertically in the air, sway him when he is carried from point to point in the home, roll him from side to side with legs flexed up on the chest, and provide other forms of playful movement input. Again, the infant's response will indicate which types of movement input are enjoyable. Of course, he still enjoys being rocked, cuddled, nuzzled, kissed, and other spontaneous actions, which are the outgrowth of interaction.

FRAMEWORK FOR ASSESSING ABERRANT DEVELOPMENTAL AND INTERACTIVE PATTERNS

The framework has a functional emphasis. It is not enough to recognize interactive and developmental patterns that deviate from the so-called norm. The intervener must also place these observations in an environmental context. The following question is posed: how do the infant's limited capacities affect his relationship with other humans and with events in his world? As emphasized at the beginning of this chapter, the intervener also maintains a holistic perspective in another way. Limitations are viewed within the context of the infant's strengths.

Effect of an Aberrant Response Threshold and a Disturbed Relationshp

If the infant is born with a developmental disability, his repertoire of behaviors and communicative signals may deviate from the expected norm, which places the evolvement of a very intimate, nurturing relationship with his caregiver at risk. This is a paradox because it is this very relationship that fosters internal homeostatic control, adaptability to stress, social responsiveness, and overall development.[90,91]

The infant's internal regulatory mechanism may be faulty, expressed by too low or too high a threshold to stimulation. If he has a very permeable stimulus barrier, the infant reacts to his environment with a high intensity response that can escalate to irritability and uncontrollable crying. Thus, state changes are unpredictable with wide mood swings. The infant lacks the ability to shut out repeating stimuli with a response decrement which can tax the autonomic nervous system. Thus, physiologic rhythms of breathing, eating, sleeping, and other vital functions may be very irregular. Reactivity may also be expressed by exaggerated withdrawal from stimuli including bodily stiffening. Or, the reactive infant may be hyperkinetic, with the arms and legs constantly in jerky motion. If the infant has abnormally high muscle tone, an extensor pattern may predominate, which also expresses disengagement and withdrawal, albeit involuntarily: head, neck, and shoulder retraction, total lower extremity extension, and even an opisthotonos position at the most extreme range. Movement is restricted, including normal movement of facial muscles. A smile may look like a grimace or sneer, and the social intent is misinterpreted.

The infant's erratic behavior and cues may project the caregiver into a disorganized state. She noncontingently is always feeding, rocking and bouncing, picking up and putting down, and talking to the infant. The disorganized state may permeate the whole household. Frequent office visits and repeated hospitalizations centered on diagnostic evaluations or illness further interfere with the provision of a contingent, rhythmic environment. Involvement in a center-based early intervention program can also be too novel and disruptive. An arrhythmic environment reinforces the infant's faulty inner regulatory mechanism. His lack of adaptability may have a turning off or distancing effect, reflected by increased isolation. The caregiver becomes conditioned to not attend to the infant's cues and even misses socially engaging cues.[92]

At the other end of the continuum is the infant with a stimulus barrier that is difficult to penetrate. The infant has a low response level and a long latency, and the usual range of stimulation may not bring him up to a state of arousal. If he evolves to a low level of alertness, there is a rapid drop back down to a drowsy or sleep state. The infant's states can be blurred and indistinct, and the caregiver is confused about whether he is alert, drowsy, or lightly asleep. If the infant has low muscle tone, there is a decrease in movement, including the facial muscles, resulting in a rather flat affect and a limp, unyoking posture. The long latency also delays an affective response, including crying, which is shorter in duration and less differentiated.

A cycle can occur in which the infant is unable to behave in ways that will stimulate his mother to behave in ways that will stimulate him. It takes a lot of effort to arouse him and to maintain a level of alertness; this can exhaust the caregiver. There is less interaction of a social nature, which reinforces the infant's limited repertoire of engaging behaviors.

As discussed in the previous chapter, if illness is superimposed on a neurologic deficit, there is an increase in competing physiologic demands. The infant has a drawn, weary look that says, "Leave me alone. My energy has to be directed to internal needs." The caregiver has to inhibit her spontaneous interactions.

Based on the above descriptions, the developmentally disabled infant may have a very limited repertoire of signaling behaviors to seek and maintain closeness with his caregiver. He is less engaging and less engaged. The caregiver may be experiencing a multiplicity of stresses due to inner emotional turmoil, health problems, or life changes, including the birth of the disabled infant, that limit her affective expressions and responsiveness to the infant's signals. Based on Barnard and associates longitudinal study,[93] mutuality requires that both members of the relationship come with certain qualities; alert responsiveness and clear signaling on the part of the infant and sensitivity and adaptiveness on the part of the mother. The caregiver may be able to draw upon the strengths within the family and social unit and carry more of the adaptive burden. If not, the pair may never get in tune with each other. One or both may derive little pleasure from close physical contact, and interaction becomes task oriented with a paucity of stimulation via talking, looking, touching, and enjoyable movement.[94] More optimistically, a close nurturing relationship between the disabled infant and his parents begins to evolve in many family units during this stage, witnessed by interveners in the field. This speaks to the innate propensity for a social relationship on the part of both infants and adults.

Effect of Sensory Impairments

The infant may not be able to receive stimulation via all the sensory modalities, or input may be distorted because of peripheral or central damage. A loss of the visual sense robs the infant of the most potent vocabulary of signs and signals in early infancy, that is, mutual gaze, gaze aversion, and eye brightening. He also misses the potent reinforcer of a smile; and his smile is more muted, infrequent, and irregular. The infant is deprived of the most economical and effective means of taking in information from the environment. He cannot watch his caregiver and other family members move toward and away from him nor can he scan his surroundings for other interesting sights. There is no visual lure to reach out toward his caregiver or an object or to raise his head in prone position. He generally prefers the supine position and prone weight bearing is delayed. With the lack of increased stability in the shoulder girdle and a visual enticement, the infant's arms remain in the primitive, stereotyped position out in the periphery versus coming to midline.[95]

The visual receptor may be intact but functioning faultily. There may be impaired conjugate eye movements and delayed evolvement of more flexible accommodation and three-dimensional vision. These impairments can interfere with monitoring the hands at close range, scanning contours and boundaries of the caregiver's face and designs, and scanning environmental activity. An abnormal nystagmus has been reported in infants with cerebral palsy and Down syndrome, which is interpreted to reflect a faulty vestibulo-ocular mechanism.[96,97] If the communication between the visual and vestibular systems remains very limited, the infant will not be able to coordinate head and eye movements to more effectively capture peripheral visual stimuli toward the end of this stage. He cannot maintain a stable image on the retina (clear visual fixation) when the head is moving. Therefore, the infant will continue to look more frequently at objects closer to the midline with eye movements alone, which limits perceptual experiences.[98]

There may be what Illingworth[99] terms dissociated visual development. The infant is able to fixate and track his caregiver and an object, but processing capacities are not comparable with normal infants, suggested by delayed preference for novel stimuli.[100] It takes longer to process familiar stimuli, which interferes with the development of recognition memory. Thus, there may be a delay in preferential responses to the caregiver. Poor health can also affect the attentional level and processing capabilities because of competing physiologic demands.[101]

If there is an auditory deficit, the infant will not hear the temporal pattern and modulated changes in the caregiver's voice. Nor can he practice movement in rhythm to sound. He, therefore, cannot begin to absorb the salient organizational features of his culture's language in terms of both the structure and emotional tone. Or, there may be processing problems reflected by sensitivity to sounds or a certain sound, an inability to shut out a repetitive sound, or an inability to discriminate his caregiver's voice and different tonal qualities in the caregiver's voice.

The dysfunction of near receptors is receiving renewed attention. An impaired vestibular system affects the development of ocular control, as discussed earlier, and possibly visual and auditory processing. The response to movement is also aberrant. If the disorder is severe, the infant will remain curled in a corner of the crib with his head down on the surface. If the tactile system is dysfunctional, the infant may resist being cuddled by stiffening. He may also withdraw from contact with the caregiver's breast, hands, and clothes. Excitatory protective reactions may remain pronounced throughout this stage, which interferes with weight bearing in prone position, the gradual waning of avoidance reactions, and possibly even self-exploration.

It is apparent that sensory deficits can interfere with the adaptive modification of reflexive responses and the coordination of schemas in primary circular reactions, such as hand-watching and hand-clasping. Some of the impairments also limit the generalization and more adaptive differentiation of schemas. Thus, the primitive internal template or referent of the caregiver and inanimate objects is being organized from a more circumscribed repertoire of experiences.

Effect of Motor Impairments

Although the effect of sensory and motor impairments is intertwined, these two parameters have been separated for organizational purposes at the expense of fully depicting the interrelationship. The reader is also reminded that although the term infant is used, the child may be at a chronologically older age but still in the infancy stage developmentally as evidenced by some of the figures illustrating the different motor impairments.

COMPENSATORY PATTERNS IN THE SUPINE POSITION. Abnormal muscle tone and reflex responses interfere with all aspects of development. If the infant has hypertonic muscles and a strong tonic labyrinthine reflex (TLR), he is pulled in exaggerated extension in supine position, which deprives him of input related to the normal flexor posture: en face orientation with his caregiver, hand-to-mouth schema, evolvement of the hand-clasping and hand-watching schemas, expanded exploration of the knees and feet, and other primary circular reactions. In the more severe form, there is head, neck, shoulder, and spinal retraction with extended, inwardly rotated, adducted, and even scissored lowered extremities. Strong tonic reflexes lock him into a holding pattern that prevents the alternate sensation of stability and mobility. An obligatory ATNR prevents free head turning to orient to sounds and visual sights and the evolvement of the hand-to-mouth and hand-watching schemas. The reflex also inhibits the development of midline head control, which is the referent point for movement and spatial orientations. The TLR and ATNR negate the evolvement of other antigravity flexor patterns toward the end of this stage: turning from supine to sidelying and assisting with head righting when pulled to sit.

COMPENSATORY PATTERNS IN THE PRONE POSITION. The abnormal tone and the influence of the TLR also interfere with the evolvement of antigravity responses in the prone position. In the young infant, increased flexion may be expressed by the following posture: The infant lies on his stomach with his shoulders and arms internally rotated, the elbows extended, and his palms facing upward. The infant attempts to raise his head with quick jerks, which elicits extension and internal rotation of the legs (Fig. 2-5A). If the infant has a strong TLR, he may resist lying in the prone position. He is pulled into a very exaggerated flexor posture that interferes with the inspiratory phase of breathing. His arms get caught under his body, and his buttocks are raised up in the air because of the flexed hips, which negates raising the head. He may not even be able to clear his nose. If he is able to raise his head, this can elicit a shift to a total extensor pattern and retraction of the head and shoulders because of the lack of the counterpart of normal flexor tone. This effort does not develop the neck muscles nor does it place his head in an optimal orienting position. Instead, the

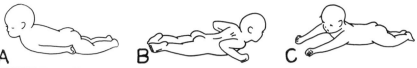

FIGURE 2-5. Prone antigravity responses are aberrant if the infant has hypertonia.

head is centered with the extended body (Fig. 2-5B). Flexor hypertonicity in the prone position may prevent sufficient extension of the spine to free the infant's arms from under his body for weight bearing. If his arms do come forward, the effort of head raising may have an overflow effect, with stiff extension and internal rotation of the arms and fisting of the hands (Fig. 2-5C). If the infant has severe extensor hypertonus in the supine position, the extensor pattern carries over to the prone position versus the exaggerated flexor pattern. The head and shoulders are retracted and the spine and lower extremities are stiffly extended, as shown in Figure 2-5B. The infant cannot bring his arms forward in a weight-bearing position.

The infant may not develop enough stability in the shoulder girdle, or extension in the midregion of the back, or inhibition of total flexion and extension to bear weight on flexed elbows in the forearms support position at the end of this stage. If he assumes this position, the arms may be internally rotated with fisting and weight bearing on the radial versus the ulnar side of the hand. The head may be retracted from the effort.

The development of antigravity responses is also impeded if the infant has fluctuating tone (athetosis) because of the influence of the ATNR and TLR. There may be exaggerated flexor tone in prone position and exaggerated extensor tone in supine position and persistent asymmetric patterns. Because there is more involvement in the upper extremities, the infant may not be able to assume a prone-propped position (Fig. 2-6A). Phasic withdrawal and avoidance responses may also persist and combine with the fluctuating tone to prevent adaptive weight bearing, if the infant attempts to assume a propped position.

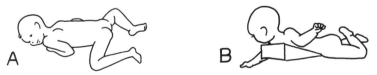

FIGURE 2-6. More involvement in the upper extremities, the phasic withdrawal response, and fluctuating tone impede the evolvement of prone antigravity responses.

The infant lacks the proximal stability necessary to cocontract muscles around a joint, and he cannot maintain contact with the surface—one or both arms withdraw, extend, and rotate outwardly (Fig. 2-6B).

The infant with hypotonic muscles lies rather limply on the surface (Fig. 2-7A). Reflexive movements are diminished in strength with a response latency, and sensory input is likewise diminished. He lacks the strength to maintain a tonic holding pattern, which interferes with the evolvement of antigravity movements in prone and supine positions. He collapses back to the surface after a short period. He also lacks the endurance for repeated practice, which delays the evolvement of more adaptive patterns. The head retracts when raised in prone position because of a lack of the opposing force of flexors. If the quality of the movement is not carefully observed, there can be the appearance of good head control. He may have difficulty moving the arms out from under the body in a propped position. When he is able to bring the arms forward, the elbows may exaggeratedly wing outward with external rotation of the arms. Thus, there is a hanging effect on ligaments and bony structures versus the use of muscles (Fig. 2-7B). The flexed elbows may not move in and align under the shoulders if he assumes a forearm support position because of the lack of stability in the shoulder girdle, and there will be the same hanging effect on ligaments versus stabilization of the muscles and normal proprioceptive sensory feedback. Because of the lack of background stability, movements are jerky and uncoordinated with overshooting, which interferes with the evolvement and quality of primary circular reactions and swiping and crude grasping schemas.

It is evident that the infant with abnormal tone does not develop antigravity patterns with the same degree of functional adaptiveness as the nondisabled infant. A comparison of some of the aberrant prone weight-bearing responses with the beginning normal weight-bearing position in Figure 2-8 further illustrates their compensatory nature.

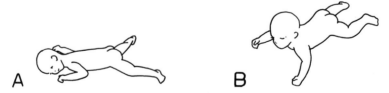

FIGURE 2-7. Prone antigravity responses are delayed and qualitatively different if the infant has hypotonia.

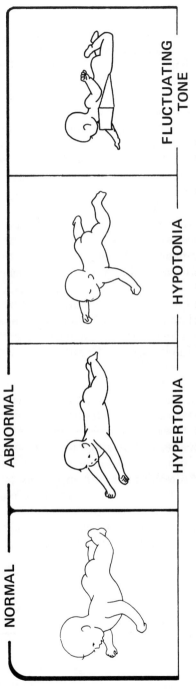

FIGURE 2-8. Aberrant weight-bearing patterns are compared with the beginning normal weight-bearing pattern.

Effect of Impairments on Oral and Respiratory Control

Many of the compensations described in the above paragraphs, including an aberrant regulatory mechanism, affect the respiratory pattern, oral control, and the nature of vocalization. The respiration rate may be faster and more variable with even a high rate and variability in the quiet sleep state. The neurologically impaired infant may spend even more time in the active REM sleep state, which increases the episodes of paradoxical respiration and the work of breathing. A higher number of apneic periods have been observed in infants with a neurologic disorder,[102] which may in part reflect increased respiratory fatigue. If the infant has a cardiopulmonary disease causing stiffer lungs, there is rather severe distortion of the rib cage even when intercostal activity is not inhibited in states other than active REM sleep. The pleural pressure has to become very negative to expand the stiff lungs, and the negative pressure also sucks in the compliant ribs. Thus, there are increased demands on the diaphragm, because of the effort required to expand the stiff lungs and the dissipation of some of the force distorting the ribs. The added work load is superimposed on the decreased ventilatory endurance typical of early infancy, resulting in diaphragmatic muscular fatigue, related hypoventilation, and possibly respiratory failure.[103,104] The infant may struggle so hard to breathe that there is no energy left for anything else. Even without cardiopulmonary problems, there may not be the typical increase in the proportion of Type I fibers and the vital capacity in this stage because of a decreased activity level. This limits the infant's endurance and affects his level of attention. There is early on the risk of being labeled lazy and stubborn when the infant's behavior is related to intraorganism demands.

If the infant remains in this stage for a long period of time and prefers the supine position, the ribs may remain flared at the side at the mercy of gravity, and the chest can appear ironed flat, especially if the muscles are hypotonic. If the infant does not develop stability in the neck and shoulder girdle, he may not develop the coordination of respiratory and laryngeal muscles necessary to gradually prolong the expiratory phase during crying, nor can be begin to maintain the thorax in a holding pattern to oppose the passive recoil forces at times during noncrying vocalization. Sounds may remain vegetative in nature related to the vegetative breathing pattern.

Weak antigravity responses also delay elongation of the neck and beginning descension of the tongue and larynx. The tongue remains more forward and less flexible, which interferes with its ability to elevate more during swallowing and to impede the air flow in particular ways to form some vowels and consonants. Head retraction related to weak neck flexors affects the apposition of oral structures and allows air to escape unrestricted. The jaw may be very lax or protracted or retracted, which limits the adjustment required to even make the frontal vowel sounds. Abnormal muscle tone interferes with oral control in other ways. Hypertonic muscles limit mobility of the tongue and lips, and hypotonic muscles limit the strength and stability of oral movements.

It is evident that the interplay of elements necessary for more productive sucking, more expressive crying, cooing, early babbling, and laughter may be lacking. The infant is deprived of communicative behaviors which so effectively fuel social interaction. Implications related to feeding will be further discussed in Chapter 4.

FRAMEWORK FOR HABILITATIVE APPROACHES

Collaborative Habilitative Focus

The intervention team can help the parents provide an environment that restores the normal integrative growth processes as far as possible. The home and family relationships are the foci of this environment; and intervention should, therefore, be collaborative in nature and in tune with the role system, values, and coping style of the family. The health and well being of the child is closely tied to the health and well being of the parents. The parents' supply of inner fuel and positive energy depends on how each of them was nurtured, the attachment and mutuality between them, social and financial support systems, and life circumstances. The birth of an infant with a developmental disability can be a significant life change, and intervention has to focus on broader ecologic factors as well as the microsystems within the family unit and the nature of the caregiver/infant interaction.

Voysey[105] contends that the professional expert influences the parents' perception of the disability. The physician and nurse are generally involved in the initial contacts with the family, and they must humbly realize this potential power. The nurse can assess the infant with an emphasis on eliciting behaviors that will engage his parents. The nurse can then help the infant display these behaviors during the initial get-acquainted sessions. The nurse can also in a sense talk for the infant and explain his lack of control over some behaviors that appear disengaging or explain the necessity of some disengaging behaviors because of competing physiologic demands. Sameroff[106] found that if parents can make allowances for behaviors, this decreases their negative effect on the relationship. The introductory sessions should be paced in accordance with the parents' stress level. There should not be forced contact, nor should the infant's characteristics be presented in an overkill fashion. This can turn the parents off or instill unrealistic expectations that can have a negative effect on the infant's later development.

The nurse and other interveners continue to help the caregiver read the infant's cues and understand his language. For example, the blind infant's hands send and receive messages to woo his caregiver. With this sensitive attunement, the caregiver can more effectively use adult strengths of flexibility and adaptability to modify her behavioral repertoire and stimulation to the infant's threshold level and modes of responsiveness. If a mutually regulating dyadic system can evolve, this will be the most potent growth-fostering source of stimulation during this stage. If there is an emphasis on the infant's deficits, which necessitate a prescriptive program, this can actually interfere with the evolvement of a spontaneous, flowing relationship imbedded in reciprocity. The parents may assume a more detached role of teacher or therapist.

The focus will then shift to a task-oriented implementation of an established curriculum program at the expense of sensitivity to affective and physiologic cues. There is the danger of overstimulation, especially if inanimate objects are a key part of the activities. Excessive environmental input taxes the infant's fragile autonomic system and interferes with the development of self-regulating behaviors, which are key elements in development. Overstimulation also elicits more extreme terminating behavior which can be erroneously interpreted as part of the disability versus the by-product of a noncontingent, intrusive environment: defensive head and bodily movements, disorganized activity level, flattened affect, staring through the caregiver, and limpness. On the other hand, there is also the danger of understimulation by not tuning in to the homeostatic curve of involvement and recovery. The caregiver may terminate the relationship when the infant only needs a brief rest period. Or, an infant may have to withdraw initially before he can become organized and orient to his caregiver. The pace of interaction may be too fast in relation to his response latency, which interferes with processing. It is an ongoing experimental process to come up with the right recipe which is not too weak, too powerful, too simple, too complex, too familiar, or too novel, or in the wrong sensory modality or modalities. The infant's cues and responses design his menu. He then senses that he has an ability to control his environment. The caregiver can also enhance his inner control by incorporating background excitatory and inhibitory approaches in the recipe to modulate the attention—excitement curve and the internal neurophysiologic state. These approaches are described in Chapter 3.

Approaches to Foster Interaction and Antigravity Responses in Supine Position

Positioning and handling approaches will be described in this section to facilitate the following habilitative outcomes:

- Assumes a more cuddly, flexed, orienting position
- Modifies reflexive movements through primary circular reactions to explore the hands
- Maintains the head in a midline position
- Expresses proximity seeking behaviors during spontaneous play periods
- Expands self exploration to the knees and feet with beginning strength in antigravity flexor muscles

Emphasis has been placed on keeping the infant with an extensor pattern in a side-lying or prone position, which disengages him from the most salient environmental stimulus—his caregiver's face. Some of the early schemas also evolve in the supine position—hand-watching, hand-clasping, and visual tracking. The hand-to-mouth schema may initially evolve in the prone position. There are ways to decrease the extensor tone in the supine position. The caregiver can facilitate a more flexed posture and face-to-face contact by placing her hand on the infant's chest or abdomen. She must monitor the effect of the pressure on breathing. When her hands are involved in diapering, some other care approach, or playful interaction, the caregiver can place a small pillow under the infant's head to facilitate some flexion. She will have to experiment with the softness and placement of the pillow, because pressure on the occipital area facilitates extension of the head, trunk, and extremities. A small pillow may also have to be placed under the low lumbar region of the back, or the infant's flexed legs can be placed up on the caregiver's thighs (Fig. 2-9A). A cuddly position in the arms is elicited by supporting the shoulders in a forward position with the caregiver's arm only in contact with the area below the occipital prominence of the head to again prevent setting off the extensor pattern she is trying to inhibit. The caregiver may also have to cross her legs to create a wedge effect with the infant's buttocks lower if he has a strong extensor pattern (Fig. 2-9B). She can carry him from place to place in a cuddled position. It is then still possible for the caregiver and infant to establish eye contact. The infant can be placed in the prone and side-lying positions to sleep when he is no longer in an alert, orienting state. If he has breathing problems, the side-lying position may be more comfortable because of the neutralization of both flexor and extensor tone.

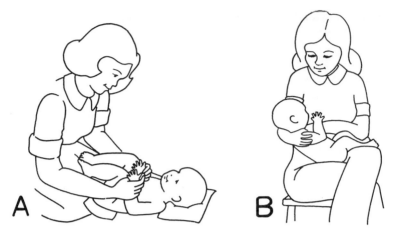

FIGURE 2-9. The caregiver uses positioning to facilitate a more flexed, orienting posture.

The following activity strengthens the neck flexor muscles to counteract head retraction and facilitate eye contact with the caregiver. The approach can be used for the infant who has either hypotonic or hypertonic muscles. The caregiver holds the infant facing her with his legs flexed and his shoulders forward by the support of her hands or the shawllike effect of a blanket. She provides necessary support to the head, avoiding pressure to the occipital area if the infant has an extensor pattern. The caregiver rocks the infant back and forth. As she feels the head actively come forward, the caregiver moves her hands down a short distance to provide less support. She uses her repertoire of interactive behaviors to motivate the infant to keep his head in a flexed, orienting position (Fig. 2-10). As the infant develops increased control, the caregiver gradually lowers her hands to decrease support to the head and increase the demand on the neck flexors, being sensitive to signs of discomfort or fatigue. She can also progress to rocking him backward to the point at which he can keep his head flexed in an orienting position. She then models the natural proximity seeking (pick-me-up) gesture and rocks him forward for a hug. He may begin to initiate the gesture on his own.

The infant with hypertonic muscles can move from one extreme to another, and too much flexion will have to be monitored in the above activities, which also disengages him from his caregiver's face. A careful rotary movement of the shoulders without pressure may relax some of the tone and help him maintain a more normal, orienting, flexor posture versus becoming too curled up. If the infant has milder hypertonicity, holding the hands together with the arms extended may be

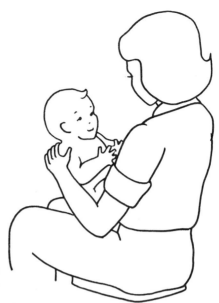

FIGURE 2-10. The caregiver uses the en face position as a catalyst to strengthen neck flexor muscles.

effective in preventing too much flexion. This approach should not be used if there is resistance to arm extension. If these approaches are not effective in decreasing excessive flexor tone, the infant should not be involved in the activities to prevent reinforcing abnormal patterns.

The diaper change can be adapted to facilitate the habilitative outcomes outlined at the beginning of this section. If the infant has a strong extensor pattern, the caregiver may initially have to incorporate the diaper change with a side-lying position and relaxing movement. For example, she can slowly and rhythmically rock the infant from supine to side-lying a number of times as described in Chapter 3. The caregiver then turns the infant to the side and flexes one leg to pin the diaper. The above approach should be repeated on the other side. After the diaper has been pinned, the caregiver slowly moves the infant on his back, applies pressure to his chest or abdomen or places a small pillow under his head, and flows into a play period which is so natural at this time. When the infant becomes very visually attentive during play periods, he may observe his hand when it is within visual range, especially if neck muscles have become relaxed in response to the slow rolling. The caregiver can move the infant's hand slightly to attract visual attention if he does not focus on the hand. If the infant does not respond, the caregiver can rhythmically move her hand in the same visual plane with his hand. He may yoke the action. If not, this rhythmic input has been found to have an organizing effect and can be used to control the level of excitement and prolong the play period. It may be that the infant will be more apt to focus on his own hand when it comes in view after pleasurable practice orienting to his caregiver's hand. Or, the caregiver can experiment with placing a rather low-intensity object (pacifier) approximately six to seven inches from the infant's eyes as a focal point in the same plane with the hand. This stimulus was felt to facilitate discovery of the hand in one study.[107] The caregiver must keep in mind that active, flexible, hand watching is dependent on the ability to converge the eyes and focus on a near object in the central visual field and move the head and arm freely. The infant may also progress to bringing his hands together in midline since the shoulders are forward. If he does not, the caregiver can clasp her hands together, experimenting with the distance of her hands from the infant's hands, which may again elicit a yoking action. She also just naturally clasps the infant's hands together during play. This natural response will have to be inhibited if the midline movement elicits increased tone and resistance. Also, lack of beginning stabilization of the neck and shoulder girdle and immature ocular control will no doubt interfere with the evolvement of the hand clasping schema. The hand-to-mouth schema should evolve in the adapted supine position or the side-lying or prone position.

When hand schemas have evolved, the caregiver facilitates expansion of the exploration to the knees. After the slow, rhythmic rocking from supine to the side, the caregiver can further relax the infant's legs by slowly and rhythmically rotating the hips from side to side, holding at the knees. Or, she can try grasping the knees and gently, slowly, rhythmically shaking the lower legs. The infant may then flex his legs up which will promote hand contact with the knees. If the infant does not flex his legs on his own, the caregiver can help bring his knees up in contact with the hands if there is no stiffness or resistance. If there is a lot of extensor tightness, the infant can be turned to the side-lying position. The caregiver places her one hand under the arm on the rib area, and the other hand on the hip and slowly and rhythmically rocks the infant's body back and forth through only a small one- or two-inch arc. As the infant relaxes, she flexes his legs, which places the knee in close proximity to the hand. The infant may also clasp his hands together in response to this input or visually monitor the movement of his hand.

The diaper routine is a little different if the infant has hypotonic muscles with legs widely abducted. The caregiver can change the diaper in the supine position with a small pillow under the infant's head to maintain an orienting position if necessary. The caregiver uses approaches described above to facilitate primary circular reactions involving the hands. Attachment of a bright ribbon to the hand may be effective in alerting the infant with a low response level, but not if the infant orients to the ribbon and not his hand or if the orientation is very demanding in terms of energy. In one study,[108] bright visual stimuli actually delayed the hand-watching schema and elicited signs of over-stimulation. The caregiver can again use her hand to try to hook the infant on hand-watching. Arrhythmic movement of the hand may be more alert-ing, and the rhythm can be adjusted to prolong the orientation. Or, the more benign pacifier approach can be tried.

A different approach is also used to facilitate exploration of the knees and feet. The caregiver lightly touches the inner surface of the thighs with her finger, a cotton swab, or a cotton ball to stimulate adductors and bring the legs in from the very wide, abducted position. She also stimu-lates contraction of the abdominal muscles by drawing an imaginary line on each side of the navel with a rather firm stroke, using the pad of her fingers. The caregiver must monitor the effect of especially light tactual input to prevent too much excitation and disorganized activity. Also, she wants the play period to elicit orienting, pleasurable sensations and not avoidance responses. The caregiver can also arrhythmically jiggle the hips, which may perk up the muscles and facilitate flexion of the knees.

During playful interaction, the caregiver just naturally provides input to the hands and feet by kissing them, fingering the fingers and toes, brushing the hands or fingers across her lips, and grasping the feet together and bending the knees up on the chest. This input can be pleasurable to the infant if he can handle the sensations. This natural stimulation may have to be adjusted some, especially if the infant is hypertonic, or has fluctuating tone, or is very tactually defensive. The infant's response will have to be the guide.

The above examples involve an interplay of the caregiver's spontaneous behaviors, positioning, and excitatory or inhibitory approaches discussed in Chapter 3 to expand the infant's reper-toire of behaviors, whereby he can explore the normal infant's sensory world as much as possible. Some very sensitive caregivers come upon many of these approaches all on their own with the above goal in mind and with the infant as their guide.

Approaches to Foster Interaction and Antigravity Responses in the Prone Position

All movement patterns involve a balance of extension and flexion, and the infant needs to experience opposing gravity in the prone position. Approaches will be outlined in subsequent paragraphs to facilitate the following habilitative outcomes:

- Raises the head to a vertically righted, orienting position with the arms in a weight-bearing position
- Combines flexion and extension to stabilize in a forearm weight-bearing position with the head in midline

- Organizes weight-bearing experiences in a primitive body sense
- Develops beginning background stability on the ulnar side of the hand
- Develops beginning coordination of respiratory and laryngeal muscles

The prone position is the starting point for the evolvement of mobility patterns; it is, therefore, important for the infant to learn to enjoy this position. The caregiver's lap is no doubt the most reassuring and comfortable support while the infant practices opposing gravity with a head movement. If the infant is hypertonic, the caregiver can slowly and rhythmically sway the infant to relax him. Or, if the infant is hypotonic, the caregiver can rather arrhythmically jiggle him to elicit increased excitation but not startles. She is right there to adjust or change his position when he signals discomfort due to breathing difficulties, fatigue, or some other reason. Also, he is becoming acquainted with the caregiver's body, which would not be possible over a bolster. A contingent response to discomfort and a lot of physical contact with the caregiver have been related to later independent exploratory play and noncrying modes of communication.[109]

If the infant has hypertonia, the effort of raising the head may increase extensor tone throughout the body. More localized neck extension may be facilitated by placing the infant at an angle with the head lower than the rest of the body for an interval, which has a relaxing effect (Fig. 2-11A). His fingers will probably also relax and open. This position aids breathing by increasing the rib cage expansion and lung volume.[110] Or, the infant with hypertonia may have difficulty raising his head in the prone position because of the influence of the TLR, resulting in exaggerated flexion. The caregiver can securely hold the infant at the pelvic level and place him in an inverted posture, gently swaying his body (Fig. 2-11B). This generally has a calming and relaxing effect, and the infant can then gently be lowered to a prone position on the caregiver's lap. This inverted position also aids breathing by expanding the neck and thoracic area and is used in some care facilities for this purpose. However, the caregiver must be careful to support the infant well, and it is safer to suspend him over a bed or other soft surface. She should also avoid holding him by the knees or ankles without orthopedic consultation, because this can be too stressful on the hip joints, particularly if there is a muscle tone imbalance, which could result in hip dislocation. The caregiver must also be alert for stress reactions.

If the infant's muscles are hypotonic, the caregiver can facilitate head extension by walking up each side of the upper spine with pressure, using the pads of the index and third fingers. Again, she must

DEVELOPMENTALLY DISABLED INFANTS AND TODDLERS

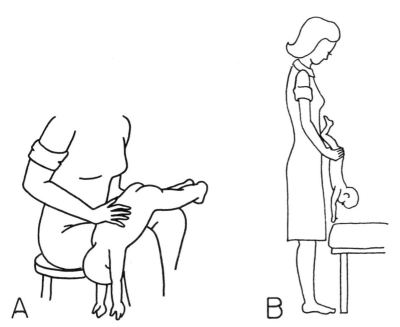

FIGURE 2-11. The caregiver places the infant in an inverted posture to relax hypertonic muscles and increase the lung volume.

observe for a negative response to this tactual input and also the elicitation of too much extension and head retraction because of weak opposing flexors. If this response occurs, the caregiver can keep the infant's shoulders somewhat forward and encourage him to focus on a bright object on the surface below to elicit a more normal head movement.

When the infant can raise his head without retraction, the caregiver encourages experimentation with weight bearing by sitting on the floor with the infant lying over her legs or by lying on her back and placing him in a prone position on her body facing her. This latter position uses the caregiver's face as a salient stimulus. Some infants with a strong flexor pattern can raise their head and breathe comfortably only with arms extended (Fig. 2-12A). Thus, the typical weight-bearing position may elicit aberrant responses and should not be facilitated. If the infant has less hypertonic muscles, he may be able to assume a more normal beginning weight-bearing position with the flexed arms in a wider base of support, if the caregiver helps him keep the shoulders and arms forward (Fig. 2-12B). If the effort begins to elicit too much extension, flexion of one leg may be helpful. The infant can be slowly and rhythmically rocked to prevent superficial holding and a static position,

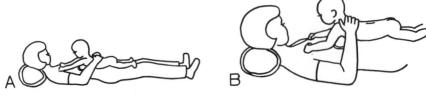

FIGURE 2-12. (*A*) The infant with exaggerated flexor hypertonia may be able to raise his head only with his arms extended. (*B*) The infant with less hypertonic muscles may assume a beginning weight-bearing position, with assistance in keeping his arms forward.

which is not typical; no infant with normal muscle tone remains locked in a position. A strong STNR can elicit abnormal extension of the arms when the head is raised. The infant is encouraged to focus on an interesting sight on the surface that limits the degree of head raising and helps him maintain a more normal weight-bearing position of the arms.

Facilitation of weight bearing has to be adapted for other manifestations of abnormal tone. If the infant has athetosis, the arms may turn outward as illustrated earlier in Figure 2-6B. The caregiver can inhibit this dysfunctional position by turning the arms inward at the shoulder (Fig. 2-13A). Also, the surface should not be rough or cold to prevent a phasic withdrawal response. The degree of head righting may have to be limited as discussed above if there is a strong STNR. If the infant has hypotonic muscles with exaggerated abduction and possibly external rotation of the arms and a hanging effect of the shoulders, the caregiver can provide pressure input to the shoulders in an inward and downward direction (Fig. 2-13B). Or, excitation may be more effectively elicited by applying intermittent pressure with a compression, hold, release, compression, hold, release rhythm. This pressure input increases stability and thus decreases the hanging effect. There will be more normal proprioceptive input to the muscles, joints, and tendons.

In all the above cases, the infant's response should be monitored to prevent compensations that will provide aberrant feedback. The goal of practice is an ability to raise the head in the midline with the face and nose vertical in relation to the force of gravity and the mouth horizontal. This is a visually orienting position and an important referent for alignment of the body and for movement all along the continuum of development. Also, the weight bearing provides sensations that are organized in a central neural template. This beginning awareness of the upper extremities is an integral aspect of the evolving primitive body sense and prehension schemas.

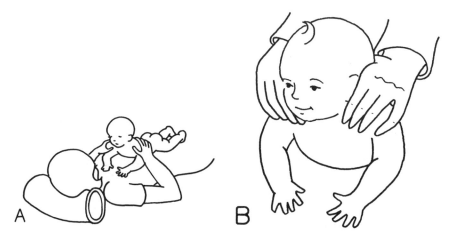

FIGURE 2-13. (A) The infant with fluctuating tone assumes a beginning weight-bearing position if the caregiver prevents external rotation of the arms. (B) The infant with hypotonia assumes a beginning weight-bearing position, with the assistance of compression to enhance stability.

Again, the caregiver is right there to respond to fatigue or discomfort so that the position is not associated with negative sensations. The infant may quickly experience ventilatory muscular fatigue, especially if he has a cardiac or pulmonary problem. Undue effort can also elicit associated reactions in other parts of the body and distorted feedback. If positions and movements are related to pleasurable bodily sensations and environmental events, the infant will want to repeat the experience. The normal infant practices motor patterns over and over. The pattern then becomes semi-automatic with less energy expenditure.

The inability to maintain his head in an orienting position may precede the infant's loss of interest in the caregiver's face or another interesting sight. The caregiver can intervene and control the infant's head for him, because the expansion of visual attention is an important cognitive goal in this stage. However, normal movement should be self induced as much as possible to enhance the infant's sense of control over his environment.

With the assistance described in the preceding paragraphs, the infant may begin to extend his arms in a slanted position, with the elbows in front of the shoulders, when he raises his head higher to orient to an interesting sight, without eliciting abnormal responses: internal rotation of the arms and fisting of the hands, disorganized movement of the arms or body, inability to maintain contact with the surface, or a hanging effect of the shoulders and arms with the elbows widely abducted. The infant may also be able to practice moving back and forth between the beginning flexed weight-bearing position and the slanted extended position, as the normal infant does.

If the infant develops increased strength in the neck, shoulder girdle, and upper arm muscles and more extension in the upper back from practicing antigravity responses in the prone and supine position, he probably can progress to a more adaptive pattern. The infant practices combining flexion and extension to bear and maintain weight on the elbows and forearms. The amount of body weight on the elbows and forearms may have to be adjusted if the infant has abnormal tone. If the caregiver and intervener do not have access to specialized therapy consultation, the following guidelines may help the infant assume the new position without reinforcing abnormal patterns. With the infant who has hypertonia and too much muscle tone, the upper body weight or less than the upper body weight will help normalize the tone in the surrounding musculature if the infant remains in the position without movement for a few minutes. He can initially try to maintain the position supporting his upper body weight, which is typical of the normal infant. If there is an increase in tone, which interferes with the maintenance of a balance between flexion and extension, the caregiver can experiment with providing support under the arms to relieve some of the body weight. If the infant has hypotonia and related lack of proximal stability, pressure in addition to the body weight facilitates increased stability. The caregiver applies inward and downward pressure on the shoulders as illustrated in Figure 2-13B. Another approach can also be used if the infant has hypotonia. He is alternately moved from side to side, which increases the body weight on one elbow and then the other elbow. This intermittent pressure may also provide enough tone to maintain the position.

As with beginning weight bearing, the goal is to experience sensations that are as normal as possible, leading to important developmental outcomes described previously. The stabilization of the neck and shoulder girdle also facilitates increased coordination of respiratory and laryngeal muscles necessary for beginning control of the expiratory phase during crying and noncrying vocalization.

Approaches to Facilitate Visual Attention

If the infant has a rather severe motor impairment, habilitative approaches very possibly will not increase head control. Yet the infant may be in an awake, visually alert state for increasingly longer periods, reflecting uneven advancement of cognitive development. It is important to focus on ways to facilitate strengths. The members of the professional team collaborate with the parents to design adaptive positioning that will substitute for the neck muscles and hold the head in an orienting, midline position. The infant can then experience the center of gravity; and, it is hoped that the stability will improve ocular control so that the infant can visually prehend his world during periods when his caregiver cannot hold him and provide support. However, his perceptual experiences may be limited by the inability to coordinate eye and head movements to flexibly turn toward objects in the periphery. An orienting position may be attained by placing the infant in a Styrofoam tub that holds drinks and floats in a swimming pool. Pillows or foam is added to provide selective support. The tub can be placed in an area where the caregiver is involved in an activity so the infant can visually monitor her movements to the extent possible. The caregiver can also gently move the tub as she goes by to provide vestibular input, which is felt to be a key component in the development of neck and ocular control. As discussed earlier in the section on normal motor patterns, there is an interplay between the vestibular and visual systems that becomes progressively more developed in this stage. If the infant has a strong extensor or flexor pattern or a strong ATNR, a more involved support mechanism may be necessary. Farber and Huss[111] have designed both a static and dynamic head support system. From a preventive standpoint, a more neutral supported position will prevent abnormal lengthening or shortening of muscles, which would result in increased weakness. The dentist is a key member of the team if a proposed approach involves oral structures.

The caregiver can experiment with other forms of vestibular input to enhance visual alertness and control. She can hold the infant facing her with his head supported at approximately a 45-degree angle. The support should allow a free turning movement. The caregiver rocks the infant and slowly tilts him from one side to the other. This may bring him to an alert state and facilitate orientation to her face. She can then slowly move her face in a bobbing action, beginning in his peripheral visual field. The infant's tracking may be a series of jerky fixations that lag behind her facial movement to let the image fall back in the peripheral region if central fixation has not evolved. Therefore, the caregiver's horizontal movement must be slow but not too slow, or the image may remain in his poorer central field too long. He may also overshoot during tracking and lose the image. The caregiver moves back across so he can fixate on the image again. She experiments with the distance to determine his accommodation capacity. Combined facial movement and continuous, soft vocalization are generally most effective in eliciting orientation and tracking. It may also help to move into an area where there is dimmer illumination, especially when the infant is very young or if the eyes are sensitive to light. If the infant has a high threshold, a stronger visual stimulus may have to be used—New Year's Eve sparkler or a battery-operated mobile toy. However, the caregiver should first try exaggerating her facial gestures and vocalization because becoming hooked to her face is so important.

Forms of vestibular input are also discussed in the section on growth-fostering environment and in Chapter 3. Of all the suggested modes, rocking is the most natural vestibular input during this stage. The position, speed, and excursion of the rocking has to be individually determined. The infant may tolerate being rocked in both a side-lying (each side) and on-shoulder position, which possibly stimulates different pairs of semicircular canals. The caregiver may be able to adapt a commercial carrier if necessary or design one herself to support the infant in a flexed posture and provide movement and tactual input next to the caregiver's body. Movement may also facilitate vocalization, since the two occur concomitantly in this first stage.

If the infant is blind, the emphasis has to be on the development of other senses to orient to the caregiver and the more immediate sensate world. As mentioned earlier, the infant and caregiver can learn to send and receive messages via the hands. All the touch input from being carressed, cuddled, wrapped, and carried around express love that the infant cannot see and helps him and all infants begin to form a primitive sense of the caregiver and themselves. The input also facilitates the beginning inhibition of protective tactual reactions toward the end of this stage. Huss[112] emphasizes that touch must be caring in nature. In other words, how the caregiver holds the infant is probably more important than how much the infant is held. Suggestions are provided in Chapter 3 to adapt touch input so that this contact can be pleasurable for both the infant and caregiver, depending on the infant's sensory threshold.

Approaches to Facilitate More Sustained Attention and Elaboration of Schemas

The quality of the overall environmental milieu is an important habilitative element. If the care approaches are organized around a consistent social base, this will support the maturation of inner regulatory mechanisms and the modulation of inner states. The infant has more distinct inner experiences which help him develop an internal set of expectations. It is hypothesized that the interplay between internal and external organization is an important biosocial foundation for memory[113] and later foresight.[114]

With the advent of more sustained periods of alertness related to better state modulation, increased processing capacities, and central visual fixation, the infant may begin to examine and enjoy dynamic visual stimuli in the form of mobiles. Gould[115] designed a Whacker Dacker, which infants have enjoyed. Lightweight arms made of braided nylon hose extend down, and objects are attached to each arm. The stimulus intensity of the objects will have to be adapted to each individual infant per guidelines in Chapter 3. The caregiver can introduce the Whacker Dacker when holding the infant so that she can support him in a position that facilitates visual orientation and awkward reaching attempts. The caregiver can also more readily observe the infant's responses, especially for signs of too much excitement and an impending overload. When he begins to reach out, the caregiver adaptively adjusts the braided arms to facilitate batting contact with a preferred object. The idea is to give the infant a sense that he can make a spectacle happen as he did with hand-watching and hand-clasping schemas. He is now coordinating the visual schema and hand movements in more complex ways and in a more outwardly direction. Suspended objects that provide auditory and tactual feedback in a consistent location help bring the blind infant's hands in out of the periphery to a more orienting position with some tactual guidance from the caregiver if necessary. If the infant enjoys the Whacker Dacker, he can be placed in an orienting supine position for a self-entertainment period to practice using his own adaptive resources. Some infants may be able to move their arm freely only in a supported side-lying position because of a strong ATNR or TLR, or an extensor pattern related to abnormal tone.

The developmentally disabled infant may not follow the pattern typical of the normal infant in this stage characterized by increased adaptability and beginning expansion of his interaction with inanimate objects and other members of the family. The intervener can again talk for the infant, explaining his response in terms of his more limited adaptive capacities. The other members of the family can be helped to modify their approach, especially if the infant needs a stimulus barrier. On the other hand, a more jazzed up approach typical of a lot of fathers may be very effective in eliciting an alert state, if the infant has a high sensory threshold. However, the infant's homeostatic curve must still be respected during the interaction. Another consideration is that even if the infant has the appearance of a high level of alertness and increased wakefulness coupled with contentment, this is not always a positive sign. The behaviors can reflect ongoing internal stress rather than typical developmental progress.[116]

Approaches to Decrease the Work of Breathing

As discussed earlier, the work of breathing can be even greater if the infant has a neurologic impairment, and this can affect his level of alertness. The expansion of the thoracic area is decreased in the supine position, because the direction of the diaphragmatic contraction tends to pull the lower rib cage inward. The lung volume is also less in the supine position because the contents of the abdomen are pushed upward, which decreases the vital capacity.[117] A change to the prone, suspended position discussed earlier or the upright position can increase the lung volume. Some primitive mothers nurse their infant in the upright position which has a sound physiologic rationale. The prone, nonsuspended position has also been found to improve ventilation by increasing the stability of the compliant chest. Thus, less of the effort of the diaphragmatic contraction is dissipated sucking in the ribs.[118] Paradoxical breathing has been decreased by constraining the abdomen. If the abdominal expansion is restricted, the increased intra-abdominal pressure from the diaphragmatic contraction has to lift the rib cage.[119] The old practice of applying a belly band appears to have a physiologic purpose other than the one intended. There is a need for more habilitative emphasis on this very vital function and a new look at age-old caregiving practices.

Alternate Caregiving Resources

Some infants will always developmentally remain in this stage of dependency and will need a protective environment which ideally will revolve around a close, intimate relationship with a caregiver. Some reactive infants will also need a strong environmental shield. It will become increasingly more difficult to provide close, nurturing input as the child's body size increases. It is also probably unrealistic to expect that a caregiver and family members can continue to maintain such intimate involvement, especially if there is limited refueling feedback. There will no doubt be a need for resources that provide surrogate caregiving: special school program, short-term respite facilities, and even possibly more long-term placement at some point in time, or possibly at birth.

It will be a challenge to provide an environment that will continue to nourish the nervous system in whatever setting the infant is in. If the caregiver recognizes the supremacy of animate stimulation in this stage of development, she will exploit periods of contact centered on care needs. There is a tendency in some programs to rush through diapering, feeding, and other aspects of care in a task-oriented manner to allow more time for a structured activity primarily involving less adaptable and more demanding inanimate stimulation.

Even with the best of intentions, the caregiver's reserve of energy, program staff ratios, and other factors will no doubt decrease the amount of animate stimulation that can be provided. Technology has not come up with substitutes for the human body, face, and voice. It is no wonder that the infant or child turns more and more to his own body for stimulation. This behavior remains very stereotyped and perseverating in nature if the infant lacks the ability to coordinate sensory input; sensations may always remain in separate spaces. Of course, self-stimulation is appropriate at this level. It is a matter of degree which expresses deprivation from other enjoyable and organizable sources.

In contrast, the dependency of the infant and emotions centered on his disability have the potential of fostering a very close, symbiotic relationship characterized by the caregiver's continuous and exclusive involvement that can be overstimulating to the infant. He may even be awakened during sleep. This engulfing relationship jeopardizes gradual achievement of autonomy to the extent possible in the subsequent stages. Also, the symbiosis can stress relationships within the family if the caregiver's life centers on the needs of this one family member.

SECOND STAGE: FIVE THROUGH EIGHT MONTHS

FRAMEWORK FOR ASSESSING NORMAL DEVELOPMENTAL PATTERNS

Description of Normal Motor Patterns

Referring to the previous stage, the four-month-old infant evolved to the first of three phases in the development of a posture and motor skill outlined in the first part of the chapter. He assumed the prone, on-elbows weight-bearing position, which involves proximal stability of the head and shoulder girdle. This cocontraction or fixation of body segments provides a reference point for movement. The infant now evolves to the second phase and superimposes bilateral proximal mobility on distal stability. His elbows remain in place, and movement occurs in the shoulder girdle, shoulder joints, and thoracic region of the trunk. The infant first rocks backward and then backward and forward with alternate flexion and extension. He shifts some weight from side to side as he freely rotates his head to scan the surroundings. When the infant rocks forward, his knees may pull up under his body and propel him a short distance in space in an inchworm fashion. These heavy work patterns increase endurance and control and stability in the prone posture to prepare him for the third phase—distal mobility superimposed on proximal stability.

In the new phase, the infant shifts weight to one elbow and reaches out toward an interesting visual sight with one arm. The unilateral weight bearing increases joint compression and thus increases proprioceptive input. There may be regression to internal rotation of the forearm and fisting of the weight-bearing hand in response to the stress of a new adaptation. The infant gradually reaches farther and higher, superimposing rotation on proximal stability in the neck and shoulder girdle: one shoulder is forward and one shoulder is backward, which prevents the infant from toppling over on his back. Thus, equilibrium responses are beginning to evolve in the prone position. The infant adapts the distal movement to alternately lift one arm and then the other arm to move forward in a modified combat (belly) crawl with shoulder rotation and lateral trunk flexion. The leg on the same side follows with little movement because of the lack of trunk rotation and immaturity of the lower extremities at this point. Increased stability and flexibility of the lower extremities are dependent on the later evolvement of proximal stability in the lower trunk and hips.[1]

The infant simultaneously practices patterns that facilitate the development of extensor muscles and proximal stability in the lower trunk and hip area. He assumes a pivot prone position which is considered to be the essential prerequisite for all weight-bearing patterns.[2] There is a total extension response except in the arms and feet. The elbows are flexed, the arms are externally rotated and adducted and the scapulae are adducted. The feet are dorsiflexed, and the extended legs are separated. When the infant sees something of interest, he excitedly waves his arms and rocks on his abdomen; and the vestibular input reinforces extension, raising the head, chest, and legs higher off the surface. He alternates between the pivot prone position with an anterior pelvic tilt (sway in the back) and an exaggerated puppy position with the head down, buttocks up in the air, and a posterior pelvic tilt. Thus, he begins to develop a flexible range of motion in the pelvis.

As extension proceeds in a cephalocaudal direction, the infant can bear weight on fully extended arms but with the elbows still in front of the shoulders. With increased stability and progressive extension, his hands and elbows align under the shoulders. The abdomen is off the surface with the hips as the anchor. The infant develops enough midline stability to shift weight onto one extended arm and reach out with rotation of the head, shoulders, and trunk. There is counter-rotation of the hips and a holding action of the thoracic and abdominal muscles to prevent the infant from toppling over. The extended weight-bearing arm flexes some at the elbow again in response to the stress. Equilibrium reactions in the prone position have evolved to a level of maturity allowing the infant to move away and back to midline while maintaining the position. The evolvement of trunk rotation also allows the infant to pivot in a circle in the prone position and combat crawl with a reciprocal movement of both the arms and legs. There has been cephalocaudal progression from neck rotation in the first stage to shoulder and trunk rotation in this stage. Figure 2-14 illustrates the evolvement of patterns in the prone position.

Because movement is dependent on reciprocal patterns, the infant practices in the supine position to develop antigravity flexor muscles further. He rights his head vertically to orient to his caregiver. There is also no head lag when pulled to sit, and the infant progresses to exerting most of the effort of pulling himself up, using flexor muscles in the neck, shoulder, abdomen, and hips. His legs begin to adaptively extend to pull himself up to standing. When the flexor muscles become stronger and extension proceeds down the back, he brings his foot to his mouth with the knees extended. The infant then progresses to also lifting the buttocks off the surface, which allows him to bring the foot to his ear. These self-exploratory movements involve shortening of flexors and lengthening of extensors, which contrasts with the shortening of extensors and lengthening of flexors in the pivot prone position described earlier. Thus, these movement patterns maintain balanced flexibility between muscle groups.

The infant also experiences weight bearing in the supine position. He turns to the side and shifts his weight to one shoulder and hip and then to the opposite shoulder and hip. The infant progresses to superimposing distal mobility on proximal stability. He reaches for a toy when in the side-lying position, which involves shoulder rotation—one shoulder more forward. With increased midline stability in supine position, rotation moves down to the trunk; and the infant can reach across midline with the arm, which involves rotation of the upper part and counter-rotation of the hips. He also moves his hips back and forth, which involves rotation of the lower part of the body and counter-rotation of the upper part of the body. Thus, more reliable equilibrium reactions are also evolving in the supine position. The infant can move away from the center of gravity and still maintain the supine position. He can also dissociate movements by completely or partially flexing one leg and extending the other leg; plantarflexing one foot and dorsiflexing the other foot. The infant develops enough strength and flexibility to assume a bridge position, raising his hips and arching his back with the head, shoulders, and feet on the surface. This elongates the flexor muscles, resulting in increased extension of the hips, knees, and the ankles; the legs move into a more neutral

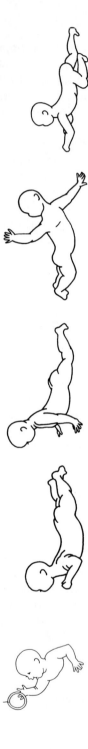

FIGURE 2-14. Motor patterns in the prone position become progressively more adaptive.

DEVELOPMENTALLY DISABLED INFANTS AND TODDLERS

extended position from the primitive abducted, externally rotated position. Figure 2-15 illustrates progressive patterns in the supine position.

The infant is simultaneously using the blend of stability and flexibility in prone and supine to move from one of these positions to the other in a segmental roll. He leads with the head, and the shoulders, trunk, and pelvis follow in a rotatory, chainlike reaction around the body axis to move from prone to supine position. There is a combination of flexion on one side and extension on the other side, with one part rotating in one direction and another part rotating in a different direction to provide a controlled movement versus flopping over. Supine to prone rolling evolves a little later with either the shoulder or hip leading and a chainlike reaction of the rest of the body. The infant lifts his head off the surface and rights the head to a near vertical position when rolling either way. With a balance between flexors and extensors and integration of vertical and rotational righting in equilibrium reactions, the infant is free to rotate away from midline, to cross midline, and to perform an activity in any position between prone and supine while maintaining his balance.[3] Thus, the infant flexibly moves with pleasurable ease on a horizontal surface.

However, when the infant moves up to a new posture farther away from the center of gravity, he must repeat the phases that evolved down on the horizontal surface. When placed in the sitting position, the infant uses the forward protective extension of the arms developed in prone position to support himself because of the lack of midline stability and equilibrium reactions. The legs also widen the base of support by abducting in a flexed, ringed position (Fig. 2-16A). He again experiments to find midline and to strengthen proximal muscles by straightening the back some and then moving back to the support position. As extension moves down the back in prone position, the infant can sit more erect with some rounding in the lower back. He practices extending the trunk to a greater degree, which elicits a pivot prone position of the arms to maintain the extension and an anterior tilt of the pelvis (Fig. 2-16B). The infant simultaneously begins to shift weight from one buttocks to the other as he turns his head to orient to something of interest, which elicits a lateral protective extension of the arm to prevent him from toppling over (Fig. 2-16C). The infant initially uses his arm to push himself back to midline, and he then progresses to pulling back to midline with a lateral flexion of the trunk. The forward, upward, and lateral adjustments of the trunk involve a proximal movement of the pelvis that both strengthens and maintains the range of motion in the pelvis (posterior tilt, anterior tilt, lateral tilt).

When extension moves all the way down the back in prone position and abdominal and lateral muscles become stronger, the infant can

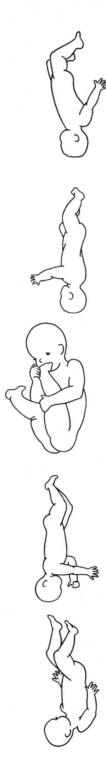

FIGURE 2-15. Motor patterns in the supine position become progressively more adaptive.

cocontract the trunk muscles and sit with the more stable pelvis in a neutral position and the shoulders aligned over the hips. The legs have to remain in the abducted, ringed position to provide a wide base of support because equilibrium reactions are still immature and evolving (Fig. 2-16D). With increased background stability, the infant can rotate at the shoulder level and begin orienting to surrounding space in a limited way. Arm movements are also less stiff and restricted as the hands become freed from the support role. The arms move farther out from the body, and there is beginning external rotation of the forearms, whereas initially in this stage the arms are internally rotated and remain close to the body.

When the infant has developed midline stability in the shoulders and trunk and beginning stability in the hips, he also moves from prone up to a quadruped position with weight on extended arms and hands and flexed knees. Since the pelvis and lower extremities are less developed, there may be a lordotic curve and hip abduction with the knees spread farther apart when the infant first begins to assume this position. The arms may also abduct wider than the shoulders and internally rotate with the stress of increased weight bearing in this new position higher from the center of gravity. The infant practices moving back and forth between the prone and quadruped position, which strengthens muscles. He also repeats the phases described earlier and superimposes proximal mobility on distal stability by rocking backward, then backward and forward, and side to side.

These work patterns further increase stability and control; the entire trunk straightens and assumes a horizontal position with cocontraction of the arms, shoulders, trunk, and pelvis. The elbows align with the shoulders, and the knees align with the hips. The weight is then more evenly distributed between the knees and hands. The evolvement of the third phase, superimposition of distal mobility on proximal stability (creeping), will be described in the next stage. The infant also begins to move from the prone and quadruped position to the sitting position by pushing diagonally to side sitting and then adjusting his leg to shift weight to both buttocks. He has to use the pushing action of the arm because of immature equilibrium reactions in this new adaptation.

As described earlier, the infant adapts the pull-to-sit movement when holding onto the adult's hands. He starts with a flexed pattern and his legs then go into extension to counterbalance the trunk coming up, and he pulls up into a standing position. Initially in this stage, the legs assume a static, protective, support position similar to the arm position in the prone and sitting postures. The pelvis is posteriorly tilted with the buttocks protruding backward out of line with the shoulders, and the toes grasp the surface for added distal stability. By

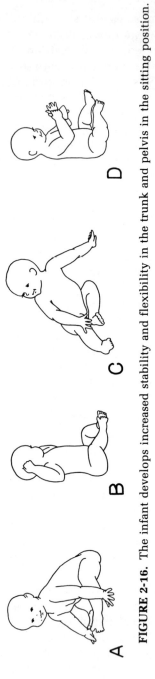

FIGURE 2-16. The infant develops increased stability and flexibility in the trunk and pelvis in the sitting position.

the end of this stage, the toe grasp is fading, the posterior pelvic tilt is decreasing, and there is less extensor tone in the legs. The shoulders are still shrugged because of lack of midline stability in this upright position farther away from the center of gravity. The phasic evolvement of motor patterns described in the above paragraphs is outlined in graphic form in Table 2-6.

EVOLVEMENT OF PREHENSION SCHEMAS. It has been hypothesized that prehension skills follow a continuum closely tied to proximal motor patterns and movement in space.[4] As mentioned earlier in the chapter, the hypothesis is being questioned. Since this is still a controversial issue, a framework will be presented based on an interrelationship between proximal and distal development.

In the last stage, even the very young infant reached out with one hand toward an interesting stimulus. The reach evolved into primarily a bilateral pattern with mirroring of the other arm. The infant also began to visually monitor the distance between the object and the hand with an alternate glance, and he awkwardly grasped the object with an ulnar-palmar orientation. The proximal and distal parts moved as a unit, and the internally rotated arm thus determined the position of the hand and direction of movement. The movement was stereotyped and ballistic in nature, with the end point remaining stable. The infant would not reach for an object if he could not see his hand, because of the poorly developed sense of the arm as an integral part of the body. This pattern is also characteristic of the first part of this stage with progression from an ulnar-palmar orientation of the hand to a palmar orientation as the forearm becomes less internally rotated.

Practice weight bearing on extended arms and hands increases stability in the elbows and wrists, and the ongoing maturation of the sensory system also provides a background for more adaptive prehension schemas. Touch and other protective receptors and pathways become modified as newer pathways are emerging and maturing. There may also be a differential diminution of receptors in the hand, which increases focal sensitivity.[5] Input is processed by the receptors and the central nervous system in a more discriminative way, which overrides the protective withdrawal response. Thus, the infant responds to a stimulus with a more adaptive, localized movement. The sensations from his movement out in the periphery are transmitted via the newer pathways and organized in a perceptive kind of memory or sensory-motor map in the central nervous system.

The way is therefore paved for the evolvement of the visually guided reach. Continual information of an ongoing motion is fed back to the central nervous system via a developing feedback system. This information is compared with previous experience, and the reach and

TABLE 2-6 Evolvement of motor patterns in phases (Second Stage)

ASSUMES POSITION	SUPERIMPOSES PROXIMAL MOBILITY ON DISTAL STABILITY	DEVELOPS INCREASED STABILITY & CONTROL IN POSITION	SUPERIMPOSES DISTAL MOBILITY ON PROXIMAL STABILITY
* (1) Prone—weight on elbows, externally rotated forearms, and ulnar side of hand	(1) Rocks backward, forward, shifts weight side to side	(1) Elbows align directly under shoulders, chest expands	(1) Shifts weight to one elbow, reaches with shoulder rotation (2) Combat crawls, reciprocal arm movements, minimal leg movements, lateral trunk flexion (3) Pivots in circle, trunk rotation (3) Combat crawls, reciprocal arm & leg movements, trunk rotation
(1) Prone—weight on extended arms, elbows in front of shoulders	(1) Rocks backward, forward shifts weight side to side	(2) Elbows and hands align with shoulders	(2) Shifts weight one extended arm, reaches with head, shoulder, and trunk rotation
(1) Supine	(1) Turns to side, shifting weight one shoulder & hip, upper arm may assume propped position	(2) Maintains side-lying position without upper arm assuming propped position	(2) Reaches in side-lying position, shoulder rotation (3) Reaches across midline in supine position, head, shoulder, & trunk rotation
(1) Sitting—arms in forward propped position, pelvis posteriorly tilted, legs flexed & abducted	(2) Tilts pelvis posteriorly, anteriorly laterally, arms assume protective position	(3) Maintains trunk in erect position, shoulders align over hips, pelvis assumes neutral position, legs abduct in ringed position	(3) Frees arms from protective role, manipulates object (3) Reaches in limited arc, shoulder rotation
(2) Quadruped—lordotic curve, arms abducted and internally rotated, knees abducted and externally rotated	(2) Rocks backward, forward, side to side	(3) Trunk assumes horizontal position, elbows align with shoulders, knees align with hips	

* (1) Beginning of stage; (2) Midway in stage; (3) End of stage

grasp are altered in flight if necessary to come in contact with the target.[6] The central map is likewise altered from the experience and so it goes. There is an improvement in the quality of the reach and grasp characterized by a more direct and accurate movement. The infant can also bring his hand in from outside the visual field. It is becoming a part of the infant's crude body sense.

A number of components coalesce to facilitate beginning dissociation of the proximal and distal segments. Weight bearing on extended arms increases wrist stability and extension of the fingers. Touch pressure input to the palm of the hand helps integrate the grasp reflex, and flexion and extension of the fingers become progressively more voluntary. Tactual stimulation to the medial side of the hand and rotation during mouthing elicit a beginning radial orientation. As described above, the sensory receptors in the hand are also becoming more discriminative. The infant begins to orient the hand to the object, grasping the object on the radial side of the palm with the thumb opposing the first two curled fingers. Reciprocity between the two hands also evolves in this stage by transferring an object from one hand to another in midline and by maintaining the grasp of an object while reaching for another object. The evolvement of prehension schemas in this stage is summarized in Table 2-7.

TABLE 2-7 Evolvement of prehension schemas (Second Stage)

FUNCTIONAL ADAPTATION	QUALITATIVE DESCRIPTION
Undifferentiated ballistic reach and grasp	Reaches and grasps object if both hand and object are in view
	Moves arm and hand in one unit, grasps object with palmar orientation
	Mirrors movements with other hand
Unilateral, visually directed reach and grasp	Brings hand in from outside visual field
	Alters reach in flight to accommodate to object
	Grasps object with beginning dissociation of arm and hand movements, radial-palmar orientation
Beginning reciprocity between hands	Transfers object from one hand to other hand in midline
	Grasps an object in each hand

Description of Normal Oral and Language Patterns

As discussed in the preceding section, weight bearing, weight shifting, and reaching with shoulder rotation in the forearm support position expand the upper chest. The infant progresses to weight bearing on extended arms, which raises the whole thoracic area off the surface. Reaching in this higher support position involves thoracic holding, which strengthens the muscles. The rotational movement in the above positions, segmental rolling, circular pivoting, and reciprocal combat crawling activate oblique muscles. This development of oblique muscles coupled with the gravitational pull in the sitting position is felt to be instrumental in initiating the gradual downward angulation of the ribs and lowering of the thorax which begins in this stage.[7]

The angle of insertion of the diaphragm becomes more oblique, which allows it to descend to a greater degree, especially in a more upright position, increasing the abdominal pressure. This pressure pushes the rib cage upward to a greater degree. The intercostal muscles become more active, which begins to tie the ribs together, providing more stiffness in the expanded rib cage. With this more stable platform and the more oblique angle of insertion, the diaphragmatic contraction is directed toward sucking in air rather than both air and the lower ribs.[8] There is also a continued increase in the size and number of alveoli in the lungs.[9] The breathing becomes deeper and slower, coincidental with the evolvement of the above structural and developmental changes around six or seven months, whereas there is little change in the respiration rate and variability during the three- to six-month period.[10]

The work of breathing is considerably less than in the earlier stage of infancy. Even if paradoxical breathing continues to occur in the active (REM) sleep state until ten months of age as observed by one investigator,[11] the infant spends less and less time in this state. The strength and endurance of the ventilatory muscles also increase because of heavier work patterns described in the previous section and the related need for air exchange. There is an increase in Type I oxidative fibers, with the proportion of the fibers in the diaphragm reaching the adult percentage at seven or eight months.[12] As described in the preceding stage, the adult value was reached in the intercostal muscles at two months of age.

Changes in the respiration pattern reflect a beginning transition to thoracic-abdominal breathing in this stage, with the upward and outward expansion of the chest resulting from an action of both the inspiratory muscles of the rib cage and the diaphragm. Wilder[13] observed a sharp increase in the percentage of cycles during which thoracic movements are present in vegetative breathing between five to eight months. There is also increased activity of the thorax during both crying and noncrying vocalization.

Wilder also observed a steady increase in the length of the respiratory cycle during crying. The duration of the inspiration remains stable regardless of the incremental increase in the duration of the expiration, and the I-fraction continues to decrease and approach the value typical of mature speech. The changes correlate with gross motor development, which implies a continued relationship between the muscular coordination required to control expiratory forces and the coordination required for motor skills.

Whereas the waveform during vegetative breathing and crying vocalization is very distinguishable again in this stage, the waveform for noncrying vocalization is still not unique. There are variations in the duration of the cycle and the I-fraction, which remains higher than the I-fraction during a short utterance in adult speech. The very important ability to negotiate a short inspiration and prolonged voiced expiration is not yet stabilized at eight months of age, as it is during crying. There are signs of progress during some utterances between the fifth and eighth month. The thoracic movements become more active to maintain the rib cage in an inspiratory phase for a longer period after the expiratory abdominal phase has begun. Thus, there is even more pronounced asynchrony to check the elastic recoil forces and regulate the force of air expulsion. By the end of this stage, the infant can prolong the expiration to produce a chain of syllables at times. Overshooting still occurs, reflected by subcycles or mini-respirations, which are not present in adult speech.

The configuration of the vocal tract continues to change with the gradual lowering of the larynx and posterior one third of the tongue in the neck. The depth of the oral cavity is also increased by the backward shift of the vertebral wall facilitated by the development of neck and upper back extensor muscles. Thus, there is an ongoing increase in the longitudinal flexibility of the tongue. The distance between the descending larynx and the oral cavity gradually increases continuing to form a pharyngeal tube, and air and liquid now share a common pathway, which results in aspiration if both drinking and breathing occur at the same time. The restructuring of the vocal tract into a two-tube system with a separate oral and pharyngeal cavity is complete or almost complete by the end of this stage.[14]

Increased neuromuscular control of the lips, tongue, and jaw is an important parameter that is intertwined with the above changes in the size and shape of the vocal tract. The sensory input from eating and mouthing of objects plays a key role in the gradual evolvement of voluntary control. The input stimulates the rich supply of receptors in the oral structures that transmit tactual and proprioceptive information to the central nervous system. The receptors become increasingly more discriminative as a function of sensory maturation and gradually provide more focal information about the position and movement of the jaw, tongue, lips, velum, and other structures. A feedback system develops similar to the system described in the previous section to guide arm and hand movements. The infant can now begin to monitor and compare the ongoing motion of oral structures with previous experiences organized in the form of a central referent or sensory-motor map and alter the movement to accommodate a novel texture (pureed food) or form a new sound.[15] The central referent is thereby modified some also.

The maturational changes described in the above paragraphs serve as the substrate for the evolvement of more adaptive feeding patterns. There is a gradual decrease in obligatory responses as primitive reflexes become integrated. The sucking reflex is no longer dependent on touch input, and the infant can voluntarily inhibit the sucking action by about five or six months. There is a less forward tongue movement with the continued backward shift of the posterior wall. The large amount of sensory input also lessens the need to seek stimulation by protruding the tongue, which Bosma[16] emphasizes is an important factor. The infant can elevate the more mobile tongue to a greater degree when guiding food back to be swallowed. The lip, jaw, and tongue movements gradually become more differentiated during sucking, versus moving more or less as a composite. The infant then progresses to closing his lips over the spoon to remove the food without a sucking action of the tongue and mandible. A diagonal munching action also evolves as the jaw becomes more stable relative to increased background strength in the neck muscles. This new adaptation allows soft food to be added to the diet, which provides a new sensory input. The sensitive gag reflex begins to wane with the increased ability to accommodate to different substances.

The repertoire of sounds also expands as an outgrowth of structural changes and the coordination of breathing and oral movements. The vowels i and a were heard at the beginning of this stage in a recent study[17] but occurred more frequently toward the middle and end of the stage, respectively. An infrequent and unstable back vowel, u, was heard at 24 weeks. Lieberman[18,19] postulates that the emergence of a right angle bend during the transition from a one-tube to a two-tube system is necessary for the production of the vowels i and u and to a lesser extent a. The infant also has to develop enough neuromuscular control to protrude and round the lips and coordinate lip, tongue, and jaw movements to form the u sound. The back vowels oo and aw were heard infrequently toward the end of this stage in the above cited study. These sounds also require more variation in the adjustment of the articulators—rounded lips and raised tongue near the palate for oo and open lips and jaw and lowering of the tongue to the bottom of the mouth for aw. The infant begins to practice more flexible readjustments of jaw, lip, and tongue movements by changing from one vowel sound to another during vocal play—oiee, ahoo. He produces the vowel sound ee within a more consistent frequency range at approximately 33 weeks, which reflects a beginning stabilization of the vocal tract.

Consonants also appear more and more frequently in the vocalization. The back consonants (k, ng, g) dominate the babbling during the first six months and then begin to decrease in frequency and continue to be heard infrequently throughout the babbling period. The labial consonants (p, b, m) evolve if they did not do so in the preceding stage, and consonants requiring a more flexible elevation of the tongue to the alveolar ridge (t, d, n, l) evolve toward the end of this stage and in the subsequent stage.[20] The infant is developing the ability to blend stability and mobility with one or two articulators moving while another holds, for example, the lips and jaw move, and the tongue holds. There is also increasing dissociation of the head from the rest of the body with less concomitant bodily movement during babbling. The infant develops the ability to babble in multiple syllables by the end of this stage, which reflects the beginning evolvement of the complex mechanisms of speech described in earlier paragraphs. He is beginning to coordinate disparate systems that will be further refined in subsequent stages.[21]

The auditory system, an important link in the complex network, is also maturing. Wilson[22] reported that the six-month-old infant can hear the same threshold of tones as the adult. A more discriminative feedback system and increased coordination of senses allow the infant to imitate babbling sounds in his vocabulary by the end of this stage. He also hears the rhythm and variation of speech during spontaneous play periods with his caregiver, and he gains sufficient control of laryngeal and respiratory muscles to vary the inflection and tone of his voice more flexibly. His vocalization repeats the commanding, complaining, declining, and questioning intonation of adults. He begins to combine vocalization with gestures of reaching and rejection, further elaborating his communicative repertoire.[23] The infant is influenced by the general interactive mood and laughs and squeals when others are laughing and boisterous, and he performs antics to get attention, for example, a fake cough.

The evolvement of oral and language patterns is a very interrelated process, encompassing structural changes, adaptations of the respiratory cycle, increased voluntary control of articulators, and increased coordination of sensations and motor movements through a feedback mechanism. This process and related maturational changes are summarized in Table 2-8.

Description of Normal Cognitive Patterns

Secondary circular reactions began to evolve at the end of the preceding stage simultaneous with increased coordination of eye and hand movements. The circular reactions herald an important transition in this stage of cognitive development; the infant is propelling his actions outward beyond the confines of his own body. He expands his world to manipulate and explore objects actively and to get to know other humans in new ways. For example, he practices the awkward reach and grasp that he acquired in the preceding stage and stumbles upon a new action—pulling the suspended object up and down. The infant repeats this new environmental effect in a circular fashion, and variations of the effect come about just as unexpectedly—pulls the object from side to side, pulls the object gently and then vigorously. As with primary circular reactions, the schema becomes modified and more adaptive through repetition. The infant also generalizes the schema to an increasing number of suspended objects.[24] Other action schemas evolve in a like manner. The infant accidentally bangs a rattle on the surface, and he repeats the hand movement to recapture and maintain the auditory effect. He then begins to adapt the schema to bang different objects on different surfaces.

Through this process a repertoire of habitual schemas evolve. The infant runs through his repertoire of acquired actions to explore the sensory-motor feedback potential of the object—mouthing, rotating, pulling, striking, banging, shaking. The infant's exploration is gross and physical in nature, adapting the object to his action schema. He responds to a novel object with increased alertness and then incorporates it in his familiar repertoire versus accommodating his actions to the unique features of the object. When the infant has exploited the feedback characteristics of an object, he becomes habituated, loses interest, and moves on to something else. Mouthing is a favorite schema during this stage, no doubt because of the rich supply of tactual receptors in the oral area, which are possibly more discriminative than the receptors in the palm of his hand based on the assumption that the myelinization process evolves in a cephalocaudal direction. Also, the infant does not develop enough distal control in this stage to explore the details of objects with individual fingers.

A progressively higher-order internal schema of objects evolves through the coordination of the action-object sequence in secondary circular reactions. The infant abbreviates action schemas habitually applied to an object, when he sees it at a distance, reflecting a motor

TABLE 2-8 Evolvement of oral and language patterns (Second Stage)

Develops increased ability to blend mobility and stability of respiratory and laryngeal muscles
  Makes beginning transition to thoracoabdominal breathing and deeper, slower respiration
  Steadily increases respiratory cycle during crying with prolongation of expiratory phase
  Regulates air expulsion to prolong noncrying vocalization at times, producing chain of syllables by end of stage
  Varies frequency of vocalization to achieve intonational effects by end of stage
  Begins to stabilize the frequency quality of the ee vowel
Develops increased voluntary control of oral movements with beginning dissociation of articulators
  Initiates and inhibits the sucking response independent of tactual input by midstage
  Increasingly differentiates the lip, jaw, and tongue movements during sucking
  Progresses to closing lips over the spoon without a sucking action of tongue and mandible
  Begins to inhibit the forward movement of the tongue
  Moves the jaw in a diagonal, munching action
  Combines back and labial consonants with vowels more frequently
  Begins to produce consonants requiring an elevation of tongue to alveolar ridge—t, d, n, l
  Begins to readjust articulatory movements to form back vowel sounds—u, oo, ah—and combine different vowel sounds—oiee, ahoo
  Decreases concomitant bodily movement during babbling
Develops increased ability to link sensory input and motor movements through a feedback system
  Imitates babbling sounds already in repertoire of vocalizations
  Imitates intonational and emotional tone of caregiver's vocalization
  Combines vocalization with gestures of reaching and rejection

recognition. Through repeated and varied contact and coordination of sensations, the infant also continues to reorganize the internal referent of his caregiver. He recognizes her specific face, voice, smell, touch, and movements when she is in sight, which Piaget[25] termed recognition memory. Also, the infant is beginning to realize that the hand that comes across his visual field, the hand that he brings to his mouth, and the hand that grasps objects is a part of him and under his control. They are not three different hands that do not exist when out of sight as was the case in the previous stage. His primitive body sense is therefore becoming somewhat more coherent.

However, the infant is in a very primitive stage in terms of the concept of an object. The underpinnings are evolving, evidenced by deferred circular reactions. The infant returns to an object he was actively involved with after a short interruption. He can also reconstruct the whole object if part of it is hidden from view. He has to be actively involved with the object when it is partially covered, because he cannot separate the object from his own actions. He perceives the two as an undifferentiated whole in this stage. The internal referent is shaky. If the infant fumbles and covers up the object, the search ends. There has to be a partial perceptual cue to internally reconstruct the object. If the object is partially covered in a new location, the infant looks in the old hiding place even though the object is visible in the new hiding place. He can conceive of an object only in one special position, and he may also expect that he can make the object magically reappear in the old location by his action of searching.

The infant progresses to maintaining an internal representation of an object for a very brief period without a perceptual cue. He crudely searches for an object he misplaced during exploration but gives up immediately if the object is not readily located by hand or eye. The infant also searches for an object that has been completely hidden by an adult, if he was actively involved with the object—manipulating it or reaching for it—and if he witnessed the disappearance. There is disagreement whether the evolving referent of the caregiver is more coherent than the referent of an inanimate object evidenced by searching for the hidden caregiver first.[26] The researchers[27] who report a disparity postulate that the infant has had more prolonged and intense association with the caregiver. Thus, the evolving concept of very meaningful human objects precedes the concept of inanimate objects.

The infant still has much to learn about the concept of objects in time and space. Although he observes the displacement of objects from one hand to the other and follows the trajectory of an object as it falls to the floor, he does not know that an object can move from one location to another as mentioned previously. Nor does he know that two objects can be in a spatial relationship to one another (in, on) or have a common boundary. If an object is placed on a platform when the infant is reaching for it, he pulls back his hand in bewilderment. If the infant accidentally shakes the object off the platform, he will then retrieve it.[28]

The infant also has much to learn about causality. Because desires, actions, and results are undifferentiated during most of this stage, the infant operates on the premise of what Piaget termed efficacy-phenomenalism. He primitively senses that his actions and desires somehow cause external happenings even at a distance (efficacy). His excitable arm waving makes the bell in the caregiver's hand ring rather than her actions, which are, therefore, subordinate to his. He also senses that one event causes another if the two temporally occur close together (phenomenalism). If the infant waves his arms just before the bell in the caregiver's hand rings, then the arm waving caused the auditory effect. He does not perceive that another object can be a causal agent acting through spatial contact.

Because of the lack of differentiation between the desire, action, and result, the infant's behavior can only be termed quasi-intentional. He stumbles upon the means to an end in the source of practicing secondary circular reactions and belatedly recognizes the connection. He does not intentionally use a string to pull an object toward him. This just happens when he distractedly explores the string. In the course of experiencing a common round of daily events, the infant primitively begins to perceive that an environmental cue signals an event outside the confines of his actions. The presence of mother predictively signals that he will be fed when hungry. The infant also progresses to pushing his caregiver's hand out of the way if it is interfering with the goal of reaching, and he removes an obstacle to find a hidden object as discussed earlier. With increased mobility, the infant swim crawls to regain an object out of his immediate reach but still in view. Thus, the infant uses locomotion as a means to an end. These behaviors mark the beginning transition from nonintentionality to intentionality toward the end of this stage. The infant is beginning to differentiate the action and result. The more flexible and intentional combination of schemas in a means-end relationship and the beginning recognition of outside causal sources evolve in the next stage.

As the infant begins to direct his attention outward, he primitively adapts schemas to reality via imitation. This is not the automatic, yoking imitation of the very young infant. He is making an effort to yield to reality with a rough accommodation or approximate correspondence of what he sees or hears. The infant attempts to copy his caregiver's highly familiar motor movements—bouncing his body on her lap after being bounced. The infant also begins to imitate sounds within his vocabulary as mentioned in the previous section. He imitates only sounds and actions that he can hear and see himself make because of the immature inner representation of body parts.[29]

The infant continues to order reality around body modes. Objects are categorized by their action relative to body actions. The infant groups a large number of diverse objects in a class of something to grasp—a prehension schema. He then progresses to running through his repertoire of schemas until he finds the one that elicits the most feedback from the object. The infant selectively applies the most salient schema first; he may then run through his repertoire to verify all the response contingent events. Thus, subclasses or subschemas evolve— things to shake, things to bang. The infant also learns that some things need to be grasped more firmly; prickly things, more gingerly. He recognizes quasi-quantitative relations between the intensity of the act and the intensity of the result—gentle shaking movement and a vigorous shaking movement. The habitual schemas are becoming more flexible and less mechanical by the end of this stage as the infant senses relationships in the real world out there in his own very primitive way, as outlined in Table 2-9.

Description of Normal Affective Patterns

At the beginning of this stage, a close dyadic relationship between the caregiver and infant is still the primary stimulus world. They have coalesced their repertoire of behaviors into an interactive fit of human relatedness that expands the infant's social behaviors. The close association with the caregiver and maturation also serve as a background for the evolvement of more differentiated affective patterns. The infant more clearly looks attentive, joyful, unhappy, quizzical, eager, dissatisfied, coy, and bored.

Awake-alert states gradually lengthen as the infant develops better homeostatic control and modulation of internal states. There is a corresponding increase in outward-directed perceptual activity and an expansion of his stimulus world. As described in the preceding section, a new dimension is added to the relationship in this stage. There is now a triadic affair between the infant, caregiver, and objects. Thus, the nature of the relationship begins to change somewhat. The infant is beginning to make the transition from a babe-in-the-arms to a separating one, a period which Mahler, Pine, and Bergman[30] term the hatching phase of the separation/individuation process.

The development of motor skills allows the infant to distance himself more actively. He perches on the edge of the lap, reducing surface contact with the caregiver's body. The infant can then observe her from a different vantage point; he explores the caregiver's face, upper body, and the objects she is wearing: he grasps her nose, sticks his fingers between her lips, grabs her hair, eyeglasses, and necklace. The infant progresses to putting the caregiver's fingers, hair, and necklace in his mouth. He also explores with excitable aggression at times, biting or pinching her shoulder. The infant gestures a desire to slide off the caregiver's lap and explores an object at her feet; he may roll or swim crawl a short distance away.

Just as he more actively distances himself, the infant also more actively seeks and achieves proximity. He rolls or swim crawls back to his caregiver and extends his arms in a pick-me-up gesture. He also uses the caregiver as a support to awkwardly pull up to a standing position and more potently gesture a desire to return to her lap. The

**TABLE 2-9 Evolvement of cognitive patterns
(Second Stage)**

Orients schemas outward beyond confines of his body
    Actively manipulates objects and comes upon a new effect
    Repeats effect achieved by chance over and over (secondary circular reaction)
Adapts schemas through secondary circular reactions
    Grasps and pulls an object up and down
    Modifies action to pull the object from side to side
    Pulls the object gently and then more vigorously
Solidifies and generalizes schemas through repetition
    Grasps and pulls the suspended object with less extraneous movement
    Applies the pulling schema to different objects
Adapts the object to action schemas
    Explores gross, sensory-motor feedback potential of object by running through repertoire of schemas
    Adapts novel features of object to familiar repertoire of actions
Performs schemas in more flexible, less mechanical ways at end of stage
    Runs through repertoire until finding schema that elicits most feedback from object
    Selectively applies most salient schema first when exploring familiar object
Forms fragile internal referent of object (action and object undifferentiated)
    Performs abbreviation of action schemas habitually applied to an object seen at a distance—motor recognition
    Relocates object actively involved with after a short interruption
    Reconstructs the whole object if partially covered while actively involved with it
    Progresses to searching for a completely covered object if actively involved with it when hidden
    Searches in old position even if sees object hidden in new position
Begins to recognize a means-end relationship ad hoc
    Gropingly pulls string attached to object, which brings object toward him
    Repeats means only after the end result is discovered accidentally—semi-intentional behavior
Relates causality to undifferentiated mixture of efficacy-phenomenalism
    Primitively senses that his actions and desires somehow cause external happenings even at a distance (efficacy)
    Senses one event causes another if the two temporally occur together (phenomenalism)
    Undifferentiates desire, action, and result initially
    Begins to dissociate the action and result in semi-intentional behavior
Begins to adapt schemas to reality via imitation
    Approximately corresponds actions to model
    Imitates only action schemas in his habitual repertoire
    Imitates only sounds and actions he can hear and see himself make
Continues to order reality around body modes
    Groups large number of objects in class of something to grasp
    Forms primitive subschemas based on the most salient action potential of an object—things to shake
    Forms a quasi-quantitative relationship between intensity of act and intensity of result

caregiver is still the center of the infant's universe from which he only gradually moves out in ever-widening circles.

As discussed in the cognitive section, the infant continues to organize affective experiences into a progressively higher order, internal referent of his caregiver. He is beginning to realize that the mother who feeds him, the mother who bathes him, and the mother who plays with him is the same mother; and he becomes upset if he is simultaneously shown three mothers in an experiment.[31] His internal referent is not coherent or stable enough to conjure an image of his caregiver when he cannot see her, but he has built up an expectancy of her reappearance to meet his needs. Thus, he does not become upset, at least early on in this stage, when she disappears while he is following her movements.

The infant may be developing an attachment to a number of persons who are actively involved in the role of caregiver: mother, father, older sibling, babysitter. There is controversy over whether these attachments all have the same meaning or if there is a hierarchy with a preference of one person over another.[32] The findings of two studies[33,34] suggest that it is the quality versus the amount of interaction that determines the strength of the attachment. Thus, even though some fathers spend less time with their infant, an attachment evolves if the interaction is embedded in sensitivity and enjoyment over the months.

There is also controversy over a reaction to strangers that may evolve during this stage. Many variables must be considered: nature of the caregiver/infant relationship, infant's characteristics, stranger's characteristics, and the context. There is general agreement that, especially toward the end of this stage, many infants respond to the appearance of a stranger with subtle negative cues: quieting, sober expression, staring, and/or averting his gaze. Communicative eye-to-eye contact is generally avoided; only familiar persons can become this intimate. Mahler, Pine, and Bergman postulate that the infant is able to modulate his arousal level and ward off a distress reaction if the initial symbiotic relationship was optimal. Contingent responsiveness created an expectancy of control, which generates to a new situation.

Curiosity and wonderment therefore predominate over apprehension during the interaction with a new person. The infant checks and compares features of the stranger's face with his caregiver's face. He may gradually warm up to the stranger enough to transfer to her lap in the presence of the caregiver. He explores the stranger's clothing and jewelry and after a while even her face. After completing his inspection, the infant generally gestures to return to the safe arms of his caregiver.[35] However, if the stranger crowds in too close too soon and violates the infant's sense of his own personal space, he can become distressed, which enhances proximity-seeking behavior toward his caregiver. He may also become upset if left with an unfamiliar person. The infant expects certain patterns of interaction. If these patterns are not forthcoming with the stranger, the mismatch may be stressful.

Just as the infant is becoming more acquainted with his caregiver, he is also becoming more acquainted with his own body. He has been bathed, dried, possibly massaged, undressed, dressed, and changed from one position to another, all of which involve many different sensations. He has also experienced a large amount of sensory feedback from evolving movement patterns and self exploration, including the genital area. The infant has sensed differences between putting his finger or a bite of food in his own mouth and putting it in his caregiver's mouth. The caregiver has also adaptively involved him in appearance and disappearance games, and to find and to be found by mother and to be mirrored by her serves to build body awareness.[36] The infant's rudimentary body map is thus becoming somewhat more coherent toward the end of this stage. If the hand is covered with a sock in an experiment[37] or is out of view, he senses it is part of his body and that the same hand is involved in a number of schemas as mentioned earlier.

The summary of affective patterns that evolve in this stage in Table 2-10 reflects the intertwining attachment and individuation process. The infant uses his new capacities to expand his exploration and to distance himself from his caregiver. He also uses his new repertoire of motor and communication skills to seek proximity and express attachment behaviors.

GROWTH-FOSTERING ENVIRONMENT

During the initial one or two months of this stage, the intimate relationship with the caregiver still provides the most optimal blend of sameness and variety, which has both energizing and regulating effects. The caregiver continues to create expectation by her responsiveness to the infant's needs. She also continues to adapt her playful repertoire of behaviors to provide a blend of repetition and variety in the tempo and intensity of different sensory modalities—visual, auditory, touch, movement. The caregiver violates the infant's personal space as she looms in to kiss his tummy, pulls out, and looms in again. It is as if she is helping the infant become less protective of his personal space in familiar, more intimate relationships.[38] The disappearance of the caregiver's face as she kisses the infant's tummy and the reappearance of her face at a distance supports the infant's exploration of his caregiver from different vantage points. The playful interaction also allows the infant to experience his vague, primitive sense of sepa-

TABLE 2-10 Evolvement of affective patterns (Second Stage)

Begins to sever a very close symbiotic relationship with the caregiver
    Expands the stimulus world with increased outer-directed activity
    Shifts the dyadic relationship to a triadic affair—infant/caregiver/object
Expresses more active distancing behaviors
    Reduces surface contact with the caregiver's body—perches on the edge of
      her lap
    Gestures to slide off her lap
    Explores at the caregiver's feet, moves a short distance away
Simultaneously expresses more active proximity-seeking behaviors
    Extends his arms in a pick-me-up gesture
    Returns to the caregiver's feet after moving a short distance away
    Pulls up to standing, gestures to return to her lap
Expresses attachment behaviors in a new situation
    Checks and compares the features of a stranger and the caregiver
    Responds to a stranger with subtle negative cues by end of stage
Organizes experiences in a primitive internal referent of the body
    Rudimentarily senses differences from exploring self and caregiver
    Relates the same hand to a number of sensory-motor schemas—something
      to suck, grasp, look at
    Senses the hand is part of him and under his control even when out of sight

rateness in a safe, enjoyable way. Peek-a-boo games just naturally follow with a rhythm of tension and relaxation. The caregiver also allows the infant to use his budding prehension schemas to explore her face, body, clothes, and the objects she is wearing when she and the infant are in a close en face position and when the infant is sitting on her lap with a little more distance between them. Imitation games evolve, with the caregiver modeling sounds and actions within the infant's repertoire of behaviors: coughing, lip smacking, familiar babbling sounds or rocking back and forth, sleepy-bye on the pillow. The caregiver's vocalization is very expressive during these interactive periods, further exposing the infant to the rhythm and cadence of language and affective exchanges. The caregiver also allows the infant to assume a more active role in initiating social interaction as his communicative repertoire expands.

The caregiver adaptively alters the nature of the interaction in another way. She gradually includes objects in the play periods. The caregiver holds the infant's plastic pants up for him to grasp, shakes a rattle, and then gives it to him, and places an object in her mouth for him to grasp. She gradually adds the appearance and disappearance dimension to objects. The caregiver partially covers the infant's hand or foot with his diaper, partially hides an object in the crevice of a blanket, partially covers an object with her hand. Progression is then made to complete coverage of the object or body part. These activities facilitate practice in reconstructing objects and also facilitate after-the-fact recognition of a means-end relationship. The caregiver ties a string on a toy, which is another way of encouraging an accidental discovery of the means-end sequence in the process of exploration. When the infant becomes engrossed in an object, the caregiver sensitively relinquishes her center stage position and moves to the wings for an interval. She allows the infant to explore the object without interference and restrictions, in accordance with his interest level, unique style, and habituation rate. The caregiver trusts and reinforces the infant's innate drive to foster his own development.

The caregiver uses her creativity in the role of Master Chef to provide the right blend of inanimate objects to maintain an optimal level of attention and motivation. The more responsive the object is to the infant's habitual repertoire of manipulative schemas, the longer he will persist in exploring the stimulus characteristics. There has to be a match between the infant's developmental level and the potential of the object to provide feedback appropriate to that level. The caregiver exposes the infant to a variety of objects within his tolerance level. Some of the objects provide information through several sensory modalities (different colors and designs, different sounds, variation in contour and texture), and some objects provide responsive feedback to the infant's actions (moving parts, change in shape, noise production). This is not to detract from the continued importance of animate stimulation as an ingredient in the recipe. Based on a longitudinal study,[39] a blend of both animate and inanimate stimulation facilitates an optimal level of attention, inner motivation, and exploratory behavior, which are potent forces in development. The ingredients for the recipe can be found in the natural environment. There are the familiar persons who know the infant's dance steps, and there is an endless variety of objects around the house. A favorite household concoction is mason jar rings placed on a large binder ring.

The caregiver provides a safe environment, which allows the infant not only to explore objects but also to practice evolving postures and movement patterns. She does not interfere with the propensity to maintain a balance between muscle groups by restricting the infant in an infant seat, jump seat, or walker. The caregiver also provides movement input during play periods: swaying the infant up in the air, tilting him in all directions, bouncing him on the knee, letting him roll around on the caregiver's body. There are excitable movement responses to the play itself. Again in this stage, there is a trend toward more dynamic modes of transporting the infant from place to place, such as a carrier attached to the caregiver's body or a pram that transforms into a suspension type stroller. These dynamic experiences facilitate maturation of the vestibular system, which is a primary homeostatic force in keeping the body oriented in space. There is also an intertwined relationship between the development of the vestibular system and the visual system and possibly other sensory systems.

Care routines are not task oriented for the most part, and mealtime is a pleasant social and sensory experience. Many infants are still content to let their caregiver feed them the majority of the food served at the meal during this stage. They enjoy the close contact, and the caregiver has become very adept at adjusting the pace to let the infant assuage his hunger in the beginning; she slows the pace toward the end to intersperse more interaction and allow experimentation with finger feeding.

A bit of restrictiveness is appropriately included in this stage. The caregiver communicates some Don'ts. For example, she pulls her body away when the infant bites or pinches her shoulder. She ends the meal if the experimentation with food gets out of hand or has gone on long enough. It is through a variety of interactive experiences that the infant develops a feel for different patterns of human behavior and attaches affective meaning to facial expressions: happiness, sadness, and anger.

Although the infant's tolerance for stimulation continues to increase during this stage, there is still a need to mediate the environment and provide a milieu over which he feels he has some control. A common round of daily events provides the basis for expectation. Excesses are avoided to prevent overstimulation and defensive adaptations: high activity level in the home, continuous or high noise level, exposure to too many objects or too many different adults, and too frequent visitations outside of the home that interfere with regular sleeping and eating patterns. The caregiver also monitors the stimulus intensity in the sleeping room. The infant may start having difficulty falling asleep, especially toward the end of this stage, or he may awaken during the night possibly because of a tension dream related to the new experience of reaching out and separation anxiety.[40]

Expanded interaction with family members is encouraged to increase the infant's adaptability within a matrix of familiarity. He is then better equipped to handle novel experiences including exposure to strangers. The infant is allowed to warm up to a stranger at his own pace with the security of his caregiver's presence. If the infant has to be left with an unfamiliar person, the stranger allows time for a warming-up period before encroaching on the infant's personal space. Also, it is best if the infant remains in his own environment with his usual routine if at all possible. A favorite object and interesting novel objects will help distract him from the worry related to an unfamiliar person. However, the infant may be low-keyed, exploring less in his caregiver's absence. His coping rights should be respected.

FRAMEWORK FOR ASSESSING ABERRANT DEVELOPMENTAL AND INTERACTIVE PATTERNS

Again in this stage the assessment focus is twofold. The intervener identifies patterns that deviate from the norm. The intervener also identifies the functional significance of these limitations in terms of the infant's development and his expanded exploration of the world of human beings and inanimate objects.

Effect of an Aberrant Response Threshold and a Disturbed Relationship

The implications of an aberrant stimulation threshold were discussed in the previous stage. It may well be that maturation coupled with a sensitive, contingent environment has facilitated increased internal state control, longer periods of sustained attention, and increased social responsiveness, which fuel the dyadic relationship. Also, the infant has gained weight at a faster rate, and episodes of illness have decreased. Thus, he has become less fragile and vulnerable, which has decreased maternal anxiety. Or, even if there has been no change in his response pattern or level of wellness, the caregiver has learned to make allowances for his behavior. The allowances decrease potentially negative effects of the behavior on the relationship. Perhaps there has been a decrease in the stress level within the family unit. It has just taken the caregiver and infant longer to get in tune with each other, which points to the importance of respecting the variable of time in any relationship. Premature, undue concern regarding the attachment process may in itself interfere with the process. Interveners must also consider elements especially in a center-based intervention program that may have a nonsupportive or even a reverse effect on the evolving relationship: disruption of the daily rhythm, exposure to illness, and dilution of the importance of animate and inanimate stimulus elements in the natural environment.

There is, however, the possibility that the relationship will continue to be disturbed. The reactive infant is still dependent on his caregiver to mediate the environment, and interaction may continue to center on stress cues, diminishing the caregiver's reserve of energy to notice or respond to positive cues. The relationship has a negative connotation depriving the infant and caregiver of the joy and pleasure of social exchange which is refueling for both of them. The infant may be isolated from family activities more and more because of escalated excitement, and the caregiver may become less and less responsive even to negative cues, leaving the infant with unresolved sensations of distress. There is also the danger of abuse.

The infant may still have a faulty internal regulatory mechanism, reflected by poorly modulated states and irregular physiologic rhythms. He may continue to be at the mercy of repeating stimuli in the environment owing to poor habituation. His periods of attention remain short, which limits focused interaction even with a very responsive caregiver. Likewise, exploration of the stimulus characteristics of objects is also limited. His internal referent of both the caregiver and inanimate objects may remain in a very low-order form. The infant's weak biosocial base compounds his low adaptability to novel experiences. His reaction to strangers may be expressed with potent versus subtle negative cues: maximal averting of his gaze, arching his back, fussing, and/or crying. A center-based program may not be a viable option if the environmental change intensifies stress reactions and fuels the cycle.

At the other end of the continuum is the infant with a high sensory threshold and a low-level response pattern. His affect remains diminished, and he may respond with expressions such as laughter to only the most intense, intrusive stimulation.[41] The caregiver cannot muster the energy required to arouse the infant to an alert state day after day. The cycle of decreased feedback and decreased involvement described in the previous stage continues, and the interaction becomes more and more task oriented in nature. The infant is left alone for rather long periods because of his undemanding temperament, which further decreases his responsiveness and perpetuates primary circular reactions centered on his own body. His low level of assertiveness and his inner directedness can sustain an image of infantile dependence.

The infant's high threshold level interferes with the expansion of his stimulus world in other ways. Whereas the reactive infant may distractingly move from one stimulus to another, the more lethargic infant has a longer response latency. It therefore takes him longer to orient to a stimulus, and he explores the object for a longer interval before becoming habituated.[42] The infant may use the same schema over and over again in a very stereotyped manner, and this in itself limits the variety of inanimate experiences. His interaction with his caregiver may also be very repetitive and stereotyped. Ironically, this may limit or shorten interaction periods when the infant actually needs more time to process stimulus dimensions of the caregiver. He may have a very weak inner referent of animate and inanimate objects. Strange situations may not elicit an anxiety reaction because of a less differential response to stimuli or a low arousal level.[43]

The infant with either too high or too low a sensory threshold may have a paucity of proximity-seeking behaviors, typical of this developmental stage, that elicit positive attention and social exchange. This places the infant at risk in terms of close, loving contact with his caregiver. Experiences may lead the infant to distrust his caregiver's accessibility and responsiveness. Thus, his internal referent of an inanimate object, albeit possibly relatively weak, may be emerging at a faster rate than his internal referent of a human object. It has been postulated that the concept of an inanimate object is less sensitively related to the affective component.[44,45] The infant may search for a covered object before he will search for his covered caregiver. He may also indiscriminately accept attention from any adult.

Effect of Sensory Impairments

The developmentally delayed infant may have a sensory impairment not discussed in the above paragraphs or a sensory loss that limits his experiences. The infant who is blind or who has very poor visual acuity cannot monitor the comings and goings of his caregiver and the displacement of objects. Contact with objects is an infrequent, chance affair because of the lack of a visual guidance and feedback system. He will not reach out to a sound cue alone because, like normal infants, he cannot yet connect the sound out there with the caregiver or object he has just had contact with. Nor will he search for an object from a sound cue. Once it is beyond his tactual range, it becomes lost in a void. Thus, there can be a delay in the emerging concept of inanimate and animate objects. There is an impoverished repertoire of facial expressions because of the lack of visual social reinforcement. The infant who is blind also stops turning to localize a sound and vocalizes less frequently than normal infants. There is a delay in the evolvement of mobility. The infant remains stalemated in the first two phases of the process of developing motor patterns. He assumes a posture and then superimposes proximal mobility on distal stability, but there is no visual lure to proceed to the third phase and superimpose distal mobility on proximal stability—combat crawl. Proximal rocking patterns can become stereotypical in nature with the infant all set to go but with no place to go. The larger environment is featureless and possibly frightening.[46]

An auditory deficit continues to deprive the infant of the feedback of his own vocalization and exposure to the temporal and intonation patterns of his caregiver's voice. He lacks a basic framework for copying the rhythm of his cultural language and perceiving affective meanings. Although the deaf infant begins to babble, his vocalization does not become further differentiated and begins to wane after approximately the first six months, which suggests that sensory feedback is necessary to maintain innate biologic tendencies.[47] His affect is also attenuated by an impoverished repertoire of vocal expressions. Environmental signals lose some of their predictive potency; the infant cannot link visual and auditory cues to form expectations and beginning means-end relationships.

The infant with a visual or auditory deficit may also have a disturbance in the vestibular system, because there is a close albeit incompletely understood interplay between these systems. There may still be an impairment of the vestibulo-ocular mechanisms that interferes with the maintenance of a stable image on the retina during movement. This impairment continues to affect visual monitoring of the environment and the evolvement or quality of the visually guided reach because of unreliable feedback. An impairment of the vestibular system also delays the evolvement of righting and equilibrium responses. The infant is fearful of gravitational shifts and rapid movements, which limits the caregiver's repertoire of playful behaviors and the infant's own experimentation moving away from midline in the different postures. He restricts his movement to primarily straight-line patterns that limit perceptual experiences. Again, if there is a severe dysfunction, the infant will avoid movement, remaining curled up close to the surface.

If the infant has a dysfunction in the tactile or proprioceptive system, the receptors may not begin to transmit more discriminative information via the newer pathways. The infant cannot respond to input in a more localized way. Generalized responses interfere with the beginning evolvement of more adaptive arm and hand movements to explore the caregiver and objects and more adaptive oral movements to accommodate to new textures, munch on soft finger foods, and possibly form new sounds. The infant remains sensitive to intermittent touch input, responding with an avoidance reaction of the hands and oral sensitivity. The protective response interferes with his ability to maintain contact in a weight-bearing position. The infant may also continue to resist cuddling and other forms of handling.

Effect of Motor Impairments

Abnormal muscle tone continues to limit normal movement and interaction with the environment. The emphasis of the following discussion will be on compensatory or habit patterns that can evolve related to the motor impairment. A disability may not be recognized or diagnosed until these patterns predominate and contrast with normal development.

COMPENSATORY PATTERNS IN THE PRONE POSITION. If the disabled infant is able to assume the forearm support position, he may not be able to proceed to the next phase and superimpose distal mobility on proximal stability. Weak stabilizing muscles cannot handle the increased demands of the unilateral weight shift. The weight-bearing arm gives way from the effort of maintaining a cocontracted support position to free the other arm. Or the weight-bearing arm regressively moves back under the infant's body in response to the stress of the higher pattern. The infant can only move the arm a short distance off the surface straight in front of him because of the fixated position he is now in, which negates shoulder rotation. The head may also be retracted.

The type of abnormal tone determines the more specific compensatory response to the stress of this new pattern. If the infant has hypertonic muscles, the effort may elicit internal rotation of the reaching arm with an ulnar orientation of the hand. The other arm is back in very close to the body (Fig. 2-17A). The stress may even elicit a traction response with increased flexion of the elbow, wrist, and hand (fisting) which pulls the arm in away from the object. Or the stress of unilateral weight bearing and reaching may cause the opposite effect: an extensor pattern with one or both flexed arms retracted or pulled back, similar to Figure 2-5B, in Stage I. Again, the infant unintentionally moves away rather than toward the interesting sight. If the infant has hypotonic muscles, there is a hanging effect of the shoulders and extraneous movements in the reaching arm because of the lack of background proximal stability. The infant immediately rolls to the side or supine position to explore the object because of an inability to maintain the antigravity weight-bearing prone position that, ironically, is so necessary to develop increased stability (Fig. 2-17B).

If the infant with fluctuating tone (athetosis) or hyperkinesis unrelated to abnormal tone is able to maintain a bilateral weight-bearing position, this can have a quieting effect and inhibit nonpurposeful disorganized movement. The position helps the infant expand periods of alertness and attention so he can visually and auditorily orient to and

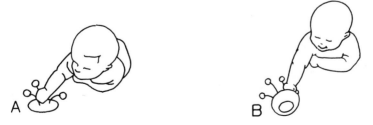

FIGURE 2-17. The stress of unilateral weight bearing and reaching elicits compensatory patterns if the infant has (A) hypertonia or (B) hypotonia.

monitor environmental events. However, if he attempts to superimpose distal mobility on proximal stability, the stress and effort may set off the disorganized movement again. He cannot maintain the unilateral weight-bearing position while he reaches for and grasps an object.

The addition of other joints to the weight-bearing pattern raises the infant farther from the base of support, which requires more stabilization. If the infant with hypertonic muscles progresses to the point of attempting to bear weight on extended arms, the stress may cause internal rotation of the arms and tighter flexion of the fingers versus a chainlike extension of the fingers. The head is pulled into the neck or pulled back, which interferes with visual orientation. There is a lack of normal extension in the midregion of the back because of shortened muscles, and extension does not move down over the hips in a normal manner (Fig. 2-18A). The infant with hypotonic muscles compensates in a different way when he attempts to raise up on extended arms. The arms may externally rotate with elbows locked or hyperextended (Fig. 2-18B). Or the elbows are widely abducted outward with the hands turned inward. He leans on lax muscles and bony structures instead of a normal use of the muscles. In either case, if the infant attempts to shift weight and reach for an object in this higher position, he topples over on his back because of the lack of a rotation and counter-rotation effect of the neck, shoulder, and trunk to maintain the prone position during movement. Mature equilibrium reactions have not evolved in the prone position.

COMPENSATORY PATTERNS IN THE SUPINE POSITION. Weak flexor muscles in supine position still interfere with exploration and proximity-seeking behaviors. If movements are influenced by the STNR, this interferes with the evolvement of the pick-me-up gesture. When the infant raises his head in supine position to orient to the caregiver, the arms flex and his legs extend which is just opposite from the extended position of the upper extremities in the proximity-seeking

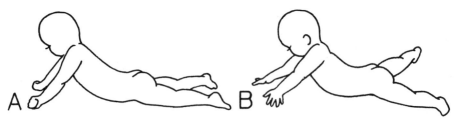

FIGURE 2-18. Weight bearing on extended arms is compromised if the infant has (A) hypertonia or (B) hypotonia.

gesture. The infant with hypotonia or hypertonia may not develop sufficient functional strength and control of flexor muscles and differentiation of flexion and extension patterns to flex the hips, extend the legs, and grasp the foot. He also cannot progress to lifting the hips off the surface so that he can easily bring the foot to his mouth and even his ear. If the infant has hypertonia, shortening of extensor muscles may also be a factor. In either instance, the infant uses a compensatory extensor pattern. The infant with hypertonia may be able to thrust the legs up, but the legs remain extended in the air with the plantarflexed feet pointed toward the ceiling (Fig. 2-19A). The infant with hypotonia and joint hyperflexibility widely abducts one of the extended legs to the side and grasps the foot (Fig. 2-19B).

Weak flexors also interfere with movement over the limb by turning from supine to side-lying to shift weight to one shoulder and hip and reach for an object. If the infant manages to get over on his side, he may always have to prop the upper arm protectively to maintain the position, and he does not experience weight directly over the shoulder. His arm is also not free to reach for and manipulate an object. Or the head and shoulder may retract (pull back) in a nonorienting position, and the weight is not directly over the shoulder. The infant is then likely to topple over on his back again; he goes with the force of gravity.

COMPENSATORY MOVEMENT BETWEEN PRONE AND SUPINE. An imbalance between flexor and extensor muscles and lack of midline stability interfere with the evolvement of rotation patterns and seg-

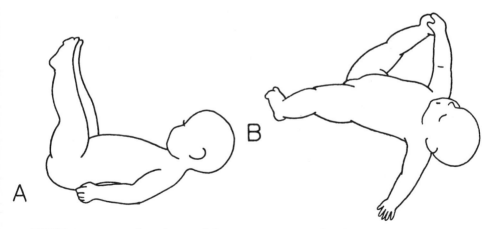

FIGURE 2-19. (A) The infant with hypertonia may not be able to flex his legs to explore the feet. (B) The infant with hypotonia and hyperflexibility uses extension and abduction to bring his foot within reach.

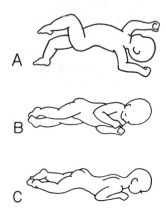

FIGURE 2-20. The infant rolls in a compensatory way if he has (A) fluctuating tone or (B) hypertonia. (C) The arms may become caught underneath the body if there is a strong TLR.

mental rolling. When the infant is in the prone position, he may retract his head, neck, and shoulders and flop over to supine or stiffly fall over if he has hypertonic muscles. The segmental movements involved with rolling from supine to prone are even more difficult. The infant with hypotonic muscles may tuck the underneath arm in close to his body and pull with the top arm and leg, which may be extended, instead of flexed, and the body turns in one unit. The tucked arm is caught under his body, because the shoulder and arm moved as one unit. Or he may arch his head and shoulders back and bring the top leg over, which then pulls the rest of the body over with minimal trunk rotation. The infant with athetosis who has less involvement in the lower extremities may also use this pattern but with more exaggerated retraction of the head, shoulders, and arms (Fig. 2-20A). If the infant has hypertonic muscles, the head and shoulders may pull back (retract) with the force of gravity, and he may not be able to move from supine to prone. Or, he may pull forward with his head, shoulders, and arms, and the overflow from the effort elicits stiff extension and internal rotation of the legs (Figs. 2-20B). Or if the ATNR has not become integrated, the underneath arm will extend as the infant turns his head and will become caught underneath his body. Or both arms may flex as he rolls over to prone because of the TLR influence and become caught underneath his body (Fig. 2-20C). Neither the infant with low tone nor one with high tone rights his head to a near vertical position during the rolling action. The head may remain on the surface.

COMPENSATORY MOBILITY PATTERNS IN PRONE POSITION. Both the infant with hypotonic and hypertonic muscles may learn to move forward in the prone position in a compensatory combat crawl pattern. The arms may be adducted and close to the body because of a weak shoulder girdle which decreases the excursion of each forward effort. The infant with hypotonic muscles may move around in a circle more than moving forward because the pivoting requires less effort. If trunk rotation does not evolve in either the combat crawl pattern or the pivot in a circle because of the lack of midline stability, the infant with hypotonia compensates by using a wide abduction movement of the legs and lateral trunk flexion. The infant with hypertonicity may simultaneously move both adducted arms to pull the body forward in one unit versus alternate arm movements. If he attempts to alternately move the arms, the weight-bearing arm becomes trapped under the chest owing to lack of stability. The head may remain flexed with rounded shoulders, and he drags the adducted, extended legs. The infant with athetosis who has more involvement in the upper extremities pushes forward with the hips and legs, and the shoulders come along. The infant with hypotonia, athetosis, or other infants who resist the prone position may get from place to place by scooting on the back in a modified bridge position. This reinforces an extensor pattern and interferes with the evolvement of head control and weight bearing in prone position and trunk rotation.

When the intervener and parents closely observe how the disabled infant moves and compare this with the ease and flexibility of the patterns the normal infant acquires on the horizontal surface during this stage, they realize the importance of interpreting the infant's behavior within a different context. He may appear distractible when all his cognitive and physical energy is being directed to changing his position in space. He may appear irritable when he is frustrated because his arms are caught under him after all that effort of getting to the new position. The infant may appear to be moving away from his caregiver when he is really trying to move toward her. It is understandable if he attempts to move and reach out to his environment less and less. The compensatory and sometimes counterproductive struggle is too effortful and unrewarding.

COMPENSATORY PATTERNS IN THE SITTING POSITION. The stress can increase considerably when the infant attempts to assume positions that provide less body surface support. Only the sitting position will be discussed in this stage. Compensations in the quadruped and standing positions will be discussed in the next stage. The infant with hypertonic muscles may assume a very flexed posture in the sitting position with a marked kyphosis and rounding of the back and a forward position of the head. He remains dependent on the forward propped position of his internally rotated arms (Fig. 2-21A). If the infant raises his head to look up or reach out, the body moves into the other extreme of extension, and he falls backward. If the infant has a lot of flexor hypertonicity, his arms flex up close to his body when he slumps forward, and he cannot sit independently. Or if the infant with hypertonia has an extensor pattern, the head, shoulders, and trunk push back when he is placed in a sitting position, which has a distancing effect (Fig. 2-21B). In time, the extension expands to the legs, and he sits on a rounded spine with compensatory rounding of the upper back and a forward position of the head. The legs are extended and internally rotated, narrowing his base of support. Again, he may have to rely on one or both propped arms for support (Fig. 2-21C). In the positions illustrated in Figures 2-21A and 2-21C, the infant's pelvis is locked into a posterior tilt. The infant with fluctuating tone (athetosis) may fix with the back to compensate for lack of midline stability, and the pelvis is anteriorly tilted. His head and shoulders are pulled back (retracted), and one or both arms are flexed and externally rotated. The legs are flexed or extended and abducted (Fig. 2-21D). The infant with hypotonic muscles initially sits in a forward, flexed position with the pelvis posteriorly tilted. His head is pulled into his shoulders and the arms are in a forward, propped position. The legs are widely abducted (Fig. 2-21E). He may not progress to fully extending his back and aligning the head, shoulders, and pelvis because of weak antigravity muscles.

The lack of midline stability and trunk and pelvic flexibility may prevent the infant with abnormal tone from pushing up from prone in a diagonal pattern to a side-sitting position and then evenly shifting weight on both buttocks. If the infant has a residual STNR, this may initiate movement to a w-shaped sitting position. The infant lifts his head in prone position, and his arms extend and the legs flex in a chainlike reaction. The hips pull straight back, and he sits between his legs or on plantarflexed feet. The infant with hypotonia and hyper-flexibility of the hips may raise up to sitting in a splitlike fashion. He spreads his legs widely apart in prone position and then pushes up and back until he is in a sitting position, pulling his widely abducted legs in front of his body.

It is evident from the above description of compensatory patterns that the infant is fixed in the sitting position. He is not free to experiment and find midline (his center), which interferes with the development of trunk and pelvic stability and flexibility and beginning equilibrium responses. Thus, the infant cannot practice shifting weight and rotating the shoulders to orient to his caregiver's voice or reach for an object. The infant very probably does not feel secure enough to perch on the edge of the caregiver's lap, and he may not be able to indicate clearly a desire to slide off the lap. In fact, the infant may involuntarily push back when he really wants to remain on his caregiver's lap. He may not be able to

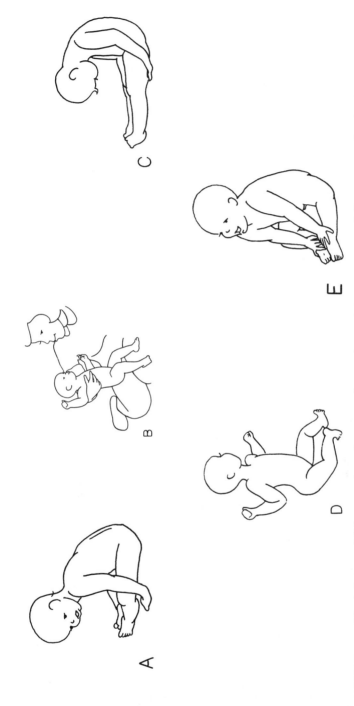

FIGURE 2-21. The infant or child responds to the stress of assuming a sitting position in different ways if he has hypertonia (*A*, *B*, *C*), fluctuating tone (*D*), or hypotonia (*E*).

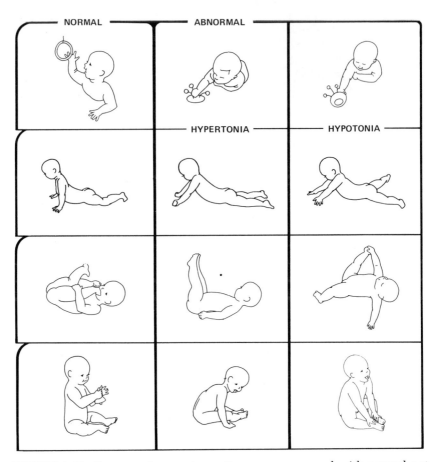

FIGURE 2-22. Compensatory motor patterns are compared with normal patterns.

freely move away a short distance and then return to his caregiver's feet and actively signal a desire to return to her lap because of impaired movement in the prone position. The infant's distancing and proximity-seeking behaviors and perceptual experiences are limited. The descriptive discussion of compensations in this section is reinforced by a comparison of normal and abnormal motor patterns in Figure 2-22.

EFFECT OF MOTOR IMPAIRMENTS ON EXPLORATIVE SCHEMAS.
If the infant does not experience sensory input from weight bearing and proximal movement over a limb, he does not have the background components for a more direct reach and beginning dissociation of the arm and hand (radial-palmar grasp) if one accepts the relationship between proximal and distal development. The infant lacks background stabil-

ity and increased sensory-motor awareness of his arm and hand. If the distal tactual receptors do not become modified with touch-pressure input, protective reactions persist in a marked or less marked form— pulls away or persistently centers on the throwing schema. The ATNR may be elicited from the stress of a new position, and the infant cannot grasp an object when looking at it or bring an object to his mouth. If cocontraction of the neck muscles is still weak, the head may drop when he reaches for a toy. If his clumsy actions do not allow him to investigate all the feedback characteristics of an object, he may lose interest more quickly.

Thus, both sensory impairments described earlier and motor impairments interfere with the evolvement of a flexible repertoire of action schemas. The infant misses out on a myriad of sensations that the normal infant experiences as he repetitively practices schemas through circular reactions. The more limited repertoire of habitual schemas and the more limited repetitive practice interferes with (1) the adaptation, solidification, generalization, elaboration, and differentiation of schemas; (2) the ad hoc recognition of means-end relationships; (3) the ordering of reality around body modes; and (4) the beginning adaptation to reality via imitation.

EFFECT OF MOTOR IMPAIRMENTS ON ORAL AND RESPIRATORY PATTERNS. Motor impairments intertwine with sensory impairments described earlier to delay the development of oral and respiratory control and expansion of the vocalization repertoire. As discussed, compensatory motor patterns are characterized by the lack of midline stability and rotation. The head, shoulders, and trunk do not become aligned with the neutral pelvis in the sitting position to provide a direct, downward, gravitational pull on the ribs. This is felt to limit the angulation of the ribs, although Wilder[48] discusses an older source that questions the relationship if the child has a disability. Lack of axial stability also limits the mobility of the ribs. The oblique muscles remain underdeveloped if there is a lack of a rotational component in motor patterns. This may be a factor in limiting the downward angulation of the ribs and the change to a more oblique insertion of the diaphragm. If there are limited ventilatory demands because of minimal repetitive practice of movements in a heavy work pattern, there will not be the typical increase in fatigue resistant, Type I fibers and muscular mass and strength.[49,50] A cycle occurs with the decreased endurance limiting activity and the need for air exchange, and the vital capacity remains smaller.

A lung disease increases the respiratory load and the work of breathing, which further increases susceptibility to fatigue. The infant has an adaptive mechanism to prevent exhaustion of inspiratory muscles, especially during hyperinflation. He alternates between using the diaphragm and intercostal/accessory muscles. This results in discoordination of movements. When only the diaphragm is contracting, the abdomen displaces outward as the rib cage expands. When only the intercostal/accessory muscles are contracting, the abdomen displaces inward as the rib cage expands. There is excessive use of the accessory muscles (scaleni and sternomastoids) in obstructive lung disease, and the upper ribs paradoxically move inward.[51,52]

If the thoracic muscles are underdeveloped there may not be the beginning transition to thoracoabdominal breathing. This interferes with the typical trend in this stage: increased activity of the thoracic muscles during crying and noncrying vocalization to check the recoil forces. Thus, the duration of the expiration during crying does not increase at the same rate, and the infant cannot control the expiration and subglottal pressure to produce a chain of syllables by the end of this stage.

Abnormal muscle tone further compounds the problem of a limited breath stream. The infant with spastic hypertonicity quickly runs out of breath when vocalizing. If he struggles to breathe in again, the effort can elicit increased bodily extension, which then interferes with breathing out to repeat the sound. The effort of breathing out may increase flexor tone, and he has difficulty breathing in again.[53] The vocalization may be weak and breathy or forced and grating.

If the infant does not develop neck and upper back extension and alignment of the head and trunk, this may delay the descension of the larynx and posterior third of the tongue and the beginning formation of the pharyngeal tube. The delayed structural changes are reflected by atypical nasality, limited variation of the vocal inflection and tone, and restricted mobility of the tongue. The posterior wall is still forward because of limited spinal extension, and the forward tongue movement persists. The forward reaching movement may also be due to sensory deprivation.

Abnormal muscle tone interferes with the beginning functional dissociation of oral movements. The lips, tongue, and jaw may fixate in one position, especially if the infant has hypertonia, or they move in a slow, clumsy, or disorganized way. This interferes with the evolvement of new sounds, including alveolar consonants and back vowels toward the end of this stage. The infant cannot flexibly readjust articulatory movements to change from one vowel sound to another. The lips cannot dissociate from the jaw and tongue to remove food from the spoon nor can the jaw move in a more flexible diagonal pattern to munch finger foods. A lax jaw may lead to mouth breathing, which affects the development of lip control, and the lack of head and trunk alignment interferes with lip closure.

It is understandable if the infant experiences physiologic stress and fatigues quickly because of immature or compensatory breathing patterns. It is also understandable if he becomes frustrated when trying to vocalize because of the inability to coordinate disparate systems. The intervener and caregiver will be less likely to misinterpret his behavior as lazy and socially indifferent.

FRAMEWORK FOR HABILITATIVE APPROACHES

The intervener continues to provide support and assistance within the framework of a colleague relationship with the parents. With this philosophy, the intervener will be less apt to intrude on the family's life style, values, and role system. The intervener also sensitively observes the stresses that the family members are experiencing on an ongoing basis; the amount of stress determines the energy that they can focus on the disabled infant's needs.

Likewise, the intervener helps the parents become more sensitive in reading the infant's signals and cues. These messages serve as the basis for flexibly adapting their repertoire of behaviors and the inanimate environment with the help of guidelines in Chapter 3. The infant expands his repertoire of sensory experiences within his ability to organize and process the input. Exploration is an active process and enhances the infant's sense of inner control during this transitional period when he is projecting outward a short distance in the environment. He is not encouraged to advance to the next level before he has developed well-integrated responses at his present level of functioning, within a context of realistic expectations in terms of his disability. This approach will decrease the likelihood that each new experience will be stressful, with one poor adaptation superimposed on another poor adaptation. The caregiver uses this philosophy as the basis for pacing the following recommended activities. A further discussion is interpolated with some of the activities as are exceptions related to a particular disability.

Approaches to Foster Interaction and Movement Patterns in Supine Position

Activities will be outlined in this section to facilitate the following habilitative outcomes:
- Develops increased strength in flexor muscles in a cephalo-caudal direction.
- Develops background proximal stability in the shoulders.
- Differentiates shoulder movements with upper thoracic rotation.

- Differentiates shoulder and hip movements with trunk rotation.
- Adapts to a gravitational shift with a beginning equilibrium response.
- Develops increased strength in thoracic muscles through diagonal movements.
- Expresses more active proximity-seeking behaviors.
- Explores the body in expanded ways.
- Modifies the reach and grasp schema through secondary circular reactions.
- Generalizes the reach and grasp schema to different objects and a new position.
- Expands the visual field and perceptual experiences.

The caregiver can continue to incorporate activities in the care routine that facilitate increased strength in the flexor muscles and orienting head and arm movements. She holds the infant facing her as illustrated in Figure 2-10 in the preceding stage. The caregiver supports the shoulders forward and rocks the infant back to the point at which he can maintain eye contact with her and not flop the head forward or backward. He is then encouraged to extend his arms in a pick-me-up gesture to be raised back up for a social reward. If the infant has flexor hypertonicity and the effort begins to pull his arms back into flexion, the caregiver can try placing her hands under the infant's arms at the shoulder joint, rotating the arms out to help the infant extend toward her with a proximity-seeking behavior. If the assistance is not effective, this part of the activity will have to be eliminated. The caregiver will also have to monitor how far back she reclines the infant with either flexor or extensor hypertonia. The effort of maintaining the head in an orienting position can reinforce abnormal tone and patterns. The infant who has hypotonic muscles may progress to righting his head to orient to his caregiver when reclined all the way back to a supine position, as does the infant with normal tone.

The caregiver can also vary the above activity if the infant has hypotonia. She rocks the infant backward to the point at which he can maintain head control and encourages him to help raise himself back up for a kiss or to perform an action in his repertoire—batting an object in the caregiver's mouth. The infant should not be required to perform a higher level manipulative activity when energy is directed to a new movement. The infant who has extensor hypertonicity with a tendency to pull back may also be able to perform this activity in an adaptive manner. Raising up against gravity provides resistance to strengthen flexor muscles and reciprocally relaxes his overactive extensor muscles.[54] On the other hand, the infant with flexor hypertonicity will very probably not respond adaptively. The effort reinforces the flexor pattern.

The infant is encouraged to propel his actions outward via a secondary circular reaction when he can maintain his head in an orienting position while being held facing the caregiver on her lap. The reach and grasp schema is facilitated by the Whacker Dacker described in the previous stage. Objects are attached to the braided arms that are easy to grasp, for example, a narrow, easily compressed squeeze toy, measuring spoons, and a yarn pompom. If the infant has a strong grasp reflex, the object may have to be larger to maintain contact with the inside surface of the palm and fingers. A narrow or very small object will provide intermittent contact and may elicit too much flexion in the grasp. The caregiver can also try grasping the elbow and gently and rhythmically shaking the hand to decrease fisting. The effort of reaching may elicit increased flexion if the infant has hypertonicity, and the caregiver can help him extend the arms as described in the above paragraph to elicit a pick-me-up gesture. He may be able to reach and grasp more adaptively in a modified side-lying or prone position, which will be described later.

The number of objects or stimulus intensity of the objects may have to be modified per suggestions in Chapter 3, especially if the infant has a low stimulus threshold. The caregiver can use her repertoire of behaviors and sensitivity to help the infant modulate his level of attention and excitement. She also tries to stay in tune with the infant's response latency and processing rate. The caregiver waits awhile for a response before she assumes that the infant is disinterested. She moves another object closer within easy reach to revive the infant's interest, if habituation occurs before he becomes fatigued. On the other hand, she does not interrupt his active exploration of an object to change to a new one. The goal is to give him the feel of maintaining a spectacle with a circular response and also to prolong periods of sustained attention. Generalization of the schema to new objects should not be rushed.

When the infant can reach and grasp an enticing object with more control, the caregiver suggests a modification of the schema by pulling up on the braided arm while the infant is grasping the object. The infant may then pull the object downward. The caregiver progresses to pulling the braided arm to the side to give the infant the feel of a new adaptation: side-to-side pulling action. However, the infant must actively expedite these actions in a circular fashion after the initial suggestion, if they are to be of value in altering his internal sensory-motor map. Animal studies[55] suggest that the infant must control his own movement and changes in sensory input.

After a period of motivating success in reaching and grasping suspended objects, the caregiver can move to the wings and let the infant experiment on his own to accidentally come upon new adaptations. The initial helpfulness on the lap paves the way for exploration fueled by internal motivation versus heavy reliance on external reinforcing cues. The infant should be placed in the supine position if at all possible, using adaptations discussed in the diapering routine of the preceding stage. This is where the normal infant begins to practice reaching, batting, and grasping, alternately glancing between the object and the hand closest to the object. However, some infants cannot oppose the gravitational force in this position, even with adaptations, because of abnormal tone and reflexes.

If the infant can functionally interact with objects in the supine position, the caregiver encourages generalization of the reach and grasp schema to the side-lying position, which elicits a weight shift to one shoulder and hip. During a spontaneous play period intermeshed with the diaper routine, the caregiver holds the infant's bootie or another article of clothing in the midline to get his attention. The bootie is then moved over to one side to elicit proximity-seeking flexion of the arms and legs, which turns the infant. If the infant has extensor hypertonia, he may not be able to turn from supine to side-lying in an adaptive way without assistance in keeping his head and shoulders forward via approaches discussed below. After the infant has turned to the side, the bootie is placed very close to his hands to let him practice grasping and exploring an object while maintaining the side-lying position. Pressure can be applied to the chest and abdomen if necessary, whether the infant has extensor hypertonia or hypotonia, to facilitate use of the flexor muscles to keep the shoulders and arms forward and the hands in midline. The infant may also practice mouthing the bootie. When he can maintain the side-lying position well with weight directly over the underneath shoulder and hip, the caregiver places the object a little farther from the infant's hand to facilitate reaching with one shoulder more forward. He should not be required to reach too far to prevent having to place the reaching hand back on the surface in a protective response. Again, the caregiver's hand is placed on the chest and abdomen, and forward pressure is applied to the shoulder if the head and shoulder begin to retract (pull back) from the stress of reaching (Fig. 2-23A). The hips should also be kept back in place. The caregiver gradually encourages the infant to reach a little farther to develop proximal stability in the entire range of shoulder movements, to elongate one side of the thorax, and to expand visual experiences. The distance will have to be monitored to prevent loss of control and compensatory extension. If the infant has flexor hypertonia, some or all of the above activities may reinforce the abnormal flexion. More specialized therapy approaches will have to be used to help the infant experience these patterns in a more normal way.

When the infant is comfortable shifting weight to one shoulder and hip and differentiating shoulder and head movements to reach in the side-lying position, the caregiver engages the infant in a game to

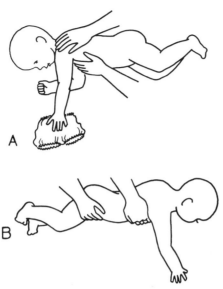

FIGURE 2-23. (A) The caregiver provides control to prevent retraction of the head and shoulder from the stress of reaching. (B) The caregiver facilitates differentiation of the shoulder and pelvis.

differentiate shoulder and hip movements. She moves the top shoulder forward and the top hip backward and visa versa (Fig. 2-23B) to elongate one side and loosen up the midsection, which is necessary for trunk rotation. This activity can be preceded with a slow and rhythmic forward and backward movement of the whole body in approximately a two-inch arc while in the side-lying position, if the infant has hypertonicity. Or the caregiver can use the slow rolling activity described in Chapter 3. The infant may progress to enjoying an adaptation of this activity in supine position. His legs are flexed and rotated to one side, while at the same time the caregiver's other hand is placed under his arm to keep the opposite shoulder on the surface. The infant with hypertonicity may resist the movement in supine position which signals a need to discontinue the activity. The infant with extensor hypertonus may not resist if positioned as shown in Figure 2-9A in Stage I. When self initiated, these activities help develop the oblique muscles and expand the thoracic area, which has significance in terms of breathing and vocalization patterns. Separation of the shoulder and pelvis is also necessary for segmental rolling.

When the diaper is changed and during and after the bath, the caregiver continues to encourage exploration of the body including the genital area. If the infant has hypotonia, she helps him develop strength in the flexor muscles so that he can bring his foot to his mouth in the more normal way, rather than using extension and wide abduction as shown in Figure 2-19B. The caregiver places the infant on his back across the changing table or her lap with legs unsupported by the surface. The head should be flexed some. She tactually stimulates the abdomen and under the buttocks to elicit leg raising. She can also continue to stimulate the inside surface of the thighs with a cotton swab or a light touch of her finger to facilitate more adduction. Light touch should not be used if it elicits adversive reactions or disorganized movement. The caregiver can suspend an enticing object above the infant's feet, which will encourage proximity-seeking hip flexion and leg extension necessary to bring the foot all the way to the mouth. The infant will also practice equilibrium responses in supine position by righting himself back to midline with encouragement from the caregiver if he begins to tip to the side when exploring his feet.

If the infant has hypertonia, it may be more a matter of helping him relax enough to curl up and grasp his feet. The caregiver rhythmically and slowly rocks him from supine fo side-lying a number of times. She then gently rolls him on his back and helps him flex his legs up by elevating his hips off the surface, keeping the head and shoulders forward. The infant should be helped to flex both legs, because if he bends only one, the other leg may straighten in a reflex response.[56] Slow rhythmic rocking in the curled position or gentle, rhythmic shaking of the legs will help ward off a tendency to stiffen and adduct the legs. The infant may discover his genitals for the first time in this curled-up position. With background, slow rhythmic rocking, the infant may also be able to flex his hips, extend his legs, and extend the arms to grasp the feet in a tripod effect, which if turned up would be the propped position that he will first assume when he sits. Thus, the combined flexion of the hips and extension of the legs in supine position helps prepare the infant for the sitting position. If the infant has flexor hypertonicity, he may not be able to use his flexion to explore the feet and other parts of his body without specialized approaches.

Approaches to Foster Interaction and Movement Patterns in Prone Position

Activities will be outlined in this section to facilitate the following habilitative outcomes:
- Develops increased strength in extensor muscles in a cephalo-caudal direction.
- Develops increased stability in the shoulder girdle, upper arm, elbow, and wrist.
- Differentiates the head, shoulder, and trunk from the hips with rotation and counter-rotation.

- Develops increased strength and flexibility in thoracic muscles.
- Adapts to a gravitational shift with an equilibrium response.
- Develops increased endurance.
- Overrides protective withdrawal responses with more localized sensations.
- Generalizes the reach and grasp schema to different objects and a different position.
- Modifies visual and manual schemas to explore the caregiver's face.
- Expands the visual field and perceptual experiences.
- Experiments with the formation of babbling sounds.

The caregiver continues to help the infant move through the phases in the forearm support position. The focus on assuming and maintaining this position in Stage I is reinforced in this stage. When the infant has developed sufficient proximal stability in the head and shoulder girdle to fixate body segments and maintain a position, he has the referent point for movement. The infant is encouraged to progress to the second phase: superimposition of proximal mobility on distal stability. In the course of dressing the infant in the morning or when he awakens in a playful mood from his nap, the caregiver places him in a prone position over her lap. Or she can position the infant on her chest and abdomen when she is lying down, which allows face-to-face contact. The infant is comfortably adjusted to bear weight on his elbows and forearms. As discussed in Stage I, the upper body weight may normalize tone if the infant has hypertonia. Or the upper body weight may have to be decreased some to prevent a superficial tonic holding pattern. The caregiver can place her hands under the infant's armpits both to regulate the amount of body weight he can tolerate and to keep his shoulders and arms forward. A small, flat pillow can be placed under the infant's elbows and forearms if the caregiver's chest or the carpet has little padding. A rough, unevenly textured, or cold surface should be avoided if the infant, irrespective of his tone, still has remnants of the primitive, phasic avoidance response.

When the infant is comfortably settled in the forearm support position, the caregiver helps him experience proximal movement in the shoulder girdle, shoulder joints, and thoracic region of the trunk by rocking backward and forward while the distal elbows remain in place. The rocking movement can be tricky when the infant has abnormal tone. If the caregiver does not have access to an intervener specialized in therapy approaches, the following guidelines may enable her to provide proprioceptive, tactual, and vestibular input similar to that a normal infant experiences during proximal movement. However, it is more difficult to come up with the right blend in a recipe when three sensory ingredients are involved. Careful observation of the infant's response by the available intervener and caregiver is very important to avoid reinforcing abnormal tone or disorganized movement. If the infant has hypertonia, a wide movement range will probably increase tone by stretching muscle fibers. The caregiver should start with a short range and gradually increase the range to the point the movement remains flexible. The rocking should also be slow and rhythmic. If the infant has hypotonia without disorganized movement, the caregiver starts out with a shorter range of movement. The caregiver can then probably shift rather quickly to a wider range and increase the speed of rocking. If the infant has hypotonia with disorganized movement, the rocking should be over a shorter range to maintain enough joint compression to increase proximal stability. The shorter arc also prevents reinforcing the infant's usual tendency for wide movement swings.

The caregiver should gradually pull back and let the infant initiate the proximal movement or just start him and then pause to let him continue, if he can. He will receive more sensory feedback if the movement is completely active on his part and under his control. The infant needs to engage in repetitive practice whereby he refines and modifies the movement. He can be encouraged to move on too quickly. The repetitive practice also increases the need for air exchange, which strengthens ventilatory muscles. Exercise has proven helpful even if the infant has a lung disease, but there has to be a more cautious attitude to prevent adding too great a respiratory load.[57,58]

When the infant can handle the input from proximal movement and has a feel of moving away and back to midline, the caregiver encourages him to move to the third phase: superimposition of distal mobility on proximal stability. She entices him to shift weight to one elbow and forearm and reach out a very short distance straight in line with the shoulder to explore her face. The caregiver may have to decrease the amount of body weight on the weight-bearing arm if the infant has hypertonia. If the reaching arm begins to rotate internally and pull back into the body in response to the stress of the new pattern, the caregiver can try grasping the upper arm at shoulder level and externally rotating the arm (Fig. 2-24). The arm may relax enough so

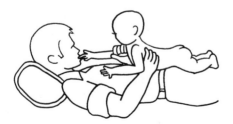

FIGURE 2-24. The caregiver may have to relieve some of the weight on the elbow and forearm and help maintain the extended arm in a reaching position if the infant has hypertonia.

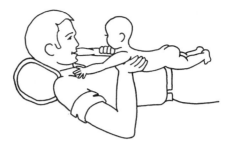

FIGURE 2-25. The caregiver provides the necessary control and position adaptations to help the infant explore his face if there is a disparity between cognitive and motor development.

that it can be rotated to a more neutral position typical of this stage. If the infant has a tendency to rotate the reaching arm externally and pull it back (athetosis), the caregiver keeps the shoulder forward and internally rotates the arm as illustrated in Figure 2-13A. If the infant has hypotonia, he may have difficulty maintaining the arm in the reaching position. Or the reach is accompanied by atypical extraneous movement because of the lack of sufficient background stability. The caregiver can provide inward and downward pressure on the shoulder as illustrated in Figure 2-13B.

These above responses can signal lack of readiness, especially if the caregiver has to provide a lot of external control. Atypical disintegration of the position of the weight-bearing arm also signals lack of readiness: collapsing, adduction back under the body, marked internal rotation and fisting, or shoulder and arm retraction.

The infant may be so motorically involved that he can neither experience proximal movement over the limb nor shift weight and reach out without a lot of abnormal compensations or associated reactions in other body parts. To compound the problem, there is no specialized therapy available. Keeping in mind the controversy over whether the distal and proximal systems are separate, the intervener and caregiver should not be rigidly tied to the normal process of development. If the infant appears cognitively ready to reach out beyond the confines of his own body via secondary circular reactions, the caregiver can help him explore her face and objects in a different pattern more suited to him. She can try supporting the infant with his weight-bearing arm in a more forward, extended position (Fig. 2-25). He should be supported so that he can reach with both hands in this position if he is still orienting in a bilateral pattern.

If the infant can reach out in space without abnormal compensations, the caregiver gradually encourages some shoulder rotation by moving her head or an object over to the side. Pressure on the chest may help facilitate the rotation movement which expands the chest and perceptual experiences.

The infant will come upon new ways to explore his caregiver's face as he lies facing her and practices secondary circular reactions. When he finds her lips, the caregiver can model a very visible, labial consonant babbling sound combined with an easy vowel—bu. The caregiver then adds another tactual cue by making the sound on the infant's chest or neck (if tolerated) so he feels her lips move in a different way. An approach that uses more than one sense to expose the infant to sounds (T-K speech) is described in more detail by Merkley.[59] The approach can be tried with all infants who have delayed expressive language, including the infant with an auditory deficit. The caregiver's vocalization should be spontaneous and relaxed, and she should not expect imitation of a new, unfamiliar sound. The modeling via a number of sensory modalities may expand the infant's experimentation when he is alone in a very quiet, relaxed environment. The intervener helps the caregiver understand all the components involved in forming sounds described in the section on normal oral and language patterns. The caregiver will be less likely to become impatient, lose her spontaneity, and take on a more formal instructive role. The intervener also helps the caregiver maintain a broader view, which helps her realize that interactive periods, movement input, and a variety of exploratory experiences are salient, facilitative forces in terms of language development.

When the infant develops increased stability in the shoulder girdle, the caregiver engages him in activities to elicit the pivot prone response, which develops the antigravity extensor muscles in a cephalocaudal direction, progressing to the trunk and the lower back and hips. This proximal stability is a very necessary background component for sitting and standing. However, the response should not be encouraged if the infant has hypertonicity or fluctuating tone, except through specialized therapy, because of the possibility of eliciting an abnormal response. If the infant has hypotonia without disorganized movement or if he has delayed motor development without abnormal tone, the caregiver can place the infant in prone position on her lap and tilt him forward with as sudden a movement as he will tolerate. His lowered head should attempt to right perpendicular with the floor, eliciting a chainlike reaction of extension down the body except for the flexed position of the arms and feet (Fig. 2-26). The infant can also be swayed up in the air facing downward, and the movement will help elicit extension (Landau reflexive response) with initially more extension in the head and trunk. The position of the head, arms, legs, and feet should be monitored in the above activities. If the head pulls into the shoulders, the flexed arms pull back too much or wing outward, the arms extend at the sides of the body or above the head, the legs tighten and adduct, or the feet plantarflex, then the activity is

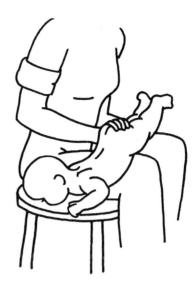

FIGURE 2-26. The caregiver tilts the infant forward to elicit the pivot prone response if he has hypotonia.

not eliciting the full effect of a normal, antigravity extension response.[60] The caregiver should not continue to elicit the response without consulting with an intervener specialized in therapy approaches.

If a more normal response, such as that illustrated in Figure 2-26, is elicited, the caregiver can progress to giving the infant the feel of raising the legs higher by placing him prone over her lap with the legs dangling. If this position does not stimulate the infant to raise his legs, the caregiver can gently jiggle the infant's body or apply tactual input to the legs. This antigravity response will increase proximal stability and extension in the lower back and hips.

When the infant develops increased stability in the shoulder girdle and upper arms, progressive stability and flexibility in extensor muscles via the pivot prone response, and beginning equilibrium reactions from shifting weight to one forearm and elbow to reach out, he is ready to progress through the three phases on extended arms. The infant assumed the propped position with his extended arms slanted in front of the shoulders in Stage I. He practiced moving in and out of the position, which the caregiver continues to encourage. As the infant develops increased background stability in the position, the arms gradually move back in line with the shoulders, and the caregiver helps the infant get the feel of moving proximal parts to rock backward and then forward again and from side to side while the distal hands remain fixed. She then progresses to encouraging the infant to practice shifting weight and freeing one distal part to reach out in space. When the infant shifts weight to one arm to reach out, he should be positioned so the weight-bearing arm can flex some under the stress. With this nuance, the caregiver avoids expecting adaptations that even the normal infant cannot come up with. The infant with hypertonia or fluctuating tone may not be able to assume this weight-bearing position farther away from the center of gravity let alone move through the phases. The stress elicits abnormal patterns which can only be inhibited through specialized therapy approaches.

For the infant who can move through the three phases, the experiences prepare him for the initial forward, propped, sitting position; facilitate rotation of the head, shoulders, and trunk, which expands the thoracic area and develops the oblique muscles; increase stability in the shoulder, elbow, and wrist; and modify receptors in the hand by continuous touch-pressure input. These last two outcomes are important background components for more adaptive prehension schemas.

Approaches to Foster Movement Between Prone and Supine

The above activities in the prone and supine position lead to a segmental movement between the two positions. Without these experiences, the infant may learn to roll in ways that do not dissociate the shoulder and pelvis. It is therefore important to focus on a flow of experiences which build upon each other. Rolling activities become a fun part of the play period when the infant joins the caregiver on her bed or down on the floor. A segmental movement from prone to supine is encouraged first, since this movement is easier. The infant is placed on the caregiver's body, and he is rolled from prone to one side and then to the other side a number of times to give him the feel of the movement. The rhythm and speed of the movement is adjusted to either relax the infant or perk him up, depending on whether he has too high or too low muscle tone or too high or too low a response level per guidelines in Chapter 3. A peek-a-boo game can be incorporated in the activity to let the infant experience finding and being found by his caregiver. The tension of the game may be too excitable for some infants. The caregiver progresses to encouraging the infant to roll from prone to supine on his own to find her. She intervenes if necessary, providing support to the shoulder to prevent it from following the head in one unit. The caregiver moves her hand on down to hold the hip back for a segmental effect. She can angle her body to let gravity help the infant initially if necessary, providing the above control. When he can roll with ease and enjoyment from prone to supine, the caregiver repeats the above series of activities with the infant in supine position. She rolls the infant to one side and then the other side a number of times, adjusting the rhythm and speed to his relaxation or excitation needs. She then encourages the infant to roll from supine to prone by leading him with the position of her face and vocalization or an enticing object. The caregiver helps dissociate the shoulder and pelvis by flexing one of the infant's legs over, keeping the shoulder back to follow segmentally. The infant with hypotonia can gradually be encouraged to roll uphill which provides resistance and encourages trunk rotation to strengthen the oblique muscles. The uphill movement also provides resistance to the adductor muscles, which strengthens them and brings the legs in from the wide abducted position. Specialized therapy approaches will be necessary if rolling elicits the TLR or ATNR response, increased tone, disorganized movement, or other abnormal compensations.

Summary of the Effect of Activities in Prone and Supine Positions

The activities down on the horizontal surface help the infant experience his body centeredness so to speak. This centeredness or midline stability is the reference point for moving away from midline in a rotational pattern and the reference point for relating to his environment. The infant practices exploring his caregiver and objects in different spatial orientations, which expands perceptual experiences and prevents the stereotyped automation of a behavior which is rigidly tied to one very specific position and context. However, the infant is also given an opportunity to practice a schema over and over, and he comes upon new adaptations through this repetition. He finds new parts of his body and becomes better acquainted with other body parts as he moves in different ways and shifts weight to reach out, using the limb as an extension of himself. The infant also develops increased endurance as he repetitively practices motor patterns. He can therefore orient to environmental input with a more alert and sustained attentional level because of a decrease in competing physiologic demands.

Approaches to Foster Interaction and Movement Patterns in Sitting Position

The infant's caregiver may be very eager for him to sit alone to further expand his world. However, if the caregiver is helped to understand all the components involved, she will realize that the new position should not be hurried. Compensatory patterns described and illustrated in the section Effect of Motor Impairments result in shortening of some muscles and lengthening of others, which weakens the muscles and can also lead to a kyphosis, lordosis, scoliosis, and a fixed position of the pelvis with all the physiologic and developmental ramifications. Some infants with more severe abnormal muscle tone will not be able to move up to independent sitting because of the lack of background components.

If the infant is less involved and expresses a real desire to sit independently, albeit in a compensatory way, the caregiver can help him get the feel of a more normal pattern and interact with his environment from a new spatial orientation. Activities are outlined in this section to facilitate the following habilitative outcomes:

- Experiences moving away and back to midline with proximal trunk and pelvic movements.
- Develops increased stability and flexibility in the trunk and pelvis.
- Develops forward and lateral protective extension responses.
- Adapts to a gravitational shift with a beginning equilibrium response.
- Actively moves toward and away from the caregiver.
- Modifies habitual schemas through secondary circular reactions.
- Adds new schemas to his habitual repertoire.
- Monitors the displacement of objects in space.
- Reconstructs the whole object from a part.
- Begins to recognize means-end sequences.
- Imitates familiar sounds and movements.

The caregiver helps the infant experiment with proximal movements in the trunk and pelvis in this new position when she is dressing him or during another daily care activity. If he is hypotonic and sits in a forward, slumped position with legs widely abducted as illustrated earlier, the caregiver places him astride one of her legs with his legs closer together and his feet on the floor. She bounces him to facilitate increased trunk extension and movement of the pelvis away from the posteriorly tilted position. If the infant enjoys this movement, he may smile or even laugh and imitate the bouncing. The caregiver rewards his imitation by repeating the movement. If the bouncing does not elicit extension, the caregiver can place her index and middle finger on each side of the infant's spine and walk up by providing intermittent pressure with the finger pads. This approach should not be used if it elicits too much extension and a nonorienting retraction of the head and shoulders. When the infant moves to a more erect position, he is encouraged to grasp a sound producing object from the caregiver's mouth. If the infant elicits a sound with a vertical arm and hand movement, he will no doubt repeat the shaking action to recapture the auditory effect. In the course of daily practice, the infant may modify his schema and shake the object horizontally. When he is contingently allowed to flex forward for a rest period, the infant may apply an old schema in his repertoire, banging the object on the surface. When he raises up again, he may imitate his caregiver's action and place the object back in her mouth. The infant may also imitate a familiar sound during face-to-face contact. The caregiver provides stability to the shoulders if necessary to help the infant maintain his head in an orienting position and control unstable, extraneous movement to complete an action (Fig. 2-27A).

If the infant with fluctuating tone fixates in the sitting position with an anterior pelvic tilt (swayback), rather widely abducted legs, and retraction and external rotation of one or both arms, he can be seated sideways on the caregiver's leg with his legs in closer together. He is encouraged to posteriorly tilt the pelvis by reaching down and grasping both feet. The caregiver internally rotates his arms if neces-

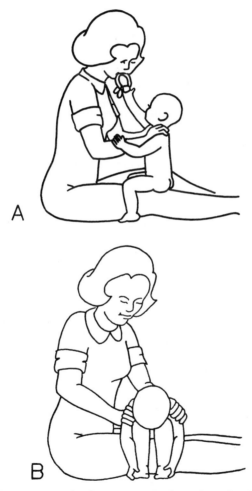

FIGURE 2-27. The caregiver facilitates proximal trunk and pelvic movements and exploration in the sitting position in a different way if the infant has (A) hypotonia or (B) fluctuating tone.

sary (Fig. 2-27B). When he raises back up, the caregiver grasps his pelvis and tilts it backward to prevent fixation with an anterior tilt again. As the infant gradually develops more proximal control of the trunk and pelvis and disorganized movement, he is encouraged to grasp a shoe by one of his feet, raise back up, and bring the shoe to his mouth. The infant may discover another schema to add to his habitual repertoire, such as shaking to elicit movement of the shoelace. The caregiver supports his actions by internally rotating the arms if necessary.

If the infant with hypertonia pushes back and has difficulty flexing the hips or has progressed to sitting back on a rounded spine with extended, adducted, and internally rotated legs, the caregiver can place him astride one or both legs to maintain a wider base of support but not too wide per the precaution of Baumann[61] from Switzerland. He stated that abduction and external rotation can place the femur in a tenuous position for dislocation. The orthopedist is an important member of the team in terms of guidelines for positioning, especially if the infant has hypertonia. The caregiver places her hand on the lower part of the infant's back and pushes him forward to bear weight on the buttocks versus the spine. She encourages him to lean forward to the point he does not lose head control and can flex the hips without resistance. He can then pull or strike a diaper off his partially covered teddy bear. The infant can also play peek-a-boo with his caregiver, swiping the diaper off her partially covered, then completely covered, face. The tension part of the game can be muted. The support to the lower back should be maintained to prevent extension of the hips and knees when he raises and moves his arm (Fig. 2-28A). On the other hand, if the infant

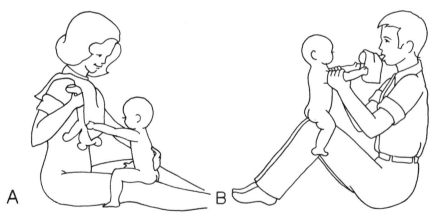

FIGURE 2-28. The caregiver facilitates proximal trunk and pelvic movements and exploration in the sitting position in a different way if the infant with hypertonicity has an (A) extensor pattern or (B) flexor pattern.

with hypertonia sits with the head and trunk flexed and the internally rotated arms in a forward, propped position, he can also be placed astride his caregiver's leg or legs in case his legs adduct under stress. She grasps the infant's hips and helps him raise up to the point he can keep his head righted. The caregiver then changes, if necessary, and grasps under his arms at shoulder level to keep the arms up, forward, and away from his body and to keep his head in an orienting position (Fig. 2-28B). Points of control described in the above paragraphs can be used by the caregiver when holding the infant on her lap at other times during the day to prevent reinforcing compensating patterns.

This may be a good time to discuss the importance of maintaining a holistic view. The caregiver should not be encouraged to place undue emphasis on whether the infant's posture is disintegrating to the point of interrupting his in-progress exploration of an object or her facial features and clothing. Intrusion is only warranted if repositioning is crucial to enable him to sustain the action and experience the means-end sequence, or if the activity is eliciting too much stress and an overflow of tone. The unpleasant sensations will then override the sensory feedback from the exploratory movements. Also the least intrusive approach should be tried first. For example, a background of slow rhythmic rocking suggested in Chapter 3 may elicit enough relaxation if the infant has hypotonia, and he can continue the movement on his own. The caregiver adapts the activity to decrease the demands the next time. She is not infallible, and the right recipe evolves from trial-and-error experimentation and sensitivity to cues.

One focus of activities described thus far in this section is facilitation of proximal trunk and pelvic movements in an anterior and posterior plane. The caregiver also helps the infant get the feel of tilting his pelvis laterally by shifting his weight and propping on the extended arm to prevent falling. It is important that the infant be sufficiently supported and assured when he first experiences this movement to allay a fear of falling and bodily tension. He can be supported at the shoulders or trunk and shifted from one buttocks to another and gradually farther to the side to stimulate protective arm extension. His attention is directed to a rhythmic song or another activity in an effort to maintain the response at a subcortical level. The stress may elicit a startle response, flexion of the arms against the body, or retraction of the head, shoulders, and arms, which signals a lack of readiness for this activity. Or protective responses can only be elicited with specialized therapy. If the infant protectively extends his arms laterally in an adaptive way, the caregiver removes her support to the shoulders or trunk. She shifts the infant's weight by lifting one of his hips, when he is sitting independently on the floor exploring an object, again to decrease cortical involvement with the response.

When the infant can sit in a functional position and protect himself from falling by a forward and lateral extension response, the caregiver facilitates a lateral trunk movement back to midline in a beginning equilibrium reaction versus the protective propping. The infant is placed astride the caregiver's leg or legs in a position that does not reinforce his compensatory tendencies as illustrated in Figures 2-27 and 2-28. The caregiver gently tilts him only a short distance to one side while he is involved in a social game with her or exploration of an object. She pauses to let the infant adjust back to midline on his own if he can. The caregiver repeats the tilt on the other side. Support can again be provided initially to prevent a fearful reaction.

Summary of Effect of Activities in Sitting Position

With practice of all these activities, first with some help and then on his own, the infant experiences moving out of the fixed sitting position. He bobs forward, upward, and to the side in a position farther away from the gravitational force. In the process, he develops increased midline stability and trunk and pelvic flexibility. The infant sits with a more direct downward gravitational pull, which coincides with beginning angulation of the ribs in normal development. The configuration of the vocal tract changes with increased neck and upper back extension and a backward shift of the vertebral wall. The tongue and larynx elongate and become more mobile, a fact which has significance for language development.

The infant also generalizes his action schemas to a new spatial orientation, and he modifies the actions and comes upon new schemas to add to his habitual repertoire. He orients to his caregiver's dynamic movements and gestures, actively moves toward and away from his caregiver and objects, visually monitors hand movements, displaces objects from hand to hand, drops and retrieves objects, and watches the comings and goings of family members from a different vantage point. Animal studies[62,63] suggest that these experiences are necessary for the maturation of visual perception. The infant organizes his experiences into a higher-order internal referent of his caregiver, objects, and environmental expectancies. Development is an intertwining process.

Adaptation of Equipment to Support Sitting Position

Some infants will not progress to the point that they can sit independently and simultaneously orient to the environment and practice schemas. Yet their responses indicate that they are cognitively ready to interact with their environment in this new position. Or, the infant may assume a w-shaped sitting position that is adaptive for him, especially if he has hypertonicity. He has a more stable base and sits with a more erect spine, more relaxed tone in the trunk and upper extremities, and more expansion of the thoracic area. The hands are also free to manipulate objects with better control. Baumann demonstrated with x-rays that the hip joints are in better approximation with the acetabulum in this position. However, the exaggerated knee flexion and foot plantarflexion have dysfunctional implications, especially if the infant has the potential of walking alone or with assistance. The professional team should collaborate with the parents to devise an alternative that is just as functionally adaptive for the infant to decrease the time in the w position. A seating arrangement should also be designed to support the infant who cannot sit by himself. The adaptive seat should preferably be on the floor and provide adequate support so the infant does not have to struggle with his position. This struggle diverts cognitive energy and limits focused attention and control of movements. Side sitting should not be encouraged without orthopedic consultation, because the infant will prefer to sit on the better side, which can result in hip dislocation.

Approaches to Foster Prone Locomotion

When the infant can comfortably sit independently, he perches on his caregiver's lap and then feels sure enough to gesture a desire to slide off, explore at her feet, and roll a short distance away. If the infant has hypotonia, the caregiver helps him adapt a pattern in his repertoire (shifting weight to one elbow and forearm and reaching out) to move away from her in a combat crawl. When he assumes the on-elbows support position, she tilts his pelvis from side to side, which propels the infant a short distance forward. She can also place a towel under the infant's chest and help him shift weight from side to side, again giving him the idea of movement toward an enticing object out in the world. The caregiver should observe for signs that the towel is causing respiratory discomfort. The infant's legs can be corraled between the caregiver's legs to limit excessive abduction if necessary. The infant may resist the harder work pattern involved in the new mode of locomotion and prefer to roll or pivot around in a circle using his abduction and lateral trunk rotation. If this is the case, stability and endurance will have to be developed in less complex patterns. Specialized approaches will have to be used if the infant has hypertonia, because the stress will no doubt pull the arms back under the body or retract the head, shoulders, and arms. The above approaches should also not be used if the infant has fluctuating tone (athetosis), because they are likely to increase disorganized movement.

The infant with hypotonia, hypertonia, or fluctuating tone may find an alternate way to move as discussed earlier. Again, the team members should collaborate with the parents to develop another source of mobility that is equally or almost as productive as his adaptation if it is reinforcing abnormal patterns. Also, they can devise a functional form of mobility for the infant who is cognitively ready to expand his world a short distance. The required energy expenditure must be considered. If the mode of forward progression is too effortful, the infant will have little energy left to direct to the stimulus he is moving toward, especially if he has limited vital capacity.

Additional Approaches to Provide Vestibular and Tactual Input

The importance of movement input has been discussed both in this stage and the preceding stage. This is expecially true if the infant's own self-initiated mobility is limited. Movement input is often preferred over visual input if the infant functions at a low cognitive level. Many of the above suggested activities involve movement. Rocking is still a very natural pleasurable input in this stage. The infant can also still be placed in a carrier attached to his caregiver's body. The carrier should be adapted if possible so that the legs are in a more adducted position if the infant has hypotonia. The team members should consult with the orthopedist to determine the appropriate position of the legs if the infant has hypertonia. The infant should also be carried from point to point in the house, facing his caregiver at times if at all possible, so he can visually and tactually explore her face and clothes and begin to learn some of the don'ts, for example, pulling the caregiver's hair. Again, the legs should be kept together as much as possible if they are widely abducted, or his legs can be placed astride the caregiver's hip if they adduct and there is no orthopedic contraindication. She can support his shoulders forward, if he tends to push back, or provide support under the arms, if they tend to pull in, and help him bring them up around her neck.

If the infant has a low tolerance for vestibular input or if this input is contraindicated because of a seizure pattern, there can be more of an effort to provide tactual input, especially at bath time. The caregiver spends more time rubbing body parts with the washcloth, including the infant's hands, which is especially important if he is blind. His body can be massaged after the bath based on an approach pictorially outlined in the book *Loving Hands*.[64] The pressure of the stroke and focused parts must be individually determined, if the infant still responds protectively to tactual input or has abnormal tone. Some guidelines are provided in Chapter 3. The tactual input may help the infant become more comfortable with vestibular input. The opposite can also be the case: vestibular input can decrease tactual adversiveness.

Adaptation of Objects and the Immediate Environment
to Foster Explorative Schemas

Vestibular input may facilitate increased ocular control because of the interplay between the two systems. If the infant also becomes less tactually defensive, he may be more apt to propel his actions outward via secondary circular reactions. Some infants may only make this important transition if objects and the immediate environment are adapted to their limitations in more specific ways. If the infant lacks endurance, the object should be lightweight and very responsive to his actions, for example, mason jar rings on large binder ring or crackly paper sewn inside pellon. A cardboard cone or other larger holding device may have to be attached to an object to provide contact with all the flexor surfaces of the fingers, as described earlier, if the infant still has a strong grasp reflex. The holding device should not be so large that it stretches the flexor muscles too much. Hiding games are also adapted to the infant's disability. The object can be partially covered with an easily grasped, semitransparent cloth to provide additional perceptual cues. A cardboard screen can be suspended with an object partially hidden behind. A simple batting action will then move it to the side to expose the object completely. Or a larger object is placed behind a smaller box that can be knocked over to expose the whole object. If the infant has poor vision, the object should be bright with sharp outlines. Food is a very motivating force for some infants. The bottle can be partially covered with the nipple exposed, or the dish of food can be partially covered. Progression can then be made to complete coverage in all these activities.

The saving grace is that the infant does not have to explore all the properties of an object actively to form an internal sensory-motor representation. He exploits the senses he has. The motor-impaired infant is positioned where he can visually observe daily activities within his tolerance level. He watches the action and displacement of his caregiver, other family members, pets, and objects. The blind infant both hears and feels his caregiver during daily care activities and playful interaction. He is also provided with objects close to his hands that provide tactual and auditory feedback. Both he and the motor-impaired infant can be positioned inside a cardboard box that has been cut off to provide a rim, or in a chair with a tray that has a rim to prevent objects from moving out of reach. As the blind infant comes in contact with objects in different locations on the table, he primitively begins to realize that an object can be displaced, and he searches in a certain arc. The blind infant also begins to reach in response to a tactual cue. He is moving along the path toward uniting tactual and auditory experiences to reach toward a sound in the next stage. The infant shows transitional tendencies by pantomiming an action he just performed (shaking action of his hand) when the bell is removed from his hand and shaken. Thus, the caregiver continues to observe the blind infant's hand signals in this stage, and they develop a ballet of hand movements to communicate with each other. Enjoyable manipulative experiences in different positions will help entice the blind infant to actively assume different positions including prone.[65]

Need for Alternate Caregiving Resources

The infant may remain in this stage for a long period of time or may never progress beyond this stage. Even though the infant is beginning to slide off the caregiver's lap, the pair are still undifferentiated in the infant's or child's eyes, and the caregiver is the central force in his world. Very probably it will be more and more difficult with the increase in his size to provide him with the close contact and emotional refueling, which he still needs, and to meet the demands for adaptation inherent in his disability. Again, the parents very probably will feel a need for surrogate caregiving at some point in time from services listed in the previous stage. There is a controversy regarding the effects of substitute caregiving reflected by conflicting research data and the paucity of longitudinal studies. There are very intertwined variables involved: physical quality of the home and substitute care setting, number and responsiveness of caregivers, and frequency of caregiver and setting changes.[66] Some observations point to the importance of a familiar caregiver. It has been noted that the infant's interaction with his parents is far different from his interaction with strangers and other infants. There is much less close, proximal contact with other infants and strangers.[67] The elementary social interaction between six-month-old infants was very brief compared with the length of the interaction period with more adaptable adults.[68] This has implications in terms of expanding intervals of sustained attention. Even with a paucity of data, it appears safe to assume that the infant should be cared for by a limited number of adults so that certain persons become significant and predictable sources of care and stimulation.

The more limited the infant's repertoire of action schemas with objects, the more dependent he will be on the caregiver's repertoire of behaviors and his own body to nourish his nervous system. If the infant is left alone for long periods because of the staff ratio, he will turn more and more inward to his own body. Some infants with a high threshold for pain and sensory input will resort to banging their heads, vigorous rocking, and other behaviors often described as self abusive. There is also the possibility that the infant is reacting to too much overall noise and confusion in the environment.

The staff is presented with a challenge to exploit the time spent with the infant and to substitute other forms of sensory input. Touch pressure from lying next to a large stuffed animal can be pleasurable. The infant can also accompany a staff person on an errand in a carrier or wagon. Caregivers in the program setting monitor any tendency to use a task-oriented approach during the daily round of events such as diapering and feeding. Instead, they take advantage of this opportunity to provide visual, auditory, tactual, vestibular, proprioceptive, and olfactory input. Rolls, bolsters, balls, and other pieces of equipment are not automatically used to facilitate motor patterns. The staff person involved in the activity uses her lap, unless the weight and size of the infant or child necessitate substituting adaptive equipment. This is a way of providing close bodily contact and reassurance.

THIRD STAGE: NINE THROUGH TWELVE MONTHS

FRAMEWORK FOR ASSESSING NORMAL DEVELOPMENTAL PATTERNS

Description of Normal Motor Patterns

In the previous stage the infant developed very flexible movement patterns down on the horizontal surface, and he also moved farther up from the center of gravity and assumed the sitting and quadruped positions. The infant progressed to the second phase in these two positions, superimposing proximal mobility on distal stability. He moved his trunk forward, upward, and laterally in the sitting position, which tilted the pelvis posteriorly, anteriorly, and laterally. His arms intermittently assumed a propped position during the shifts to compensate for immature equilibrium responses. Likewise, the infant rocked forward, backward, and from side to side in the quadruped position. These work patterns increased proximal stability. The infant's shoulders aligned over the neutral pelvis in the sitting position with the flexed legs still abducted to provide a wider base of support. His hands aligned under the shoulders and the knees under the hips in the quadruped position.

With increased background proximal stability, the infant now progresses to the third phase and superimposes distal mobility on proximal stability. The hands are completely freed from the support position when the infant is sitting, and he practices shifting his weight to reach out and grasp his caregiver's ear or an object more to one side, which involves upper thoracic rotation. He then progresses to reaching across midline, which involves rotation of the head, shoulders, and trunk, and counter-rotation of the pelvis to maintain the sitting position and not topple over. Surrounding space is opening up now that the distal part is free to reach out in different orientations.

The infant integrates midline stability with vertical and rotational righting reactions, which allows him to adapt to a gravitational shift with a more mature equilibrium response. The infant flexes and rotates the head and trunk away from the direction of the tilt, and he abducts the arm and abducts and externally rotates the leg on the side opposite the tilt. This antigravity response brings the infant back to midline, and he then vertically aligns all the parts again. The rotation component has been added, whereas the infant adjusted with lateral head and trunk flexion in the previous stage.

A backward protective response also evolves. The infant extends his arms if he falls backward, and then pushes himself back up to midline with his hands. By the end of this stage, the infant can right himself back up to midline if he is tilted only a short distance backward by moving his head, shoulders, and arms forward and extending his legs. He also rights himself to midline when tilted forward in sitting position by moving the head, shoulders, and arms backward and flexing the legs. The infant can always fall back on the protective extension response of the arms if he is tilted too far in any direction.

The process down in the prone and supine positions has repeated itself. The infant has discovered the midline orientation in a higher position, which serves as the reference point for flexible movement. He moves away from the center and back, tilting his pelvis in all planes and differentiating body segments to rotate one part and hold with another part as a counterforce.

With a background of increased midline stability and more mature equilibrium reactions, the upper extremities continue to move to a more functional position from adduction and internal rotation typical of early infancy to more outward abduction and external rotation with the radial fingers oriented upward and more active. The legs move in from the flexed, abducted, externally rotated position. They extend and assume a more adducted, neutral position in line with the hips. The functional directional change is thus opposite with the upper extremities moving outward away from the midline of the body and the lower extremities moving inward toward the midline of the body.

The infant also progresses to the third phase in the quadruped position. As he develops increased proximal control and stability, the infant feels secure enough to shift weight to one upper extremity and reach out to his caregiver as she approaches. The infant adapts the reach to move forward with the arm, and the leg on that side flexes and moves forward. He shifts weight on that arm and moves forward with the opposite arm, and the leg on the same side flexes and follows. The infant has come upon a new form of mobility—homolateral creeping. This pattern is soon adapted to a reciprocal movement of the extremities. When one arm moves forward, the leg on the opposite side flexes and moves forward. In fact, the caregiver may not be aware of the initial homolateral movement because it is so short-lived. The stress of this new mobility pattern elicits regression. The arms and legs move out of alignment with the shoulders and hips to provide a wider base of support. The elbows abduct out beyond the shoulders and the arms internally rotate. The legs likewise revert back to an earlier position— abduction and external rotation. The initial creeping pattern thus involves wasted movement with a wider side-to-side weight shift because of the extremity abduction. There is also a lateral movement of the trunk versus rotation.

The added demands of a unilateral weight shift up farther from the base of gravity increase the stability in the extremities. The extended arms and flexed legs gradually move back and align under the shoulders and hips as the muscles strengthen. Practice creeping also increases the stability of proximal muscles in the shoulder, trunk, and pelvis, which provides a background for more mature equilibrium reactions involving a rotation and counter-rotation component. The shoulder of the leading arm is forward, and the opposite hip is back in a diagonal orientation, which rotates the trunk. The movement is directly forward versus the wider weight shift from side to side. The infant gets from place to place faster and more efficiently with less expenditure of energy. This integrated pattern depends on higher level sensory processing to plan, execute, and monitor the movement of each body part and adjust movements in space. The central nervous system is receiving more discriminative visual, tactile, proprioceptive, and vestibular input. Thus, the intertwined nature of sensory and motor function becomes even more apparent as movement patterns become more complex.

While the infant is refining his posture and movements in the sitting and the quadruped positions, he is also practicing moving up a little farther from the center of gravity in a semi-standing position on his knees. The infant's hands initially move back to a support role, the knees abduct to widen the base of support, and the pelvis anteriorly tilts, with the hips farther back than the shoulders. When the infant begins to feel more secure in the new position, he superimposes proximal mobility on distal stability and bounces up and down and shifts weight from one knee to the other. This provides the first rudimentary experience of maintaining the body weight on one lower extremity, which is required in walking. The infant begins to rotate his head and shoulders to orient to the caregiver's voice as he shifts weight more to one knee. He progresses to moving laterally on his knees toward an interesting object at the other end of the low table. As the infant develops increased midline stability, the shoulders, trunk, and hips again align with each other; and he experiments with freeing his hands from the support role to manipulate objects. The stability also provides the background for a rotation component. The infant rotates his trunk and maintains a counter-rotation of the pelvis to visually orient to a wider surrounding space. He also reaches down and retrieves a toy more to one side, but his one hand moves back to a support position. The infant may progress to walking forward on his knees at the end of this stage.

The infant adapted the pull-to-sit by extending his legs and pulling up to a supported standing position in the preceding stage. When the infant moves up on his knees, he begins to adaptively assume a half-kneel position and to pull himself up to a piece of furniture. His movements are awkward initially. The leg that is brought forward is abducted and externally rotated, which places the weight more on the lateral surface of the foot. The opposite knee is also rotated outward, and the hip is not fully extended on that side because of the inability to completely dissociate movements. The infant relies more heavily on his upper extremities to pull himself up, because the wider position of the legs decreases the leverage of lower extremity movements.

As the infant practices assuming an upright position even more removed from the center of gravity, he repeats the process in the kneeling position. His hands move back in a support role, his legs abduct to widen the base of support with more weight on the medial surface of the feet (flatfoot position), and his pelvis anteriorly tilts. With practice sitting, creeping, and knee standing, the infant develops enough midline stability in the shoulders, trunk, and hips to inhibit the strong positive support reflex. The static standing position gives way to a little flexion in the knees as some muscles are freed from cocontraction. This provides the looseness to superimpose proximal mobility on distal stability when the infant gets his bearing in the new position. He bounces up and down, rocks back and forth, sits down and pulls up, and shifts weight more to one foot to rotate his head and shoulders and orient to his caregiver's voice.

Weight shifting propels him into the third phase: superimposition of distal mobility on proximal stability. The infant frees one arm and hand to reach for an object, an action which involves shifting his weight to one leg. The other leg is then free to move, and the infant steps laterally in a righting response to realign his body. A new mobility pattern thus evolves—cruising. The extra demands of unilateral weight bearing fosters increased stability in the legs just as was the case with the arms. Also, the weight shift to one foot provides pressure on the lateral surface, which arches the foot.

As the infant develops increased midline stability from all the above experiences, the legs gradually adduct; and the knees and feet align under the hips. The weight of the body is directly over the legs and feet by the end of this stage. More direct weight bearing over the limb facilitates increased awareness and control of movements in the leg and foot and is therefore an important precursor to walking, just as it was related to the development of arm and hand control in reaching and grasping, that is, if one accepts a proximal-distal relationship.

Increased midline stability also provides the background for more flexible movements. The infant rotates his trunk one way and maintains the pelvis in counter-rotation, which opens up surrounding space from a new, upright vantage point. He reaches down and picks up a toy in different positions on the floor. The infant then raises up and stands on his toes in an attempt to reach an object or to signal more actively that he wants to climb back on the caregiver's lap. The infant uses rotation to cruise diagonally around the corner of a piece of furniture, whereas a wider base of support and weight shift with lateral trunk flexion allowed him to cruise only in straight-line planes initially. The infant also uses rotation to assume a more mature half-kneel position. The knee of the forward leg is aligned horizontally with the hip, which places weight on the whole surface of the foot. The knee of the other leg is aligned with the completely extended hip. Thus, there is dissociation with hip flexion on one side and hip extension on the other side. The lower extremities now play a more active role in providing leverage when pulling up.

Increased midline stability, more mature equilibrium responses, and trunk rotation allow the infant to freely change positions in space. I counted how many times an 11-month-old infant changed positions in a 30-minute interval, and the number was surprising—52 changes. By the end of this stage, the infant eliminates some wasted motion during position changes in the lower postures. He does not have to roll all the way over to prone to move into a sitting position. He rolls to the side, props his arm, and then moves the trunk up to side-sitting with rotation.

The infant adapts the creeping and pull-to-standing patterns to crawl over, under, on, in between, and around the other side of objects. Sometimes he gets caught under an object or between objects. The infant uses past experiences organized in central structures and a feedback mechanism to plan movements and to figure out how to adapt the movement of body parts to get where he wants to go. The movement patterns and accommodations open up a whole new panorama of spatial and sensory experiences.

The above descriptions exemplify the rather phenomenal refinement of motor patterns during the first year. Even the meaning of stability is being expanded to include dynamic holding during movement. There is no longer fixation of portions of the body to the same degree as was the case with the earliest positions.[1] Figure 2-29 illustrates the evolvement of motor patterns in this stage, and Table 2-11

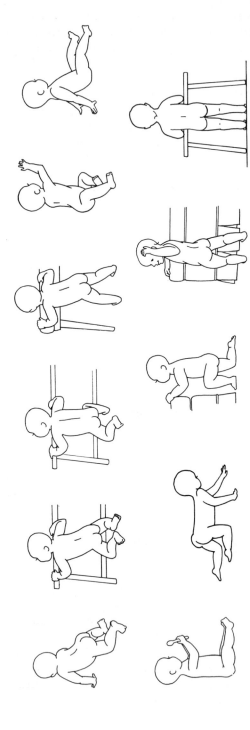

FIGURE 2-29. The first four figures illustrate the quality of motor patterns at the beginning of this stage, and the remaining figures illustrate the quality of motor patterns by the end of the stage.

TABLE 2-11 Evolvement of motor patterns in phases (Third Stage)

ASSUMES POSITION	SUPERIMPOSES PROXIMAL MOBILITY ON DISTAL STABILITY	DEVELOPS INCREASED STABILITY & CONTROL IN POSITION	SUPERIMPOSES DISTAL MOBILITY ON PROXIMAL STABILITY
* (1) Sitting—trunk erect, shoulders aligned over hips, pelvis neutral position, legs abducted, ringed position	(1) Continues practice tilting pelvis anteriorly, posteriorly, laterally	(3) Trunk maintains erect position, pelvis assumes neutral position, legs extend and align with hips, arms assume more abducted and externally rotated position	(2) Reaches across midline, rotation head, shoulders, and trunk
(1) Quadruped—trunk horizontal, elbows aligned with shoulders, knees aligned with hips	(1) Rocks diagonally	(3) Arms align under shoulders, knees align under hips when creeping	(1) Shifts weight to one arm, reaches (1) Creeps, arm and leg on same side move forward (1) or (2) Creeps, reciprocal movement arm and leg (3) Creeps with more differentiation of shoulder & hip, trunk rotation
(1) Knee standing—arms in support position, shoulders shrugged, knees abducted, pelvis anteriorly tilted	(1) Bounces up and down, shifts weight from knee to knee	(3) Knees align with hips, pelvis assumes neutral position, arms free from support role	(1) Reaches with one arm, shoulder rotation (1) Cruises laterally on knees (2) Reaches—head, shoulder, trunk rotation (3) May walk forward on knees
(2) Standing—arms in support position, shoulders shrugged, legs abducted, pelvis anteriorly tilted	(2) Bounces up & down, rocks back and forth, shifts weight side to side	(3) Knees & feet align with hips, pelvis assumes neutral position	(2) Reaches with one arm, shoulder rotation (2) Steps laterally—cruises (3) Reaches—head, shoulder, trunk rotation (3) Cruises around corner, trunk rotation

* (1) Beginning of stage; (2) Midway in stage; (3) End of stage

graphically outlines the process as the infant moves through the three phases in each position.

EVOLVEMENT OF PREHENSION SCHEMAS. With all the practice of changing positions in space, shifting weight to one extended arm and then the other while creeping, reaching in different orientations including across midline, and practicing a repertoire of manipulative schemas, the infant is exposed to a variety of sensory input that challenges the organizational capacities of the central nervous system. Neuronal networks continue to develop, which facilitate integration of sensory input. Newer dorsal column pathways continue to mature and become more heavily myelinated and thus transmit more localized sensations to the central nervous system. Skin receptors continue to become more discriminative; and the protective, more diffuse touch sense is inhibited except in response to more intense input—prickly object. Unilateral weight bearing in the higher quadruped position challenges the stabilizer muscles in the shoulder and arm, which become stronger. With a background of increased stability, elbow, wrist, and finger movements become more flexible. The infant also becomes increasingly more aware of his arms and hands and their linkage to other parts of his body.

The above components provide the background for continued refinement of prehension schemas via the same process described in the preceding stage. The infant draws upon past experiences organized in a central map or template to plan his reach and grasp of an enticing object. He uses discriminative proprioceptive, tactile, and visual feedback to modify the plan and further accommodate his hand to the object. The infant also changes the position of the hand and fingers to take in more sensory information. The modification of the initial motor plan and the new sensory information are integrated in the dynamic, ever changing central template.

The above refinement process is reflected in more adaptive explorative schemas. The infant visually orients his hand to the object, which he then grasps with a radial-digital accommodation. This places the object between the thumb and fingers with no palmar contact. He also progresses to grasping a very small object between the tip of the thumb and index finger with a facile pincer movement. The infant flexibly differentiates finger movements to explore the surface of the object, and he can even flex one finger to poke at details. He also flexibly differentiates the elbow and wrist to move the object in closer and farther away, to rotate the object, and to examine it from different distances and angles. He supinates the hand to grasp a cube and then pronates the hand to release the object voluntarily, controlling flexion and extension movements of the fingers. The infant independently uses one hand, and he can cross midline with that hand to reach for an object. He also coordinates the movements of his two hands to clap them togehter in midline or bang two objects together. The accuracy and rhythm of the bilateral actions improve with practice.

The infant practices adjusting the timing of his grasp to the speed of a slowly moving object. He can therefore engage in ball play in a rudimentary way. If the ball is slowly rolled toward him in a horizontal plane while he is sitting with his legs spread apart, he will attempt to grasp or trap it against his legs. The trapping is a delayed reaction when he cannot adjust his grasping movement to the speed of the ball.

It is evident that the infant has also come a long way in refining and coordinating the movements of his smaller muscles during the first year. The accomplishments in this stage are summarized in Table 2-12.

Description of Normal Oral and Language Patterns

Although Wilder[2] followed infants only to eight months of age, it is reasonable to assume that there is a continued relationship between gross motor development and the coordination and control of respiratory and laryngeal muscles. Two forces are probably instrumental in angulating the ribs in this stage: the increased activity of the oblique

TABLE 2-12 Evolvement of prehension schemas
(Third Stage)

FUNCTIONAL ADAPTATION	QUALITATIVE DESCRIPTION
More refined visually directed reach and grasp	Visually orients hand to object
	Grasps object with radial-digital orientation, no palmar contact
	Grasps very small object with pincer orientation—thumb-index finger opposition
Beginning differentiation of elbow and forearm movements	Moves arm and hand to inspect object at different distances and angles
	Supinates hand to grasp object, pronates hand to release object
Beginning differentiation of finger movements	Explores surface of object with finger
	Flexes one finger to poke at details
Beginning bilateral coordination	Bangs two objects together in midline
	Grasps or traps slow moving ball with both hands
	Crosses midline with one hand to reach and grasp object

muscles during rotational movements and the gravitational pull in the progressively more well-aligned sitting, kneeling, and standing positions. The rib cage also becomes more mobile with a background of increased midline stability. These maturational changes no doubt influence the evolvement of a complex interaction between thoracic, abdominal, and laryngeal muscles and the recoil forces of the lungs to maintain a relatively constant subglottal pressure during vocalization. As discussed in the preceding stage, Wilder proposed that this interplay is evident when the infant begins to babble in multiple syllables, which is a more prevalent form of vocalization in this stage.

It is easy for the adult to take the above complex mechanisms for granted, since they are so automatic. It is therefore important to review the different types of respiratory adaptations to appreciate the relationship between speech and breathing. The infant very possibly approaches the adaptations described in research studies of adult subjects toward the end of the first year when there is a rather marked increase in costal activity.[3] Some investigators[4,5] emphasize that specific muscles cannot be categorized as inspiratory or expiratory, because the functions of breathing are not that simplistic. This is no doubt the reason there is disagreement concerning the role of specific muscles in the literature. There is a growing tendency toward the use of more generic terms—rib cage muscle and abdominal muscles.

During quiet breathing there is a nearly equal ratio of airflow in and out, with the inspiration only slightly shorter than the expiration. The expansion of the rib cage is predominantly affected by a diaphragmatic contraction. The intercostal muscles serve in the role of fixators to provide some stiffness to the rib cage, which prevents distortive sucking in of the intercostal spaces as well as air by negative pleural pressure.[6,7] The thoracic muscles may play a more active coordinated role with the diaphragm to expand the rib cage in the upright position.[8] The expiratory phase of quiet breathing is a passive phenomenon resulting from the force of gravity, untorquing of cartilage, and the elastic recoil of lung tissue and extended viscera in the abdomen.

Adaptations of the quiet breathing pattern during vocalization is determined by the rate, length, and loudness of the utterance. If the utterance is short and soft, the inspiration does not have to be modified to increase the lung volume. There is also no need for a braking or checking of passive recoil forces, because the relaxation pressure does not exceed the necessary subglottal pressure for phonation. There may be a need for the thoracic expiratory muscles to become active and supplement the relaxation pressure exerted by the passive recoil forces as the utterance proceeds. If the utterance is lengthened and the volume is increased (less soft), the respiration cycle has to be adjusted with a more rapid and deeper inspiration and a more prolonged expiration.

The initial relaxation pressure is greater than the subglottal pressure desired for vocalization, and the inspiratory muscles remain active in a holding maneuver to resist the passive forces of expiration, as discussed in the preceding stages. There is balanced gradual reduction of the inspiratory braking action as the volume of air in the lungs decreases and the relaxation pressure also decreases. If the utterance extends to the point that the relaxation pressure is insufficient, the expiratory muscles come into play and become progressively more active to maintain the pressure and steady flow of the air stream necessary to complete the utterance.[9,10]

Some of the above respiratory adaptations have significance in further decreasing the work of breathing in this stage. The fixation of the rib cage muscles counteracts the distorting forces of the diaphragm and increases the efficiency of the inspiratory contraction. The vital capacity continues to increase because of a number of factors: enlargement of the thoracic cavity due to angulation of the ribs, increased need for air exchange relative to the evolvement of mobility skills, and the growth of new saccules in the lungs. The volume of the lungs is four times that at birth by 11 months of age.[11] Thus, the respiration rate continues to decrease with less energy-consuming muscular contractions per unit of time. As the rib cage and abdominal muscles become progressively more developed, they are capable of assuming a larger share of the work load when ventilatory requirements increase. There is also an increase in the mass of the respiratory muscles with use. All of these factors intermesh to increase the infant's resistance to respiratory fatigue.

Moving on to other aspects of the complex interplay of mechanisms discussed at the beginning of this section, the adjustments of the larynx and articulators play an important role in modulating the air stream into specific speech sounds. More refined adjustments are dependent on structural changes in the oral and pharyngeal cavities and neuromuscular control. Increased extension of the spine elongates the neck and stabilizes the posterior pharyngeal wall. There is continued descension of the larynx and the posterior third of the tongue in the neck, which expands the pharyngeal tube. The structural expansion continues to be reflected by increased mobility of the palate, larynx, and tongue, and the lips elongate and become more mobile.[12] The evolvement of more dissociated tongue, lip, and jaw movements also correlates with increased separation of different parts of the body, such as head and shoulders, elbow, wrist, and fingers.

Sensory maturation continues to be an important component relative to the increased neuromuscular control of articulators. Refinement of oral movements involves the same process as the refinement of prehension schemas discussed in the previous section and is especially dependent on two elements: more discriminative proprioceptive and tactile sensations and higher order integration of sensory input. There is also the acquisition of new sensory receptors in the alveolar area with the eruption of teeth.[13] The infant can more effectively monitor movements of the lips, tongue, and jaw and differentially respond to textures of objects and substances in his mouth. He draws upon past experiences organized in a central template and a feedback mechanism to plan and modify movements to accommodate to a new input.

These background components provide the framework for more adaptive oral and language patterns. The infant becomes more aware of the articulators, and he is especially intrigued by his tongue. The infant playfully reaches into his mouth to grasp the tongue, and he also adaptively moves it in different directions: licks food off the lower lip and corner of the mouth, sticks the tongue out and in. The varied movements involve protraction, retraction, lateralization, elevation, and depression. The bite is functionally prehensive, and the infant begins to move his jaw in a rotary excursion and his tongue laterally to perform a chewing action. The diet is expanded to include large pieces of finger food, such as chunks of canned fruit. The lips accommodate better to a glass or cup with less associated jaw movement (pumping action). The infant's vocalization repertoire expands considerably. There is an increased incidence of one back vowel (oo), but front and middle vowels still dominate, possibly because stabilization of back vowels is dependent on the lowering of the larynx and rear portion of the tongue into the neck, which takes several years. The front vowels a and ae and the middle vowel ʌ become more stabilized in terms of pitch quality around 38 to 40 weeks, coincidental with the complete restructuring of the vocal tract into two separate cavities. The vowels i and I also become more consistent and easily differentiated by the end of this stage.[14] The front, alveolar consonants (t, d, n, l) begin to dominate, but there is still incomplete dissociation of articulators; most infants move the jaw up and down when making the "la" sound. The infant flexibly varies his babbling by placing the consonant at the beginning (bu-gu), medially (abu), or at the end (ub-ab). The babbling chain expands to six or more syllables in one expiration because of the longer breath stream and increased respiratory control.[15]

The infant's response to sounds also becomes more refined. He localizes sounds in space more quickly and directly, no doubt because of increased experience moving himself in space. He orients to sounds above ear level as well as to the side and below ear level. The infant also turns and orients to more subtle sounds outside his peripheral field. Thus, sound has become a more predictable environmental cue.

With increased sensory maturation, the infant can form rudimentary auditory-visual associations to connect certain words with a gesture, person, or object—no-no, da-da, bye-bye. He will selectively look at, touch, or hand one or more familiar objects to an adult when labeled. According to the results of one study,[16] the amount of his verbalization is not related to receptive recognition of an object. The infant who made the most accurate selections did not vocalize. Comprehension appears to be related to functional meanings that the infant has come upon through active exploration of the properties of an object and involvement in routine events.[17,18] The infant's comprehension is initially limited to a stereotyped response in one setting. He will look at or crawl to a certain location in the room in response to "Where's daddy's shoe?" However, he will not identify the shoes otherwise. The infant does not realize that the shoes can move from place to place. By ten months of age, he begins to associate a word with a familiar person and less often an object in nonroutine contexts in which the time and place are unusual.[19] The identity and existence of a person and possibly a familiar object are becoming less rigidly bound to a specific context. This will be discussed further in the section on cognitive patterns. The infant also begins to express a selective sense of humor by laughing at progressively more subtle and complex social and visual stimuli, whereas laughter was initially a response to more elementary stimuli—bouncing, touching, nuzzling. The infant laughs if the caregiver sucks on his bottle or crawls on the floor.[20]

The infant may move on to being not only a decoder but also a budding encoder. This is a gradual process, and the infant practices forming rudimentary auditory-motor associations to imitate more closely the inflection and rhythm of the caregiver's speech. Thus, his intonational patterns become more distinct, expanding to as many as seven different expressions at the end of this stage, such as exclamation, delight, and placidity.[21] He also imitates an increasing number of familiar sounds in his repertoire. The caregiver is very instrumental in helping the infant begin to modify his familiar sounds. For example, he has heard himself and felt himself say mu-uh-muh many times. His mother picks up on this and refers to herself as ma-ma. The infant begins to modify his babbling sound to imitate her syllable combination. Through this interaction certain syllable combinations are connected with a visual stimulus. On sight of the object, person, or gesture, the infant associates the visual input with his internal referent of a sound and pattern of vocal movements. He executes the motor pattern and says ma-ma, da-da, or bye-bye without verbal prompting. There has to be a concrete perceptual cue—actual presence of the person, object, or gesture. It is evident that encoding is quite a feat and is dependent on the background components described in the initial paragraphs of this section. The infant may learn to approximate only one or two words that label a person, object, animal, or gesture that he is in contact with each day. Familiarity and social connotations are therefore very salient forces. The infant very probably will not accommodate to a word that requires a more novel combination of sounds (cracker) during this stage. He imitates with familiar sounds that may not be at all similar to the word. Accommodation to novelty via trial-and-error experimentation evolves with cognitive advances in the next stage.

Even though the infant's vocalization is still highly repetitive in nature by the end of the first year, his modes of communication have expanded considerably. A close, intimate relationship with his caregiver and active involvement in a common round of daily events have served as the basis for forming matches and expressing himself in different ways: sound and object (names a familiar person or object in view), gesture and object (waves bye-bye when he sees a door open), and gesture and sound (waves bye-bye when someone says bye-bye). As the infant's vocalization increases, the caregiver's vocalization decreases. She gives the infant more of an opportunity to assume the role of initiator. The expanded repertoire of oral and language patterns is outlined in Table 2-13.

Description of Normal Cognitive Patterns

The infant propelled his exploration outward in the preceding stage through secondary circular reactions. He repeated an interesting effect that he came upon in the course of interacting with an object. There was a dim awareness of the connection between the behavior and the result. His interest was primarily centered on nourishing his habitual repertoire of schemas in a very action-oriented way. The infant stumbled upon new schemas to add to his repertoire, but they existed as separate response sequences. He banged to reproduce a certain sensory effect or shook to reproduce a certain effect. The practice solidified the schemas, and they were becoming more flexible and less mechanical by the end of the stage.

This beginning flexibility paved the way for the evolvement of more versatile and exploratory adaptations in this stage. The infant begins to unlock the schemas from the habitual repertoire and combine them in different ways, which Piaget[22] termed coordination of secondary schemas. For example, in the course of interacting with his stimulus world, the infant sees an enticing object out of reach. When he attempts to obtain the object, he grasps the attached string. The action has a pulling effect, which draws the object closer. He continues to employ the pulling action until the object is within reach. Unlike in the preceding stage, the infant more clearly begins to recognize the connection between the means action and the end result, and he intentionally coordinates the schemas to repeat the goal-directed behavior. In

TABLE 2-13 Evolvement of oral and language patterns (Third Stage)

Develops increased ability to coordinate and adapt thoracic, laryngeal, and abdominal muscular movements
    Prolongs the expiration and regulates the subglottal pressure to babble in a chain of six or more syllables
    Varies the pitch to effect more distinct intonational patterns
    Produces front and middle vowel sounds with less variation in the pitch quality
Develops increased ability to dissociate and adapt oral movements
    Flexibly protrudes, retracts, elevates, depresses, and lateralizes the tongue
    Chews with a rotary movement of the jaw and lateral movement of the tongue
    Drinks with better accommodation of the lips to the rim and less associated jaw movement
    Babbles with predominantly alveolar consonants
    Flexibly varies the babbling by placing the consonant at the beginning, medially, and at the end
Develops increased ability to integrate local sensations, perceptions, and motor performance
    Forms rudimentary auditory-visual associations to connect words with a gesture, person, or object within a specific context
    Progresses to associating a word with a familiar person and less often an object in an unusual context
    Forms auditory-motor associations to imitate more familiar sounds in his repertoire
    Begins to modify familiar sounds to imitate a similar syllable combination—muh-uh-muh to ma-ma
    Associates visual input with his internal referent of a sound and pattern of vocal movements to form a word or approximation without verbal prompting—ma-ma
Develops increased ability to localize sounds in space
    Orients to more subtle sounds outside his perceptual field
    Localizes sound in space more quickly
    Localizes sound above ear level

the course of practice, he recombines the schemas in different ways to pull in either a horizontal orientation across a surface or a vertical orientation to obtain a suspended object. The object must be in view.

Thus, in this stage the infant becomes progressively less keyed to the raw sensory-motor feedback provided by the object, and there is a gradual waning of repetitious manipulation that is more grossly physical in nature (mouthing, banging, swiping, shaking). The schemas gradually become more object centered than action centered, as the infant focuses on combining and recombining habitual schemas to achieve a goal. To be characterized as intentional behavior the goal must be in mind before the means to achieve the goal is put into action. The behavior is not intentional when the goal is discovered in the midst of the activity as in primary and secondary reactions in the two previous stages. The schema used as a means to achieve the goal must be clearly defined from the schema applied to the goal. The infant's exploration of a bell characterizes this transition. He is less apt to run through a repertoire and mouth, shake, and bang the bell. The infant grasps the bell by the handle, shakes it, and then pauses, as if he is applying a different schema to the end result of his action. He is listening to the sound effect. He also explores the details of the bell.

There are limitations to the extent that the infant can accommodate his actions to achieve a goal. He is able to coordinate only those schemas already in his repertoire. The infant cannot devise unfamiliar means when faced with a new situation. This is evident when a toy is out of reach, and he is given an intermediary tool (spoon). He unsuccessfully applies a familiar means—bangs on the object with the spoon and then reaches for it as if the banging action in and of itself will magically bring the object closer. Or he strikes the object, which pushes it off the surface. He cannot detach from the immediate perceptual cue and accommodate for a gap in space. It is in the next stage that the infant comes upon new means schemas through trial-and-error experimentation.

The caregiver's contingent responsiveness throughout the stages of development has been very instrumental in the evolvement of goal-directed behavior.[23] Some of her actions become very predictable over the course of time. In the last stage the infant began to realize that a signal announced an event outside the realm of his actions. It is in this stage that the infant more clearly begins to recognize that the behaviors of another person are independent of his actions. When the caregiver goes into the kitchen and removes a certain dish from the cupboard, the infant anticipates that a certain event will follow and creeps over to his high chair. He also actively elicits his caregiver as a means in this stage; for example, he places her hand on the toy radio to rewind it. An outside source can cause an effect only if the infant is a part of the action in some way. He has to place the caregiver's hand on the toy.

With a more goal and object-oriented focus, increased dissociation of arm, hand, and finger movements, and higher order discrimination and integration of sensory input, new exploratory schemas evolve. The infant begins to behave as if he wants to know how the object works and what he can do with it. Thus, there is an increased interest in the novel features. The infant uses his fingers to explore surfaces and feel contours especially projections, holes, and intersections. He visually examines the object, tilting it one way and then another at different heights and distances from his body to study the constancy of size and shape. He also views an object as three-dimensional, rotating it to examine the other end.

The increased control of his own body and action schemas allows the infant to experiment with space by moving himself and objects in his environment via what is often termed displacement schemas. The infant releases an object on one side of his body, on the opposite side, and behind himself to study the movement. The infant may not turn to recover the object behind him unless it happens to drop in sight. This spatial orientation is just evolving. He also moves objects away and toward his body with the pulling and pushing schemas and deliberately drops objects and watches their vertical trajectory. The infant tracks a moving object, creeping after his caregiver, a ball, or a pet. When his creeping pattern becomes more mature, he carries an object from point to point. Now that sensations are more discrete and localized, tactile, proprioceptive, and visual impulses give the infant more information about the size, texture, and shape of objects and the movements of his own hand. He begins to compare and relate schemas to visually guide his hand inside a container to grasp an object and bring it out. Initially the infant is an undoer, which frustrates his caregiver. He then progresses to adapting the voluntary release schema to place an object inside a container. The infant is beginning to primitively perceive the spatial relationship of one object to another—contents and container. However, the primary focus of displacement schemas in this stage is to discover the relationship between his action and the object. It is in the next stage that the infant more actively experiments with object-object relationships.

The concept of an object continues to change in the course of all the above experiences. Initially in this stage, the infant begins to recognize that an object is separate from his actions. He searches for the hidden object even though he was not reaching for it or manipulating it when it was covered. The results of one study[24] suggest that his recollection is of a specific object. There is a differential reaction when the infant uncovers the same or a different toy than the one hidden. The infant will also search for a longer time if the object is not easily seen when he removes the covering. However, his memory is still short, and he loses interest if he confronts too many difficulties. The object is still position bound and only continues to exist if it is located in some particular point in space. If the object is hidden under point A and then in full view hidden under a different cover at point B, the infant will search where he found it the first time, although he watched it being hidden somewhere else. Piaget postulated that the internal image of the object is still dependent on a particular action context; the internal image still lacks mobile freedom. There is a recollection of a spoon being placed under a particular diaper in a particular spot, and the image cannot be unlocked from the context. If the alternate hiding game is repeated a number of times during one play period, the infant may begin to search under the cloth where he last saw the object disappear; but the more adaptive response is generally short-lived. During a subsequent play period, he very probably will revert back to searching the spot where the object was just found. As discussed in the preceding section, the infant will look for his father's shoes only in the usual location.

By the end of this stage, the infant begins to develop a sense of invariance. He is coming upon the realization that he remains coherent when moving in space and that other persons and objects remain coherent or constant. His caregiver looks larger when she is up close and smaller when farther away, but the infant's senses also tell him that she is the same caregiver. As animate and inanimate objects more clearly come to have a degree of independent existence external to the infant and his actions, he realizes that his search behavior does not magically make the object reappear in a privileged position. If the infant finds an object under cover A, and it is then placed under cover B, he appropriately searches under cover B where the object was actually hidden. The infant progresses to finding an object alternately hidden under A, or B, or C. However, the ability to follow a series of events independent of his actions is still very shaky. The infant cannot follow sequential displacements: object under A, back out where it is visible, and then under B. This ability evolves in the next stage.

The infant continues to order reality within the context of his own actions. He does not yet know that there are also rules and categories that emanate from outside his body. Meanings are constantly being restructured and reorganized and linked to other meanings being formed from actions brought to bear on objects. The infant continues to categorize objects that respond similarly to a certain action as he did in the previous stage, and new subclasses are formed as new schemas evolve— things to poke, things to push. The object either belongs in the class or it does not belong; his categorization is black or white. As the infant begins to accommodate his actions to the potential of the object, it becomes endowed with certain properties that place it in a rudimentary functional class. He will bring a comb and brush up to his hair and a cup and spoon up to his mouth. There can be only a certain degree of discrepancy between an object and his internal representation to be included in his functional class. In one study, all nine-month-old infants smiled and hugged a big doll that had realistic features, but they did not react similarly to a small doll.[25] The evolvement of goal-directed behavior in this stage also elicits a new category: the undesirable obstacle and the desirable goal.

Many functional meanings are the outgrowth of imitation, which becomes the vehicle whereby the infant more seriously attempts to copy reality. With the increased flexibility of schemas and coordination of sensory input, the infant attempts to imitate actions and sounds that he has not performed before. However, the sound or movement has to be perceived as modifiable to his schemas and what is known. The infant practices to find a combination of familiar schemas that correspond to the observed action. His effort may be a gross approximation; the infant brings the comb up to or close to his hair but does not imitate the actual combing action. There is gradual improvement in his approximation with practice. The infant will probably have difficulty imitating a novel movement that he cannot see himself perform (facial gesture) because of an immature representation of his own body. His attempt may be a similar visible action; he opens and closes his hand instead of blinking.

The functional exploration of objects is a precursor to symbolic play, which evolves in a later stage. There is also another precursor that appears in this stage. The infant begins to ritualistically run through a habitual pattern of concrete behaviors that are a well-established part of his routine and environment. For example, if he spots a pillow, he will lie down with his head on it, place his thumb in his mouth, stay in the position for a few minutes, and then get up. He is not pretending to go to sleep, because he is not capable of representing an action that is not consciously experienced by his senses and body movements.

The more typical play behavior in this stage is expressed by light-hearted experimentation with schemas. The infant may change his focus from a goal and playfully interact with the obstacle. As Piaget emphasized, there is no intent to solve problems or achieve a goal in play behavior. The infant is merely celebrating his increased control of schemas and what he knows. The carefree playfulness can frustrate parents at times, because they view the behavior as regressive or attach a meaning: "He is doing this to annoy me."

During the first year the infant has developed a repertoire of explorative schemas that have become more versatile, object centered, and intentional. He is also beginning to recognize that a world of objects exists independent of his actions and that these objects have functional properties. This ongoing adaptation of cognitive patterns is summarized in Table 2-14.

Description of Normal Affective Patterns

As discussed in the preceding section, the infant is beginning to sever the umbilical cord that ties the self, objects, and actions. Each exchange with his caregiver over the months has involved a sensory-motor-

**TABLE 2-14 Evolvement of cognitive patterns
(Third Stage)**

Intentionally combines habitual schemas to achieve a goal (coordination of
  secondary schemas)
   Recognizes the connection between an action and the end result
   Intentionally coordinates schemas to repeat the goal-directed behavior
   Recombines familiar schemas in different ways to achieve a goal
Begins to adapt action schema to object
   Becomes progressively less keyed to raw sensory-motor feedback of object
   Adapts schemas to explore novel features of object—tilts, rotates, pokes
Discovers relationship between his actions and objects
   Displaces objects in different positions relative to his body
   Tracks moving object or person, creeps after it
   Carries object from point to point when creeping
Begins to view object as an independent entity separate from his actions
   Searches for longer period if misplaces an object
   Searches for object hidden when not actively involved with it
   Begins to unlock internal image from particular spatial and action context
   Searches for object where actually hidden if alternately placed under two
     and then three screens
Begins to recognize independent causal sources outside himself
   Places caregiver's hand on wind-up toy to activate it
   Perceives external causal source as instrumental only if he remains part of
     the action somehow
   Clings to elements of efficacy-phenomenalism
Adapts self to reality in expanded ways
   Attempts to imitate unfamiliar actions and sounds
   Imitates only unfamiliar actions he can see himself perform
   May attempt to imitate unfamiliar actions he cannot see himself perform
     with a similar visible action
Adapts reality to self in lighthearted and presymbolic play
   Playfully interacts with obstacle rather than focusing on goal
   Ritualistically runs through concrete behaviors related to a familiar rou-
     tine—sleeping
Orders reality in expanded groupings within context of his actions
   Groups objects into more and more subschemas, e.g., things to poke, push
   Groups objects into a rudimentary functional class—spoon and cup relate
     to eating
   Rudimentarily categorizes obstacle as undesirable and goal as desirable

affective experience that Mahler, Pine, and Bergman[26] and Stern[27]
postulate is necessary for the formation of an internal representation of
an animate object, whereas an internal representation of inanimate objects can evolve from sensory-motor experiences alone. The internal
referent of the caregiver is altered somewhat during each interactive
experience and becomes progressively more coherent. The inner refer-

ent is still not stable enough to allow the infant to evoke an image of the caregiver when she is absent. However, he immediately recognizes that her characteristics match the inner referent when she returns and progresses to recognizing the match even when he sees his caregiver in an unusual context.[28] She becomes increasingly more coherent in space and time.

At the same time that the infant is rudimentarily becoming aware that his caregiver is a separate person, he is also continuing to become more attached to her, reflected by very observable differential behaviors in this stage. Schaffer's findings[29] support the view that it is the affective component and not physical care per se that is the important element in the relationship. This implies that the infant may or may not be attached to a person in the caregiving role. If he forms an attachment to more than one person, it is still questionable in this stage whether he has a hierarchical preference. Ainsworth and associates[30] reported that some but not all infants show a preference for one parent over the other.

Simultaneous with attachment to a significant person or persons, the infant is also in the process of separating himself out as a distinct entity. Increased mobility allows him to evolve to the early practicing phase of the separation/individuation process, using the framework developed by Mahler, Pine, and Bergman. The infant views his caregiver up close and then ventures farther away from her feet to view her from a distance and from the many different positions that he can now assume. The infant is just beginning to separate into his own being, and he is not sure where his body begins and ends. He, therefore, needs his caregiver as a reference point to provide meaning to distance and as a home base for emotional refueling. When the infant is in a good mood, he is quickly recharged and goes off again. The infant begins to venture farther away for longer periods of time, because he does not have to bother with actually touching base all the time. He can use the distance receptors—vision and hearing—to accommodate for the gap in space and verify his caregiver's presence. Mahler, Pine, and Bergman found that the infant who could use distance receptors to re-establish contact with his caregiver ventured the furthest away.

If the infant has experienced responsive caregiving, he will not become upset when his caregiver leaves the room in a familiar environment. His past experiences have engendered confidence that she is accessible to him even when out of sight. He only becomes distressed if she is gone for too long a period or if his efforts to establish proximity with her are frustrated. The infant still needs to confirm his budding belief that the caregiver has some measure of permanence. He very probably will also not become distressed if left with familiar persons. The infant has worked out a dialogue with them that he can count on. He also senses a bit of the presence of his caregiver because of her comfort with these persons in a surrogate role.

However, most infants in this stage immediately recognize and experience anxiety when confronted with a stranger. There are many variables that determine the degree of anxiety: characteristics and behavior of the stranger, length of exposure to the stranger, previous experience with strangers, the nature of the infant's attachment with his caregiver, and the context.[31] If the infant senses the security of his caregiver's presence, he may gradually warm up to the stranger and come within close enough range to inspect a toy offered to him, especially if the toy is novel. He then creeps back to his familiar caregiver to touch home base. The infant may gradually interact with the stranger in a play activity centered on an object. As in the previous stage, he very probably will avoid intimate eye contact, especially initially. With his caregiver as a safe anchor and a more mature inner regulatory mechanism, the infant can reach out and explore the novelty in a wider stimulus world.

However, if he is left with the stranger, especially in an unfamiliar environment, this is too much novelty, and the infant's anxiety level increases. He may be able to contain his reaction to more subtle tension behaviors: shrugging his shoulders, raising his hand behind his head, fingering his clothing, looking toward the door, or decreasing exploratory behavior. The distress may escalate to the point that he cries. Ainsworth and associates reported that most infants in their study did not cry immediately or become highly distressed. The upset infant most generally will resist any attempts by the stranger to console him. He may ignore his caregiver upon her return or respond with ambivalence, approaching her and then turning away. However, research findings[32,33] suggest that the securely attached infant is more likely to initiate contact with his caregiver and respond positively to being held and comforted. After an emotional recharge, he is willing to leave the caregiver's lap and explore the new environment again.

The infant's budding autonomous function in no way supplants his enjoyment of interactive periods with his caregiver when they are in close proximity to each other. These play periods become more frequent because of the infant's emerging capabilities. As discussed in an earlier section, the infant's repertoire of gestures and vocalization expands, and his expression of emotions and other communicative signals becomes more differentiated and thus easier to read. He has more definite and new ways of eliciting his caregiver's attention, which places her more often in the role of responder. The proportion of time that interaction centers on physical caretaking gradually decreases with age, and spontaneous play periods increase.[34] New twists in the spontaneous play reflect the adaptability of the caregiver's and infant's repertoire of behaviors. The pair continues to play peek-a-boo, but with the infant assuming a more active role. He covers his head and then varies the tempo by removing the cloth immediately one time and prolonging the disappearance another time, as if he is now playing back his caregiver's pattern to control her level of attention and excitement. Other appearance and disappearance games are added to help the infant deal with the idea of separation—throwing and caregiver retrieving or catch me with the caregiver in pursuit of the creeping infant. The caregiver also models new actions which the infant attempts to imitate—"so big!"

Some interaction in this stage is more indirectly initiated by the infant. His increased mobility leads to situations in which the caregiver intervenes to prohibit or redirect the infant's activity. He begins to relate a sharp rise in the voice or even the word "NO!" to certain objects such as enticing buttons on the television set. However, the infant tests the limit over and over again. His caregiver's consistent response helps him determine that some expressions of action schemas are not permissible. Researchers[35] have related compliance with the caregiver's sensitivity to the infant's signals and behaviors over the months. A strong attachment evolves, and the infant has a biologic propensity toward obedience.

This does not imply that the infant is passively obedient. Through experimentation with holding on and letting go, he begins to attach value to his autonomous will. The infant wants to be more actively in charge, which is evident from his gradual resistance to being fed. He begins to communicate a desire to handle the food himself with his fingers, choosing what he eats, what he squishes in his hand, and what he throws on the floor. When the infant is hungry, he will permit his caregiver to feed him appropriate foods with the spoon, but he helps guide the spoon or simultaneously brings some of the cereal to his mouth with his fingers, up to his hair, and elsewhere. He also experiments with the spoon by sliding it across the surface, jabbing it vertically in the dish, and then licking it. The infant also experiments with the cup, which is introduced to initiate the weaning process. He does not understand the relationship between the angle of the cup and the flow of liquid. The infant may miss his mouth initially; and even when he brings the cup in contact with the lips, he tilts it too much and spills liquid down his bib. He has much to learn about spatial orientations, his own body, and the use of intermediary tools.

However, his internal representation of self is becoming more coherent. The infant is beginning to develop a sense that the head, arms, legs, and trunk are linked up and belong together somehow. He is also beginning to define the boundary of his body—what is me and not me. This awareness evolves from interacting with his caregiver and moving his body in space. The infant bumps into objects or gets stuck underneath them and finds that he has to make the adjustment versus the unyielding obstacle. Sensations from contact with objects and bodily movements are becoming more localized and discriminative as discussed in the earlier section on motor patterns. The infant can more sensitively monitor where his legs are in relation to his arms, where his head is in relation to his trunk, and other relationships.[36] The infant uses the poking schema to explore the ear, navel, vulva, or scrotum. He also uses the pulling schema to tug on the penis. Goldberg and Lewis[37] suggest that parents subtly reinforce behaviors appropriate to the gender of the child, reflected by differences in the personality and interests of the male and female infant by the end of this stage. There is a lot of controversy about gender identity and sex stereotyping. Probably most importantly as Kaplan[38] emphasizes, "A baby gets to know what he is by what is mirrored in the faces of those who look at him." If the look is very loving and positive, this will become part of his self image. The infant will have pleasurable inner feelings toward himself and other persons, reflected in social responsiveness. He trusts that other persons are an accessible means to meet his needs. The infant has a sense of power, and he is also developing a very primitive recognition of independent causal sources outside himself.

Just as is the case in other areas of development, there is a dynamic adaptation of patterns in the affective domain during the first year. Interaction behaviors become progressively more elaborate and differentiated, and the infant becomes attached to a significant person or persons. He simultaneously becomes aware of his own coherence and body boundary in a rudimentary way. The adaptations that culminate in this stage are described in Table 2-15.

GROWTH-FOSTERING ENVIRONMENT

The Master Chef expands the familiar menu to include novel dishes with which the diner is free to experiment at his own pace. Transposing the symbolism, the caregiver adapts her repertoire of behaviors and the environmental milieu to strengthen the intimate bond between her and the infant and foster his budding autonomy. She sensitively allows the infant to venture out in the stimulus world at his own pace. When he returns to home base, the caregiver confirms the constancy of her emotional availability with a pat on the head, a hug, or a snuggling period in the lap, depending on the type of battery recharge that the infant needs. The caregiver is also very attuned to the infant's signals from a distance, responding to his bid for a loving look or encouraging vocalization, which provides the impetus to venture further away and for a longer period before coming back for proximal, emotional refueling.

The caregiver provides a safe environment by removing as many potential hazards as possible and by monitoring the infant's explora-

TABLE 2-15 Evolvement of affective patterns (Third Stage)

Begins to differentiate self and the world of animate and inanimate objects
    Begins to recognize that he and his caregiver are coherent in space and time
    Begins to recognize that the caregiver's behaviors are independent of his actions
Uses mobility skills to expand distancing behaviors
    Ventures farther away from the caregiver for longer periods of time
    Views the caregiver at different distances and angles
    Increasingly uses distance receptors to verify the caregiver's presence
Begins to place a value on autonomous functions
    Expresses a desire to feed himself with fingers and experiment with intermediary tools (spoon, cup)
    Squirms and resists passive handling at times
    Tests limits over and over
Simultaneously expresses more definitive attachment behaviors
    Views the caregiver as an emotional anchor, periodically returns to home base for refueling
    Responds very differentially to the caregiver in the presence of a stranger
    Becomes more anxious if left with a stranger, may cry
Assumes a more active role in the relationship with his caregiver
    Places his caregiver in the role of responder more frequently
    Uses emerging capabilities to elicit more frequent spontaneous play periods
    Assumes a more active role in mediating the level of attention and excitement during spontaneous play periods
Organizes experiences into a more coherent inner referent of body/self
    Senses the movement of body parts more discriminatorily
    Senses the linkage of body parts in a primitive way
    Begins to sense details and crevices of the body
    Begins to imitate gender appropriate behaviors

---

tion in an unobtrusive way. He is then free to creep across more and more thresholds. There is more to see, feel, touch, and smell to nourish his sensory system. The mobility also increases the need for air exchange and develops the ventilatory muscles. As the infant experiments with his new skills, he encounters environmental obstacles that exceed his adaptive capacity at times. The caregiver responds to the infant's distress signals by getting down at his level if at all possible to offer encouragement. With emotional support, the infant may be able to come up with the right motor plan to solve the problem on his own or with just a little help, and he more actively senses the boundary of his body.

The caregiver places interesting objects in familiar places and also at new thresholds. The infant in this stage of development is generally attracted to toys that have more intricate configurations to examine visually and to explore with the fingers (three different geometric shapes attached together that move out of alignment). He may also enjoy toys that are responsive to varied action schemas (Surprise Box), toys with unique properties that lend themselves to a specific action schema (xylophone to bang, ball to roll), and toys that suggest imitation (toy telephone, necklace). The above examples do not imply a need to purchase a lot of expensive toys. There are a variety of objects in the home, and an appropriate level of novelty can be maintained by allowing the infant freedom to explore, by rotating the presentation of objects, and by adding new ones on a serial basis. A drawer is filled with odds-and-ends that feed into the infant's new interest in displacement (mostly out). He comes upon objects with details or a novel movement (garlic press) which foster more adaptive examination schemas. A string is attached to one or more objects and draped out of the drawer to encourage a means-end discovery. The infant experiments with spatial displacements by taking pans and other utensils out of the kitchen cupboard and placing them in different positions relative to himself. He again comes upon an object with interesting details to explore, such as a flour sifter. The infant also rudimentarily begins to experiment with the relationship of one object to the other by attempting to put the lid on a pan, place one pan inside the other, and place his hand and then an object in a pan. During the course of the day, an object disappears under a table, couch, or pillow, and the infant learns how to push the obstacle aside or adjust his body to retrieve the object in an intentional goal-directed manner. He is also practicing search behaviors.

The caregiver observes what types of objects match the infant's perceptual-cognitive level and elicit a high degree of interest. She uses these observations as a guide when making objects around the house more available and when purchasing a toy. A good match helps maintain the infant's level of alertness, attention, and excitement in more optimal ranges during exploration. This does not imply that in reality there is always a perfect stimulus match. There are times when the infant becomes overexcited, and there are times when he becomes bored.

The caregiver does not substitute toys and objects for herself. Her contingent response to the infant's refueling needs and her excited response to a discovery encourage his exploratory behavior. The infant also places a high value on the spontaneous play periods in the course of the daily routine. As discussed in the preceding section, the caregiver adapts her repertoire of behaviors to the infant's developmental level. She allows the infant to practice autonomy by assuming the more active role in a familiar game—peek-a-boo; the caregiver responds with mock surprise. Imitation becomes an integral part of the play period, which promotes communicative turn-taking and practice in combining and recombining schemas. The modeled actions are as varied as the infant-caregiver dyad—la-la sound in two contrasting tones, shrugging the shoulders, bouncing and rocking to music, or rolling a ball back and forth. The caregiver encourages imitation of functional actions with an object by giving the comb to the infant after grooming his hair. The infant is also exposed to the functional meaning of objects by being included in the mainstream of family activities within his tolerance level and by experimenting with a cup and spoon at mealtime.

Hiding games continue to be intertwined in spontaneous play periods and elicit a high level of interest. The caregiver adds novelty by changing the obstacle and gradually increasing the complexity. She hides the object under a box, in a sack, and in a L'eggs container. The caregiver progresses to making the object a little less easy to find: loosely wrapped in a tissue and hidden under a cup or box or under two pillows. Progression is also made to alternating the hiding place: the object is covered in one hand. When the infant finds the object, it is covered in the other hand. Likewise, the object is hidden under a napkin (A). When the infant finds it, the object is hidden under a cup (B). A third alternative is gradually added; the object is hidden under a bib (C). The order is then varied. The object is hidden under C (bib). When the infant finds it, the object is hidden under A (napkin). After a successful search, the object is then hidden under B (cup). The object can be hidden under B again if the infant is still interested in the game. The object is always hidden in view of the infant. The focus is not always on goal-directed behavior during a play period. The caregiver shares the pleasure of the infant's lighthearted and even what appears to be silly expression of schemas.

The caregiver's spontaneous verbalization is associated with routine environmental events and actions during the day to emphasize the functional meaning of words. She names very familiar persons and objects when the infant is attentively involved with them and labels needs when he gestures. Her vocalization also reflects different emotional tones: delightful "Look at you!" when the infant accomplishes a new feat, a sharp "No!" when he tests a limit. On the whole, communication has a positive meaning, which facilitates the expansion of the infant's communicative repertoire according to the results of a longitudinal study.[39] The findings from another study[40] suggest that the infant's sociability influences his cognitive performance more so than his innate competence. The sociable middle class infants in the study had sociable mothers.

The environment still reflects physical and temporal organization in this stage. Recurring events facilitate an awareness of the constancy of animate and inanimate objects and means-end relationships.

The noise and activity level is modulated to prevent stress on the infant's adaptive capacity and diversion of his attention from more focused exploration. Familiarity is balanced with novelty, which elicits heightened interest in this stage. In addition to the rotation of objects discussed earlier, interaction with different family members adds variety. Following the pattern discussed in the first stage, the infant's play periods with his father may be more romping and jazzed up in nature. The father may also not adhere as closely to the schedule while the mother is away on an outing, if he does not regularly assume a caregiver role. The infant will have a great time but may become overtired, overhungry, and irritable. He is ready for his mother to put him back together again with a resumption of his usual schedule.

The caregiver also plans regular outings, which may involve a visit in a relative's or neighbor's home, a ride in the stroller to the park, or a grocery shopping session when the infant is in a good mood. The experiences expose the infant to new sights and help him become more and more familiar with persons in the social sphere. However, the caregiver provides a safe base and allows the infant to initiate interaction with other persons at his own pace. If she must leave him with an unfamiliar person for emergency reasons, the caregiver uses the distractive value of novel objects. She also leaves a very familiar object that will maintain a bit of her presence. When the caregiver returns, she sensitively responds to the infant's proximity-seeking behaviors. She calmly remains accessible if he initially ignores her or is ambivalent.

Although the environment is adapted to minimize explorative restrictions and interaction with a negative connotation, the caregiver continues to expose the infant gradually to the real world, which does not completely revolve around his egocentric needs. She establishes limits centered on his safety and the needs of other family members. The limits are kept at a minimum to maintain a skewed balance of positive experiences. The infant is not allowed to stay up late and intrude on his parents' special time together, nor is he allowed to interrupt a sibling's engrossed play. If he becomes upset when his desires are thwarted, the caregiver remains intact and serves as a pacemaker with her calm manner and voice. She thereby helps the infant pull himself together again. The caregiver also exploits the infant's short memory and his interest in novelty to divert his attention to a permissible activity. This diversionary approach decreases distress episodes.

The practice of mobility skills provides a lot of vestibular, tactile, proprioceptive, and visual input, which gives the infant a sense of his own body and where he is in space. The caregiver and family members enhance the input with motor play which becomes a little more romping in nature—riding the horsey on the back or foot, being tossed a short way in the air, or being turned upside down. The infant may also enjoy riding a rocking horse and swinging in a chair suspended from the doorway. He can be carried in a backpack on outings and may even enjoy a ride on the bicycle in the backpack, which involves turns, stops, and starts. All these experiences facilitate gravitational adjustments and the evolvement of equilibrium reactions. Many infants also engage in spontaneous crib rocking, which provides vestibular input. Again in this stage, the activities must be individually adapted; what is enjoyable input to one infant is not necessarily enjoyable to another infant.

FRAMEWORK FOR ASSESSING ABERRANT DEVELOPMENTAL AND INTERACTIVE PATTERNS

As in earlier stages, the assessment is placed within an environmental context. How does an identified disability limit the infant's capacity to attend to and process environmental events? What alternative routes does he use to compensate for impairments? How does the infant's aberrant patterns affect his relationship with the primary caregiver(s) and other family members?

It may be that the infant and other members of the family have developed a very positive relationship over time. The infant has become even less fragile and vulnerable, which lessens the need for very close, vigilant caregiving. With decreased physiologic demands and inner stress, he is continuing to find new sources of pleasure through social interaction and the exploration of objects. The caregiver can more easily read the infant's cues, partly as the result of trial-and-error experimentation. She has learned ways to hold and care for the infant that enhance the enjoyment of close, proximal contact. The caregiver has also learned how to mediate the infant's response threshold. Her sensitive adaptability has increased the infant's adaptability, and the pair have developed a unique interactive style. The infant is becoming an integral part of the family with all members feeling more comfortable in their relationship with him.

Even if the infant's relationship with his caregiver and other family members started off on a rather negative note, this does not foreordain a continued troubled relationship in subsequent stages. The results of a longitudinal study by Barnard and associates[41] suggest that the parenting style is dynamically affected by the inner emotional state of the caregiver, outer life circumstances, and changes in the behavioral pattern of the infant. The style of the caregiver may also change from one context to another during the day. The intervener's impressions likewise must not remain static. To emphasize an earlier statement: intervention must be based on an ongoing assessment of all aspects of the infant's environment from both a micro- and macro-system perspective.

Effect of an Aberrant Response Threshold and a Disturbed Relationship

There is again the possibility that the relationship is not evolving in a manner that provides pleasure, satisfaction, and growth-fostering experiences for both the infant and his caregiver. If the infant has a low sensory threshold, the premature distancing that was described in the preceding stage may continue. The caregiver has not been able to read and respond effectively to the infant's unpredictable cues. She feels inept and more or less gives up, becoming less attuned and less responsive to the infant's signals. She is more frequently angered and irritated by the infant's behavior, and these feelings may again escalate and be expressed by abuse. Or the caregiver may attempt to control the negative feelings with a rather rigid, compulsive demeanor and approach to caregiving.

The infant may experience chronic, inner anxiety from being pushed out of a protective nest prematurely, which fuels his poor adaptability to stress. He may react by enhanced proximity-seeking behaviors. The infant anxiously monitors his caregiver's whereabouts or clings to her feet or her favorite chair, and he frequently whines and cries. Or the infant may sense a need to seek close contact and reassurance, and yet he avoids this contact to divert his anger or protect himself from experiencing a rebuff. He possibly has not experienced pleasant sensations when being held because of an impaired tactual system. This sensory impairment may have been a very significant factor in setting off what is now an aversion to physical contact by both the infant and caregiver. The infant may turn more and more to the world of inanimate objects, but his exploration lacks orientation. He does not have a stable base to leave or return to, because he does not have confidence in his caregiver's accessibility or her responsiveness to his emotional needs. Or his caregiver may be inconsistent, intrusively interrupting his activity when she feels a need and avoiding contact when the infant signals a need. He is confronted with his own vulnerability and has little energy to direct to more focused explorations. The infant's affect may be stilted with infrequent smiling, vocalization, and laughter. Or he may venture out in a scattered, disoriented manner because of the lack of internal and external stability, moving from one object to another.

It is difficult to sort out the relative impact of a disturbed relationship and aberrant processing capabilities associated with organic damage. Because of a lack of stabilizing forces, whether weighted more so or equally to outer or inner influences, the reactive infant may explore objects in a more global, physical way. He alternates between recklessly banging and throwing objects and sucking his thumb and engaging in other body-directed schemas. The infant may be easily distracted by extraneous environmental stimuli because of poor habituation, which shortens his attention span and focused exploration. An erratic shift of internal states may vary his awareness and response to stimuli to the point of causing perceptual inconsistency. The impatient infant's mobility skills may be disparately ahead of his perceptual/cognitive level, and he is confronted with too much novelty that he cannot process and make sense of. He avoids exploring novel objects or warily inhibits exploration for a prolonged period. Thus, the infant may timidly venture out no matter how supportive his caregiver is, because sensory experiences are very unstable, unpleasant, or even painful owing to dysfunctions that alter his perception and organization of input.

It can be difficult for the caregiver to view any aspect of the infant's exploration as positive in nature. For the most part, the infant's disorganized and reckless manner increases his vulnerability for negative interaction and physical contact. This is especially true if he has a decreased propensity for compliance because of limited internalized control. The infant's behavior may lead to increased restrictive intrusion, frequent confinement in a crib or playpen, and possibly physical punishment.

The infant may respond to the novelty of a stranger and a new environment with immediate and intense distress, especially if the stranger encroaches on his physical space too soon, or if he is left with the stranger. Anxiety increases the need for proximity to a familiar person, regardless of the strength of the relationship with that person. The infant may also resist being left with anyone except a certain caregiver. He is very difficult to soothe when his caregiver returns, and she may exacerbate his reaction by insensitively attempting to hurry the consolation and put him down again. Or the infant may ignore his caregiver or react with ambivalence and seek and then resist proximity. If the infant has a very weak inner representation of his caregiver because of a paucity of affective experiences, he may not be wary of strangers.

In contrast, if the infant has a high sensory threshold, the caregiver may have more or less given up trying to perk up his arousal level, especially if he is very lethargic. The cycle of decreased responsiveness described in the preceding stage continues. Physical care is primarily task oriented in nature with limited affective expressivity.

If the infant develops mobility skills, he may also feel adrift with lack of confidence in the accessibility of his caregiver as a beacon to provide meaning and orientation to his exploration. The infant may respond in a more resigned manner than the reactive infant—sitting and stroking a blanket, rocking, or humming in an attempt to recreate a feeling of human contact. He may sit in front of a mirror and rock his body and gaze at the reflected face. The infant may turn more and more to his own body as a source of stimulation, expressed by stereotyped repetition of autoerotic activities. He may reach an extreme, giving up and not tuning in to his environment and losing all desire to explore. The stimulus intensity is not great enough to elicit a level of excitation.

Even if the caregiver is supportive of explorative ventures, the infant with a relatively nonpermeable stimulus barrier may remain focused on manipulative schemas that elicit a high level of raw sensory feedback from the object—shaking, banging, mouthing. He continues to repeat the same action with slow habituation. The infant does not respond as differentially to novelty as the normal infant. His interest centers on nourishing habitual schemas versus the typical elaboration of explorative behavior.

The infant's slow processing of incongruities results in an arousal lag that diminishes the intensity, variation, and selectivity of affective responses.[42] His more undifferentiated communicative signals are still difficult to read. He may not laugh at more subtle visual cues in this stage—mother sucking on a bottle. The selectivity of the laughter response was very predictable of the level of cognitive functioning in a study of infants with Down syndrome.[43]

The infant may not react with anxiety to a stranger because of the processing impairment, a low reactivity to stress, or a weak attachment to his caregiver. Or the infant may express attachment behaviors in a more attenuated way.[44,45] It may be that attachment expressed by stranger anxiety will be delayed compared with the normal infant's timetable.[46]

If there has been a paucity of affective experiences in the infant's stimulus world because of a disturbed relationship with his caregiver, regardless of the causal influences, it is evident from the above discussion that the infant's budding autonomous function is in jeopardy. The interaction may be characterized by a predominance of reciprocally ignoring states. The infant loses confidence in his ability to restructure his environment in ways that meet his needs, and he even loses the desire to communicate. If there are no meaningful humans to separate from, the infant's own separation/individuation process will be impeded.

At the other extreme is the infant who is smothered with affective attention. He is not allowed to explore and practice his budding autonomy. The infant can have a delusion of invulnerability. His caregiver is right there to maintain a high level of closeness and meet his every need. The infant is confined to the lap, crib, playpen, or other protective space. Or he may attempt to venture out but senses his caregiver's anxiety, which influences the infant's behavior. He becomes timid and hesitant. Or the caregiver swoops the infant up and directs his attention back to herself. He also lacks the support to move along the separation/individuation path.

Effect of Sensory Impairments

VISUAL IMPAIRMENT. It is evident from the above discussion that sensory impairments can limit or distort the infant's stimulus world. If he is blind or has minimal vision, the infant continues to be deprived of the most efficient receptor for acquiring information about animate and inanimate objects and mapping space. Without a visual lure, he has no incentive to move from one position to another. The infant cannot actively distance himself from his caregiver and visually monitor her movements with all the related perceptual variability. He cannot form visual-auditory associations to attach a sound or label to certain very familiar persons or objects. The infant's expressive and possibly receptive language may be delayed, and his affect is still muted with the lack of social, visual reinforcement.

If the creeping pattern does not evolve in this stage or is delayed in evolving, the infant does not sense the movement of distal parts and touch-pressure and proprioceptive input from unilateral weight bearing to the same degree as the sighted infant. This lack of input may impede the maturation of the sensory system, reflected by less discriminative processing of stimuli. The muscles in the shoulder girdle and arm are also hypotonic from lack of exercise. More refined manipulative schemas do not evolve because of the lack of background stability and discriminative visual and possibly tactile feedback to refine arm, hand, and finger movements. There is the possibility that hand movements will remain very primitive: scratching, clawing, pinching, protective throwing. With the absence of important background components, mouthing may remain the dominant form of exploration. The infant may resort to body rocking, twirling, jiggling, eye poking, and other behaviors because of boredom or as an outlet for tension. The limited exploratory repertoire and self-initiated, functional movement interfere with the construction of a world of animate and inanimate objects that are beginning to exist independent of the infant's actions and move from place to place.

If there is no organic damage and the infant's environment has been enriched, he will probably coordinate tactile and auditory sensory input in this stage just as the normal infant does. The infant then begins to reach toward a sound cue alone such as the caregiver's voice or the sound from an object. He seeks proximity to the sound by self-initiated movement (creeping) and position changes either in this or the next stage. The world out there is no longer a void.

If there is a dysfunction of the visual system, instead of complete loss of function, the impairment may be expressed by the faulty coordination of eye movements and the lack of flexible accommodation described in the preceding stage. Or the infant may have difficulty making sense of visual input or integrating visual sensations with other sensations. Although it can be difficult to pinpoint the exact nature of an impairment, there is an impact on explorative behavior. The infant may have difficulty guiding and modifying his arm and hand movements to accommodate to an object more deftly. He also has difficulty altering his plan to adapt to a change when the object moves. The infant may not be able to coordinate visual and somatosensory feedback to move the arm and hand and examine objects from different distances and angles. Nor can he insert the hand in a space (container) to grasp an object, progressing to releasing the object in a circumscribed space. The infant may have difficulty discriminating the object from the background or perceiving details of figures, which affects the evolvement of visual examination schemas. He may not be able to maintain a stable image on the retina to monitor the whereabouts of his caregiver and follow the trajectory of a moving object, creep after it, and push it again. The infant may avoid eye contact because the visual stimulus is too potent, or he cannot look and listen at the same time, which affects interaction with his caregiver and the imitation of sounds and actions. It is evident that dysfunctions can affect development in many of the same ways that a complete or severe visual loss does.

AUDITORY IMPAIRMENT. If the infant has a hearing loss, he cannot associate visual and auditory input to link a sound with animate and inanimate objects and gestures. The infant's communicative repertoire remains limited even if he has an intermittent loss. He lacks a sufficient amount of consistent auditory feedback to experiment with differentiating his babbling sounds.[47] The infant cannot compare the hearing of his own utterance with the tactile and proprioceptive feedback from his tongue, lips, and jaw. Nor can the infant compare his sound with the sound that comes from the caregiver. He therefore cannot experiment with recombining sounds to form a new babbling sound or approximate a word. The infant's muted affect and limited communicative repertoire prevents him from assuming a more active role in initiating and maintaining interaction with his caregiver in a positive way.

If the infant cannot hear intonations and stress patterns, he misses the fueling expression of delight over his discovery and an encouraging word to prolong his explorative venture. The infant also misses the restrictive no from a distance. He cannot hear temporal regularities that serve as the basis for forming expectations and a rudimentary sense of this occurring before that. This lack of temporal rhythm can affect the infant's self regulation. The noncompliant behavior so often associated with deaf children may be emerging in this stage, which can elicit a higher level of restrictive intrusion from the caregiver. There is often an associated vestibular dysfunction that can be expressed by restless movement. This superimposed behavior also has the potential of eliciting negative interaction. The attachment and separation/individuation process may be jeopardized.

As with the visual system, there may be a dysfunction rather than a complete loss of the sense. If the infant still has difficulty habituating to a repetitive sound or background noise, this distracts from focused attention on speech sounds and the unique sound of an object. If the auditory link does not provide accurate information, the infant may have difficulty capturing the temporal sequence and blending of sounds. Or certain sounds may be painful, evidenced by the infant placing his hands over his ears. A dysfunction may interfere with localizing the source of a sound in space.

VESTIBULAR IMPAIRMENT. The relationship of visual, auditory, and vestibular dysfunctions has been discussed in the preceding stages and in the above paragraphs. The importance of the vestibular system is especially evident in this stage because of the infant's expanded mobility and exploration. There are three primary senses that synergistically provide input to monitor the infant's position and movement in space: vestibular, visual, and proprioceptive. The senses tell the infant if he, the surface, or objects are moving; how well and where he is moving; and the position of his joints in relationship to one another. If there is a dysfunction in the feedback from these senses, this interferes with the evolvement of equilibrium and righting reactions. The infant tensely fixates in a position and avoids weight shifts and movement from one position to another. The proximal area may become inflexible or woodenlike, and the infant moves as a block in straight-line patterns. He may quickly change his position when he senses instability. For example, the infant moves to quadruped when there is a gravitational shift in the sitting position versus adjusting away from the shift to maintain the sitting position. He has to keep moving to maintain his balance reflected by a restless demeanor. Or the infant may not be able to respond to the shift quickly enough, and he topples over.

On the other hand, vestibular input may become a primary source of nourishment. The infant spends a lot of time rocking and waving or shaking his head and hands. This emphasis on vestibular input is often manifested by infants who respond very minimally to visual stimuli.

TACTILE AND PROPRIOCEPTIVE IMPAIRMENTS. If newer pathways do not mature or mature more slowly, impulses are not transmitted at a faster speed with less spread and influence on other areas. The central nervous system does not receive more localized proprioceptive input, which increases the awareness of subtle joint movements. The cutaneous receptors in the hands and feet may be incompletely modified from the initial role of protection. The refinement of explorative schemas and movement patterns is dependent on more focal input as the basis for devising and modifying a motor plan through a continuous feedback loop. The infant cannot guide the hand and finger movements to explore the details and novel features of an object and his caregiver's face. The infant continues to explore objects with more gross action schemas, or he may avoid manipulating objects.

Other motor patterns remain clumsy and uncoordinated. If a protective response persists, the infant may bear weight only on his fingertips and knees when he creeps. He flexes his knees so that the lower legs and feet are not in contact with the floor, and the infant may resist creeping on rougher surfaces. He also moves up on his toes in a supported standing position. Likewise, oral receptors may not become increasingly discriminative, which negates the evolvement of more dissociated and refined movements of the jaw, lip, and tongue. The infant may avoid placing objects in his mouth, and he resists textured foods.

The infant may continue to respond to physical contact in a protective manner when being held, dressed, bathed, and during other care routines. He is especially reactive to light intermittent touch such as nuzzling. The infant may be more comfortable when body surfaces are covered with long pants and long sleeved shirts, but he expresses discomfort when wearing clothes made from a fabric with a particular texture. On the other hand, if the infant has a very high receptor threshold, he craves more intense tactual input. He may intentionally bang his head or pinch, bite, and hit himself.

Summary

Sensory impairments affect all aspects of development and to a greater degree if there is more than one dysfunctional system. If the infant is not able to perceive and integrate input accurately and systematically, and if he cannot insert an object in a number of different schemas, the inner structural network may be more loosely interwoven. A less elaborate and complex internal schematic organization affects the emergence of a more coherent representation of the caregiver, inanimate objects, and the infant's own body. The infant may not begin to realize that there are things out there independent of his actions. If the infant has difficulty coordinating sensory input, this hampers combining and recombining schemas to intentionally achieve a goal, copy reality in a more adaptive way, and begin to accommodate his actions to explore the novel features and unique properties of objects. The infant may overreact to novelty, or he may be slow to recognize and thus be aroused by novelty. In a general sense, the infant may experience a sense of both inner and outer instability that diverts energy from expanded exploration of the stimulus world.

Effect of Motor Impairments

Although the content has been organized to discuss sensory and motor impairments separately, it is more and more evident that the two systems are functionally intertwined. An intact sensory system is essential for the development of motor patterns and skills, and a visual stimulus is the primary catalyst of movement evidenced by the delay in the evolvement of mobility patterns if the infant is blind. As in the preceding stages, an older child may still be in this stage in terms of motor development. Thus, infant refers to the developmental level rather than the chronological age in the description of motor impairments.

COMPENSATORY PATTERNS IN THE SITTING POSITION. The infant with a motor impairment may not move through all the phases and assume a more functional sitting position. If his pelvis does not become flexible and he does not develop balanced strength in the flexor, extensor, and lateral muscles, the infant lacks the background components to sit in a well-aligned position with the shoulders over the neutral pelvis and the legs extended in line with the hips. The lack of midline stability also interferes with the evolvement of more mature equilibrium reactions, and the infant will continue to feel unstable in the position. He cannot freely rotate the head, shoulders, and trunk one way with counter-rotation of the hips to reach out in different spatial orientations, including across midline.

If the infant with hypertonia has had a tendency to push back in extension over the months, he may assume a poorly aligned position, as was the case in the preceding stage. When the infant extends or incompletely extends the legs, he has to sit back on his spine because of lack of flexibility in the pelvis and hips and tight hamstrings secondary to this. The legs are adducted and internally rotated, which provides a narrow base of support. The infant compensates by flexing his head and trunk forward over the sitting base to prevent falling backward. His neck is still hyperextended but to a lesser degree than in the preceding stage, and he maintains his head in a less forward position, albeit stiffly. If the infant tries to free one or both hands to manipulate an object, this causes increased tone in the trunk and one or both upper extremities (Fig. 2-30A).

The W-sit position (Fig. 2-30B) may continue to provide the only stable base for infants with hypertonia and for other disabled infants

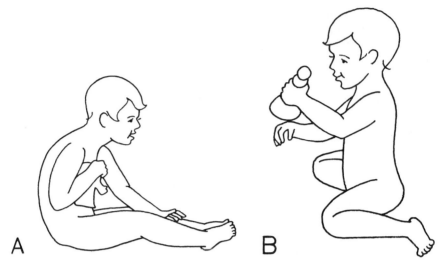

FIGURE 2-30. The infant or child with hypertonia may assume a (*A*) compensatory long-legged sitting position or (*B*) use the STNR to assume a W-shaped position.

who lack the background components that have been described. As discussed in Stage II, Baumann[48] demonstrated that the hip joints are in better approximation with the acetabulum. However, the knees are markedly flexed and the ankles are extended, which are not functional positions for later walking. Thus, a functional adaptation in one position is not always a functional prerequisite for a higher position. This is just one example of the habilitative dilemma.

If the infant with fluctuating tone (athetosis) sits with legs extended, he may fixate at the pelvis with an anterior tilt to compensate for lack of proximal stability. The infant may also fixate with the medial border of one or both feet, which internally rotates the abducted legs. His head is pulled back, and the arms assume an aberrant pivot prone position with one flexed arm externally rotated and the other flexed arm internally rotated, which negates the functional use of the hands (Fig. 2-31A). Or the infant may compensate in another way if hypotonicity predominates as the tone fluctuates. The infant sits with the back rounded, the pelvis posteriorly tilted, and the head pulled into the shoulders. One of the extended abducted legs may be externally rotated, and the other leg is somewhat internally rotated. The arms are in a propped position (Fig. 2-31B).

When the infant with hypotonia sits more erect, he may also fix in midline with an anterior pelvic tilt to compensate for the lack of midline stability. The arms assume a modified pivot prone position to help maintain the more erect posture, and the extended or hyperextended

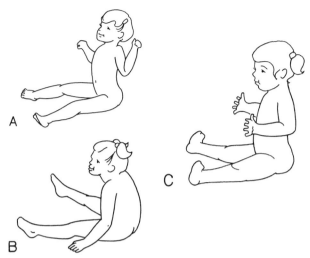

FIGURE 2-31. The infant or child with (*A* and *B*) two forms of fluctuating tone and (*C*) hypotonia compensates for lack of midline stability in the long-legged sitting position in different ways.

legs are widely abducted and externally rotated (Fig. 2-31C). There is intermittent regression to a slumped posture with rounded shoulders and back.

If equilibrium reactions remain very immature, the infant may always have to catch himself with protective extension of the upper extremities when he attempts to shift weight; and the reaction may be slow because of a response latency or because of unreliable sensory feedback. Or a weight shift may elicit a persistent Moro response, and the infant cannot extend his arms to catch himself. The infant has a strong drive to develop, evidenced by the use of strengths. He may evolve to the point at which he can adjust to a gravitational shift with less involved parts, which somewhat frees him from a fixated position. If the infant has hypertonia and more involvement in the lower extremities, he adjusts himself back to midline by an exaggerated lateral movement of the head and trunk and abduction of the arm. The infant with athetosis relies on his less involved lower extremities. He rights himself by abducting the leg on the side opposite the weight shift.

If the infant cannot sit with the proximal body parts in good alignment and rotate in different spatial orientations, he will not be able to flexibly move in and out of the position. The infant may continue to move straight up in a W-sit position as described in Stage II. Or he may widely abduct the legs in a full split position and push up to sitting if he has hypotonia and a hyperflexible range of motion. However, if the infant develops reliable lateral propping reactions in the sitting position, he may progress to turning from prone somewhat to the side and pushing himself up to the sitting position with his arms, but he primarily uses lateral trunk flexion versus trunk rotation to help raise himself up.

COMPENSATORY PATTERNS IN THE QUADRUPED POSITION. Abnormal tone also interferes with the evolvement of more functional mobility patterns. The infant may continue to move in space on his stomach with an immature or aberrant combat crawl pattern as described in Stage II. Or he may scoot around on his back or buttocks. If the infant with hypertonia attempts to assume the quadruped position, he may lack sufficient proximal stability. The head and spine are flexed with one or both arms also flexed, and the hips may collapse and rest on the feet (Fig. 2-32A). He cannot even maintain the position, which negates progressing through the phases leading to a skilled movement—creeping. Or it may be that the STNR still influences motor patterns. When the infant assumes the quadruped position and raises his head, this elicits too much extension of the arms with internal rotation and fisting of one or both hands. In contrast, the legs exaggeratedly flex with a tendency toward adduction and internal rotation, and there is a lordotic curve. The coupling influence of the STNR and excess tone places the infant in a static versus a dynamic holding pattern (Fig. 2-32B). If he lowers his head, the arms and spine flex, and the legs adduct, internally rotate, and extend, sliding the infant forward on his nose. The STNR also interferes with superimposing proximal mobility on distal stability. When the infant rocks backward, which involves extension of the arms, this flexes the hips. The flexion of the hips and knees will not release to allow him to rock forward again. The infant may learn to use the STNR to move about in a homologous pattern—bunny hop. There is a simultaneous forward movement of the extended arms followed by a simultaneous forward movement of the flexed legs (Fig. 2-32C). Or the infant with hypertonia may use another aberrant movement pattern—homolateral creeping. He shifts weight to one shoulder and arm and moves the opposite arm and leg forward with lateral trunk flexion. The infant then shifts weight to the other shoulder and arm and simultaneously moves the extremities on the opposite side forward. The hips stiffly sway back and forth with the lateral trunk flexion, and the leg more or less gets pulled up in tandem because of poorly dissociated pelvic and leg movements (Fig. 2-32D). The infant may turn his head from side to side to use the ATNR response functionally. The arm extends in a support position when he shifts weight to the face side.

The infant with fluctuating tone may not be able to assume the quadruped position because of lack of proximal stabilization or an inability to flex one part and extend another part in a differentiated way.

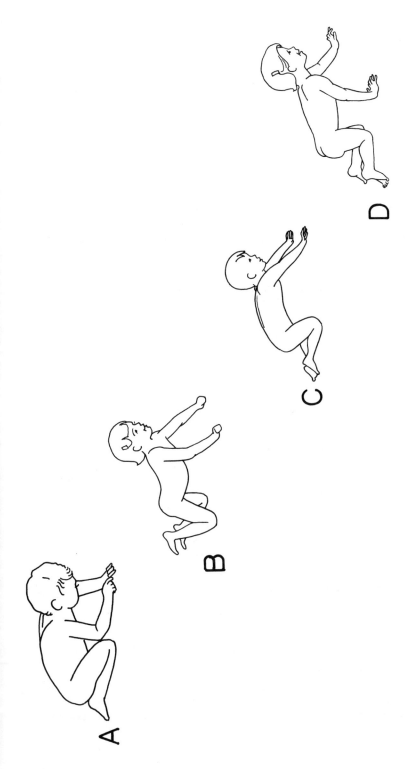

FIGURE 2-32. The stress of attempting to assume the quadruped position and creep elicits compensations in various forms if the infant or child has hypertonia.

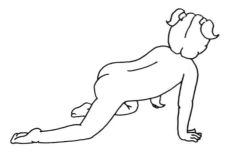

FIGURE 2-33. The child with fluctuating tone creeps with an aberrant pattern influenced by primitive reflexes.

He may also adaptively use the STNR to move up to a W-sit position and move forward with a bunny hop pattern illustrated in Figure 2-32C. If the infant is able to assume the quadruped position and attempts to creep, he may move the extremities in a homolateral pattern described above. Or the movement in the lower extremities may be aberrant in another way if the primitive crossed extension reflex has not been integrated. When the infant brings the one leg forward into more flexion, the other leg almost extends (Fig. 2-33). The arms may intermittently collapse into a more flexed position with increased rounding of the shoulders because of weak proximal stability. Arm flexion may also result from a STNR influence when the infant lowers his head to orient to the surface.

The infant with hypotonia may adapt the sitting position to scoot forward on his buttocks. If he assumes the quadruped position, the lack of proximal stability may again be evident by a hanging effect. The elbows are abducted, the hands may be turned inward, and the knees are abducted and externally rotated. There is a lordotic curve in the back because of weak abdominal muscles. The infant has a tendency to fix the trunk and arms, which provides enough stability to maintain the position. The fixation interferes with practice in superimposing proximal mobility on distal stability. Initial attempts to rock may be restricted. Or the movements may be poorly graded with overshooting; the hips collapse on the feet as the infant rocks backward, and the arms collapse as he rocks forward. He may also fixate his trunk to provide enough stability to move the arms and legs when he begins to creep. There is a wide weight shift to one abducted arm. The infant then moves the lower extremity on the opposite side with lateral trunk flexion (Fig. 2-34A). Or the infant may initially move the arms and legs in a homolateral pattern. There is frequent interruption of the sequence because of the lack of background dynamic stability to regulate the smoothness and timing of movements. He has to stop to regain his bearings, so to speak, and there is also the fatigue factor. The infant with Down syndrome may have a tendency to move from sitting to quadruped with one leg extended and abducted, which can contribute

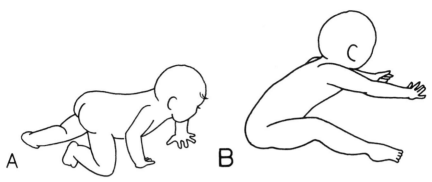

FIGURE 2-34. The infant or child with hypotonia (A) exaggeratedly abducts the extremities when he creeps and (B) moves from sitting to quadruped with an aberrant, wasteful movement.

to joint alignment problems (Fig. 2-34B). The shift also involves more wasted movement and energy expenditure compared with the normal infant's position change.

COMPENSATORY PATTERNS IN THE KNEELING POSITION. If the infant with hypertonic muscles pulls up to knee standing, he may have difficulty dissociating patterns to extend the hips fully when the knees are flexed. Thus, he stands with partially flexed hips, and the shoulders and back are rounded. The head flexes forward, the arms pull into flexion, and the legs may adduct and internally rotate narrowing the base of support (Fig. 2-35A). Even if the infant has used an extensor pattern in lower positions, he may compensate by assuming the more flexed position described above. Or the infant may attempt to maintain the knee-standing position with static extension. If the head and shoulders retract, he falls backward (Fig. 2-35B). If the infant with fluctuating tone is able to pull up on his knees, he may compensate with exaggerated extension of the hips and an exaggerated anterior pelvic tilt (lordotic curve). He may also compensate for lack of proximal stability by fixating with the medial border of one or both feet. The infant internally rotates and extends the arms forward to prevent falling backward (Fig. 2-35C). If hypotonia predominates as the tone fluctuates, the infant may lean into the support with rounded shoulders and some flexion in the hips. The arms are flexed and rest on the support or the hands grasp the surface (Fig. 2-35D). If the infant has hypotonia that is not associated with fluctuating tone (Down syndrome), he compensates for lack of stability by using midline fixation and extension to maintain the position. The pelvis is anteriorly tilted, and the knees are widely abducted and externally rotated. There is compensatory shrugging of the shoulders with neck shortening (Fig. 2-35E).

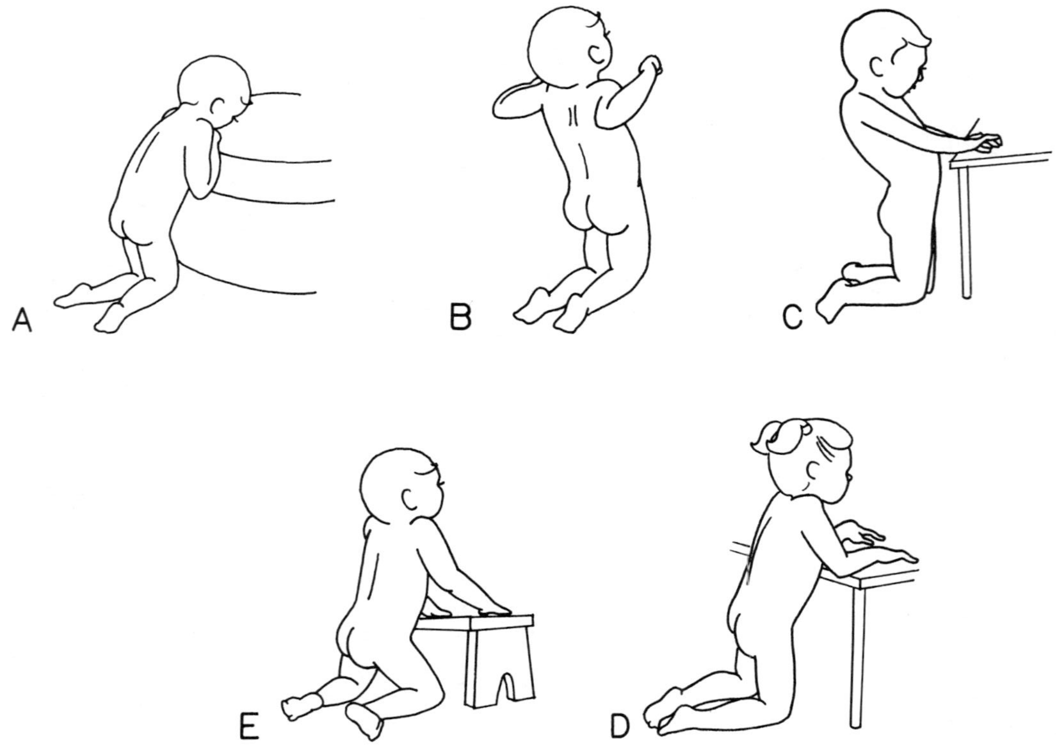

FIGURE 2-35. The knee-standing position elicits varied compensatory patterns if the infant or child has (*A* and *B*) hypertonia, (*C* and *D*) different forms of fluctuating tone, or (*E*) hypotonia.

DEVELOPMENTALLY DISABLED INFANTS AND TODDLERS

The infant with abnormal tone may not develop sufficient midline stability to shift weight and walk laterally on his knees, or the movement may be relatively stiff. The infant with hypertonia, hypotonia, or fluctuating tone may have difficulty reaching down and retrieving an object. If the infant with hypertonia reaches down to pick up an object, flexion may begin to dominate, and he cannot raise up again. Or his effort to move back up may bring the extensors into play again. This tendency to move between extreme total patterns with no grading in between interferes with the development of functional adaptations in the knee-standing and higher bipedal positions. The infant cannot blend flexibility and stability. If the infant has hypotonic muscles, he moves in a stiff, straight-line pattern without rotation. When the infant reaches down, he may sit between his feet because of lack of stability to grade movements, and he has to pull himself back up to the knee-standing position again. The infant with fluctuating tone also has difficulty grading movements. He may collapse into flexion when he reaches down or the stress sets off disorganized movement. With these limitations and compensations, the infant with abnormal tone may not be able to superimpose flexibility on stability and rotate the trunk to retrieve objects in different locations.

COMPENSATORY PATTERNS IN THE STANDING POSITION. The infant with a high degree of abnormal tone may never be able to pull up to a bipedal position. If the infant with hypertonia is supported by the caregiver in the standing position, the lack of functional midline stability high above the surface may elicit a total extensor pattern: retraction of the head, shoulders, and arms; anterior pelvic tilt (lordotic curve); and a strong, positive support response with exaggeratedly extended legs and heels off the surface (Fig. 2-36A). Or the infant with hypertonia may react to the stress of being held in a standing position with flexor compensations. The shoulders and trunk are rounded; the pelvis is posteriorly tilted; the hips are incompletely extended; and the head is flexed forward. The arms are flexed, internally rotated, and pulled in or downward, and the legs are internally rotated with the knees together and the weight on the toes, which provides a narrow base of support (Fig. 2-36B).

If the infant has less severe hypertonia throughout the body and is cognitively in this stage, he will be very motivated to expand perceptual experiences by pulling to a standing position. The infant very probably cannot dissociate the legs from the pelvis or one leg from another to assume the half-kneel position. He pulls himself up with internally rotated arms, and the legs remain extended, adducted, and internally rotated. They are more or less pulled up in tandem. The infant may assume a more flexed position very similar to Figure 2-36B,

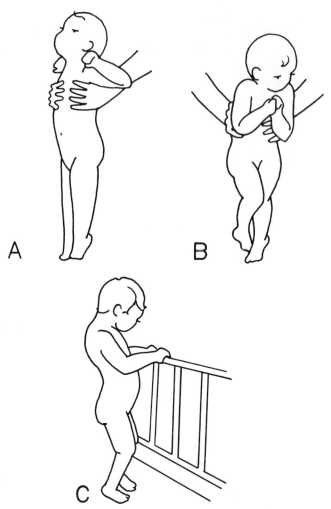

FIGURE 2-36. A supported standing position may elicit (*A*) an extensor pattern or (*B*) flexor pattern if the infant or child has hypertonia. (*C*) The child with less involvement in the upper extremities maintains a compensatory standing position with heavy reliance on a support.

leaning into the piece of furniture just as he did in the kneeling position. He may be able to bring the heel down and place the whole surface of one foot in contact with the floor, whereas the heel of the other foot remains off the surface. The infant with hypertonia who has less involvement in the upper extremities than the lower extremities will probably also be able to pull up to the standing position but in the same compensatory manner described above. The infant cannot fully extend his hips in the upright position, which sets off a chain of compensations. The pelvis is anteriorly tilted to help him remain upright, which increases the lordotic curve, and the upper back and shoulders are rounded forward toward the base of support to prevent him from tilting backward too far. The neck is hyperextended with a forward jutting of the chin. The infant relies heavily on his flexed, internally rotated arms to hold onto the support. The legs are internally rotated with the knees close together and weight on the toes (Fig. 2-36C).

The infant with hypertonia, expressed by either of the above patterns, may not be able to free himself from the static, bilateral standing position to superimpose proximal mobility on distal stability or shift weight from one leg to the other. If the infant attempts to cruise, this exaggerates the stiffness, and one foot may cross over the other. Or he moves sideways with a small, stiff lateral step, and weight remains over the medial border of the foot. The infant may rely even more heavily on the support, moving forward into more flexion.

If the infant with fluctuating tone cannot sustain contact with a grasped object because of a residual, phasic avoidance pattern, and if the lower extremities are more involved, he very probably will not be able to hold on to a support to pull himself to standing and maintain the position. When the caregiver supports him, the pressure from contact with the surface elicits total extension, adduction, and possibly internal rotation of the legs, which may scissor. The weight is high on the toes. The head and shoulders also retract, which would thrust him backward if the caregiver were not holding him (Fig. 2-37A). However, if the lower extremities have remained mobile and abducted and the avoidance response has diminished, the infant will be very motivated to assume a new position. He pulls himself up in an undifferentiated way similar to the pattern described for the infant with hypertonia. He may fixate the medial border of one foot to help push himself up. The infant compensates for the lack of proximal stability by maintaining the upright position with exaggerated extension of the hips and legs and an exaggerated lordotic curve. He further compensates by adducting the knees and by fixing with the medial border of one or both feet, which places them in a pronated position. The infant is generally able to keep his feet dorsiflexed and in contact with the surface, but the toes may claw in an attempt to increase distal stability. The infant adaptively balances the extensor pattern that thrusts him backward by extending the arms forward, with one or both in an internally rotated position (Fig. 2-37B). He has difficulty freeing himself from the fixated position because of the lack of stability and difficulty grading movements between two extreme ranges. If the infant flexes his knees, the whole body may go into flexion and he will collapse. The infant adaptively learns to cruise with a stiff shuffling gait to maintain the extension.

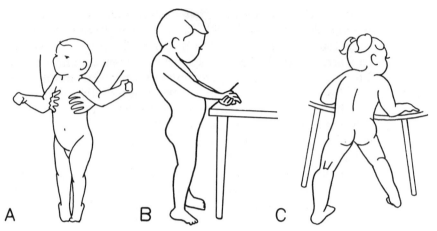

FIGURE 2-37. (A) The supported standing position may elicit an exaggerated extensor pattern if the infant has fluctuating tone, necessitating adult support. (B and C) The infant or child may adapt his particular form of fluctuating tone to maintain the supported standing position.

There is a minimal weight shift and lifting movement of the foot. If hypotonia predominates in the tonal fluctuation pattern, the infant may compensate in a different way. He flexes his hips and heavily leans into the support to remain upright. The infant widely abducts one leg to cruise laterally, bringing the other leg over to meet it. (Fig. 2-37C).

If the infant has hypotonia, he may also pull up to standing with the arms, keeping both legs extended. He uses an extensor pattern to compensate for lack of midline stability in the upright position, which is characterized by an anterior pelvic tilt and hyperextension of the knees. The legs are widely abducted, the ankles are pronated, and the toes are curled. The infant more or less stands on ligaments (Fig. 2-38A). He cannot release muscles from the fixated, extensor pattern to practice proximal mobility freely. Bouncing, rocking, and weight shifting movements are relatively stiff. The infant cruises with stiff widely abducted leg movements and a lateral flexion of the trunk. The weight does not become evenly distributed on the foot because of the malalignment of the knee and ankle. Thus, the foot may remain pronated even during the weight shift in cruising.

The infant with hypotonia will no doubt progress to assuming a half-kneel position to pull up to standing. The forward foot and knee are abducted and externally rotated similar to the immature pattern of the infant without a disability. The pattern may persist if the infant has hypotonia. He has to rely heavily on the hands to pull himself up, and there is a lateral twist of the pelvis and trunk versus rotation (Fig. 2-38B). The infant with hypertonia or fluctuating tone will likewise

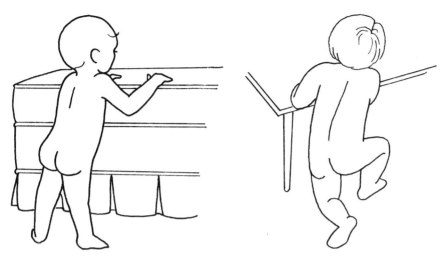

FIGURE 2-38. The infant or child with hypotonia fixates with hyperextended legs to maintain a standing position and pulls to standing with minimal leverage in the abducted legs.

have minimal leverage in the legs if he progresses to pulling up from a half-kneel position, and there is the same lateral twisting effect in the pelvis and trunk. The rotation movement may not evolve.

Summary

The disabled infant's innate drive to develop and interact with his environment is impressive. The infant adapts his patterns to gradually move up farther from the supportive surface until he reaches the pinnacle—the bipedal position. The compensations are functional from this standpoint but dysfunctional in other ways. He gets only a taste of all the available experiences in the upright position. The infant cannot freely move away from midline with rotation and counter-rotation of body parts, which limits his ability to view the caregiver and objects from different angles and reach out in surrounding space. He cannot shift weight to one extremity in a normal way to facilitate the same degree of stability, and the legs do not become aligned with the rest of the body to transfer weight directly over the knees and feet. The infant, therefore, does not experience a direct gravitational force and a sense of his anatomic midline or centeredness in the same way as the infant with normal tone. With a lack of proximal lower back and hip stability, leg movements remain stiff and poorly differentiated.

Compensatory patterns are effortful and wasteful and may at times elicit unpleasant sensations. It is no wonder that the infant fatigues quickly, and this affects his ability to venture out progressively farther in the stimulus world. A cycle evolves with low endurance begetting low endurance. It is also understandable if there are rather wide swings in his affect and attention level. The infant may have an immature inner regulatory mechanism that is further compromised by an incoherent sense of his body and where it is in space in relationship to his caregiver and objects. The implications of compensatory patterns become more evident when aberrant and so-called normal motor patterns are compared (Fig. 2-39).

INTERTWINED EFFECT OF IMMATURE PATTERNS. The infant who does not have abnormal muscle tone, but who is in a hurry to sit, stand, and cruise, has to compensate in many of the ways that have been described. He also has to fixate to maintain the position. This postural tension or wooden effect interferes with the evolvement of flexible patterns as illustrated in Figure 2-40A. The infant still has a strong positive support reaction characterized by stiffness of the legs and toe curling, and there is related stiffness in the shoulders and trunk. The infant cannot free some muscles from cocontraction to dance with his caregiver in the same flexible, light-hearted manner as his twin sister in Figure 2-40B. The stiffness also prevents him from rotating his trunk to orient to the caregiver's voice behind him (Fig. 2-40C). The infant's upper extremities are not free to move in different orientations farther away from his body in the sitting position, and he cannot adapt his action schemas to the unique properties of the object as his twin sister does. The male twin still adapts the object to his habitual actions— bangs the pegboard (Fig. 2-40D). The compensations stem from an intertwined immaturity of both sensory and motor functions.

EFFECT OF MOTOR IMPAIRMENTS ON EXPLORATIVE SCHEMAS. It is evident that the sensory and motor systems cannot be differentiated in terms of their impact on the evolvement of more refined and adaptive manipulative schemas. However, it is impossible to fully reflect this interrelationship within the confines of static words and separate pages. For organizational purposes, the primary focus of the following discussion will be on the effect of aberrant motor patterns.

Some effects of weak midline stability are illustrated in Figure 2-40D. If the infant cannot shift weight from one extremity to another in a normal way during creeping, he will not develop optimal background stability in the shoulder and arm as discussed in the section on sensory impairments relative to blindness. The infant cannot grade arm and hand movements with the refinement typical of this stage to reach and grasp a slow moving object nor can he dissociate arm and hand movements to adapt to an object with a radial-digital orientation or ex-

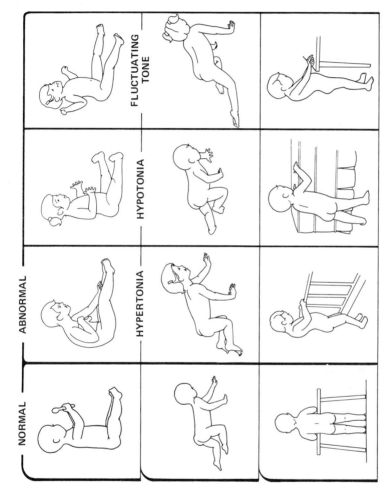

FIGURE 2-39. Compensatory motor patterns are compared with normal patterns.

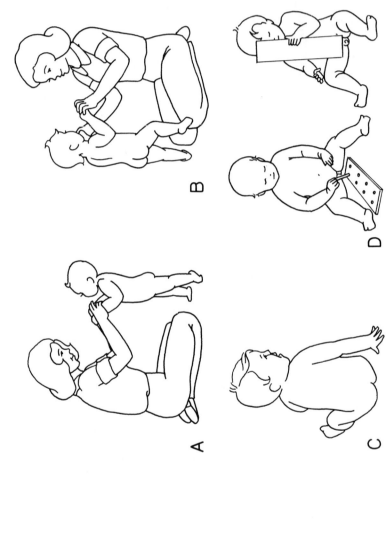

FIGURE 2-40. Proximal fixation and a strong positive support reflex does not allow the (A) male twin to dance with his caregiver with the flexibility of (B) his twin sister. Lack of midline stability in the sitting position prevents him from (C) rotating his trunk to orient to his caregiver's voice or (D) adapt his action schemas to an object as does his twin sister.

plore details with his fingers. If the arms and hands are in a protective or tense position and the head is retracted or in a stiff position, the infant is not free to move an upper extremity flexibly and examine objects visually from different distances and angles. Or the infant may lack the necessary muscular strength to lift his arm and look at an object from above or reach for a higher object. If the infant cannot experience reaching out in different directions and angles, he will not construct the relationship of his arm and hand in space in the same way as the normal infant does. Nor can he study the constancy of size and shape and dimensionality of objects in the same way. It is understandable if the disabled infant remains dependent on more gross action schemas (mouthing, shaking, banging) to obtain sensory feedback from objects and nourish his developing nervous system.

The stress of new positions may elicit the ATNR. The infant has to turn his head to the right to extend the fingers and rest them on an object. He then has to turn his head to the left away from the object to flex his arm and fingers to grasp and pick up the object. He has to turn to the right again when he wants to extend his fingers and release the object. His fingers may have been fisted so long that the extensors are very weak.

EFFECT OF MOTOR IMPAIRMENTS ON ORAL CONTROL. It is evident that compensatory patterns in the higher positions are still characterized by poor alignment of body parts and the lack of a rotational component which may interfere with the optimal sinking of the abdominal organs in the upright position and the angulation of the ribs. The thoracic volume remains smaller, which delays the typical trend toward deeper and slower breathing. The respiratory muscles may be weaker because of a low activity level, which increases the susceptibility to fatigue. If there is an unstable midline platform and poor alignment of body parts, this interferes with increased mobility and control of thoracic muscles. The infant may not be able to inspire enough air, or he may not be able to adjust inspiratory and expiratory muscle activity to maintain a steady outward flow of air. He therefore cannot babble in a chain of six or more syllables by the end of this stage. Anxiety from the stress of new positions can also affect the control of respiratory muscles and may elicit excessive sighing and hyperventilation.

The neck muscles may still be weak, even though the infant is assuming higher positions. Lack of stability and flexibility in the neck can have a chainlike effect. There is also lack of stability and flexibility in the jaw, which in turn affects the control and coordination of tongue movements (retraction, elevation, and lateralization).[49] The tongue is therefore restricted in its role as modulator of the air stream into specific speech sounds. The infant may not be able to dissociate articulatory movements to form alveolar consonants, vary his babbling by placing the consonant at the beginning, medially, or at the end, or recombine sounds to approximate a word. Or the infant may be able to babble within the normal timetable, but there is a difference in the quality. In one study,[50] infants with Down syndrome vocalized with a greater number of easier labial consonants and bilabial trills (raspberries) than normal infants.

If the shoulders are shrugged and the head and chin are forced forward or the head is pulled back, this changes the configuration of the vocal tract and movements of the larynx. The vocalization will lack the resonant quality of vocalization produced with the head in a neutral position. If the infant has hypertonia, the effort to communicate may increase muscle tone in the oral area and the whole body, which further decreases the ability to vocalize. Or the infant may be so engrossed in trying to coordinate his oral movements and respirations to form a certain sound that this affects his ability to listen simultaneously to the caregiver's utterance and modify his movements to imitate her babbling combination.

If the caregiver understands the very complex nature of speech in terms of both sensory and motor functions, she will be more appreciative of the infant's attempts to communicate and more empathetic when he cannot communicate. The caregiver will be less likely to pressure the infant, which is counterproductive in terms of both breathing and oral control. She will also be less likely to pressure the infant to engage in physical activity and work patterns beyond his endurance level. The caregiver recognizes that the infant cannot continue to meet the heavier demands for air exchange, especially if he has an increased workload from associated lung disease. The infant's level of alertness and sustained attention can be affected by an immature breathing pattern and the lack of inner physiologic stability.

FRAMEWORK FOR HABILITATIVE APPROACHES

Habilitative Focus

The intervener continues to collaborate with the parents to help them use the strengths and resources within the family unit and community to cope with stressful situations. As the intervener becomes more acquainted with the individual style of the parents and the value system and organization of roles within the family unit, she becomes more sensitive and responsive. The intervener provides support and suggestions that build upon and reinforce the positive attributes already in each parent's behavioral repertoire. This intervention approach fosters the parents' self-confidence and trust in their own common sense and intuition. The intervener avoids creating an aura of expertness and the right way, because there is no generalized right way. Her suggestions are presented as only one of many alternative ways the daily routines can be adapted to meet the unique needs of the disabled infant and his caregiver at that particular point in time. This places the infant and caregiver at the helm.

The parents may sense the importance of quadruped locomotion during this stage when gradual expansion of the sensate world is a key developmental focus. However, they can be helped to realize that if the infant is pressured to assume positions and perform movement patterns before he is ready, this approach can foster compensatory adaptations with all the described dysfunctional costs. The infant may also meet up with stimulus events that he is not emotionally, cognitively, and perceptually ready to handle. On the other hand, the infant should not be stressed by discouraging him from assuming postures and locomotor patterns that he has initiated on his own. This interferes with the budding expression of his autonomy and hampers his development in other ways. The caregiver can involve him in activities that improve the quality of the pattern. She also serves as a buffering force when the infant becomes overwhelmed by all he is seeing, hearing, and touching. He is changed to an area where the complexity and diversity of stimuli are more muted. Or it may be that he needs to be fed or quieted for his nap if he is experiencing competing physiologic sensations. The caregiver's responsiveness strengthens the infant's expectancy of her accessibility, and her refueling and environmental adaptations help him to become organized and feel whole again.

This philosophical view applies to all the subsequent activities and will be further elaborated. However, it is recognized that no human is infallible. The environment will not always meet the infant's needs nor should it, because he will have an illusion of invulnerability. Also, the infant's signals can be very difficult to read. Or the caregiver may be experiencing inner stress, which decreases her responsiveness. Her needs move to a high priority status in terms of the intervention focus. This is a time to lessen caregiving demands.

Approaches to Foster More Adaptive Patterns and Interaction in the Sitting Position

Activities will be outlined in this section to facilitate the following habilitative outcomes:
- Develops increased proximal stability and flexibility.
- Differentiates body segments to rotate away from midline with counter-rotation.
- Moves from prone to sitting with rotation.

- Adapts to a sudden gravitational shift with a protective response anteriorly, laterally, and posteriorly.
- Adapts to a less marked anterior, lateral, and posterior gravitational shift with an equilibrium response.
- Further develops thoracic muscles and exerts a downward and diagonal pull on the ribs.
- Assumes a more active role in spontaneous play.
- Orients to visual and auditory animate and inanimate stimuli from different spatial perspectives.
- Displaces objects in different spatial orientations relative to the body.
- Constructs the relationship of the arm and hand in surrounding space.
- Combines and recombines schemas to achieve a goal.
- Searches for a hidden object not tied to his actions.
- Groups objects in a rudimentary functional class.
- Imitates alveolar babbling sounds and intonations.

An erect posture maximizes the gravitational pull on the ribs and helps the infant experience his anatomic midline. The better alignment of body parts is dependent on two important elements that are often overlooked. The pelvis must become more stable to remain aligned with the shoulders. However, the pelvis must also be flexible so that the abdominal muscles can help maintain it in the neutral position. There has to be a focus on the interplay of proximal stability and flexibility and different muscle groups. The infant may still need to engage in some or all of the activities in prone, supine, and side-lying positions described in Stage II to improve the quality of background components.

The caregiver also continues to engage the infant in activities described in the preceding stage to elicit a faster and more reliable protective response, both forward and laterally, which increases the infant's confidence in his ability to prevent himself from falling. Related precautions and contraindications for the activities are followed in this stage. The caregiver simultaneously engages the infant in activities that facilitate equilibrium reactions to adjust back to midline after a weight shift versus going with the force of gravity. When the infant feels comfortable adapting to unstable movements astride the caregiver's leg or legs per the activities described in the previous stage, the caregiver gradually reduces her support and the assistance of the infant's feet resting on the surface. She places the infant in a sitting position on the floor to undress him. The caregiver engages the infant in a peek-a-boo game during this daily care activity, placing him in a more active role as the one who hides. While the infant is engrossed in pulling or striking the shirt off his head and dictating the tempo of the game, the caregiver tilts one of his buttocks up and then the other. She progresses to lifting and flexing one leg to pull his shoe off, repeating the action when she pulls the other shoe off. The caregiver also progresses to placing the infant on a more unstable surface, such as a piece of foam or pillow. When he adapts to the new support, the caregiver completely covers the infant's shoe or another more enticing object when he is not reaching for it or manipulating it. As the infant becomes engrossed in removing his shirt to find the shoe or object, the caregiver lifts one side of the foam or pillow and then the opposite side. The infant may also enjoy sitting in a Styrofoam tub that is used in a swimming pool to hold drinks. The tub confines objects to a space within his reach, and the caregiver gently tilts the tub to one side and then the other to elicit an adjustment back to midline. The caregiver observes the infant's behavior to detect increased tenseness, which inhibits or decreases the flexibility of the antigravity response. She responds by adapting or eliminating the activity. As an example, it may be that the tension of a peek-a-boo game is too excitatory for some infants, or the tilt is too abrupt.

There is a social game that even infants with hypertonia enjoy in a relaxed manner. In fact, the activity may elicit the infant's first attempt to help right himself back to midline. Familiar, trusted family members surround the infant and act as baby catchers. The infant is tilted to the side by one person and is caught by the person on the other side before he tilts too far. He is then tilted back to the first person (Fig. 2-41). The catchers progress to gently nudging the infant forward and backward if this is not too stressful. A diagonal forward and backward movement may be tolerated better. Any directional tilt should be avoided if it elicits fear, increased tension, disorganized movements, or a Moro response. The infant's secure sense that he will not be allowed to fall helps him overcome the fear of falling. He gradually begins to make antigravity adaptations, and the activity also elicits increased flexibility in the pelvis.

Other forms of movement stimulate receptors in the inner ear and facilitate antigravity adaptations. Suggestions were provided in the section on a growth-fostering environment. However, caution must be exercised when involving the disabled infant in more romping movement activities typical of this stage. He may not be able to process the more rapid input and may be limited in his ability to clearly signal that there is a mismatch. Movement input should also be cautiously provided if the infant has a seizure problem, even if controlled with medication. Some types of input may elicit seizure activity and are therefore contraindicated.

The infant with abnormal tone may enjoy some forms of input if his position or the rhythm and tempo of the movement is adjusted. If the infant has an extensor pattern, he may enjoy and tolerate being

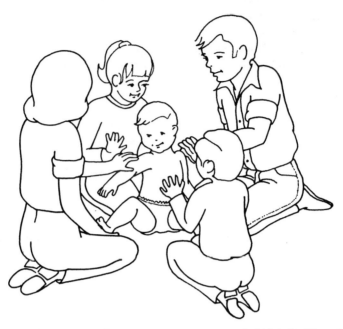

FIGURE 2-41. A beginning adaptation to a gravitational shift is facilitated with a Catch the Baby game.

slowly swayed up and down and back and forth if he is supported in a flexed position. The excursion of the sway will also have to be adjusted. If the infant has flailing disorganized movement, he may enjoy being swayed if his extremities are corralled. Bouncing can be enjoyable and arousing for the infant with hypotonia. However, the intermittent movement elicits increased tone, disorganized movement, or other aberrant patterns if the infant has hypertonia or fluctuating tone unless the intensity of the bouncing is skillfully adjusted and intertwined with inhibition via specialized therapy.

The infant may also enjoy being placed in a wagon or a carrier attached to his caregiver and taken around the house in the course of daily chores. These movements involve acceleration and deceleration and different orientations with stops, starts, and turns. The infant's world is expanded if he has a limited ability to move about on his own. He can observe the common round of daily events, which involve displacement of animate and inanimate objects, means-end relationships, and the functional use of objects. For example, the infant sees clothes disappear in the washer and other clothes reappear from the dryer. If he has a visual defect, the infant can feel the clothes and then hear and feel the washer and dryer. The infant is sensorially nourished by the contrasts of temperature, texture, and sound. This helps maintain and sustain the infant's level of arousal and attention, whereas he becomes more and more sensorially deprived remaining in one place. However, the infant's involvement in the mainstream of events must be paced in accordance with his tolerance level, regardless of the nature of his impairment.

As the adjustment to a gravitational shift becomes more reliable in response to the facilitative activities described above, the infant feels secure enough to begin orienting to surrounding space, which expands perceptual experiences. The above activities, therefore, foster the evolvement of rotation, which eventually allows the infant to reach across midline. The caregiver also engages the infant in activities that more directly elicit rotation when he becomes more stable in the sitting position. The caregiver initially facilitates head and shoulder rotation by vocalizing when she approaches the infant from one side. If the infant is blind, the caregiver immediately touches his arm or another body part on the side corresponding with the direction of her voice. She also uses touch to initiate visual orientation if the infant has a hearing loss.

The caregiver facilitates rotation and expanded spatial experiences in another way by encouraging the infant to reach out and bat or grasp an object a little to one side and then to the other side. The infant should be required to turn only a short distance initially. It is better to progress slowly and maintain a good pattern. The caregiver gradually entices the infant to rotate more as he develops increased midline stability. She places her hand on the abdominal muscles if necessary to facilitate involvement of these muscles. The caregiver may have to move her hand to a progressively higher position if the shoulders begin to retract under the stress of a new pattern (Fig. 2-42).

The infant is encouraged to experiment with spatial displacements relative to his body by swiping an object off a surface into a larger container to one side of him, to the other side, and in front. The infant can release the object in the container if the action is a well-established part of his repertoire. As discussed in the previous stage, he should not be required to perform a new manipulative task when he is learning a new motor pattern. The object should initially have a round shape, for example, a cloth ball. A circular object does not have a common boundary with the surface and is easier to differentiate and topples over easily.

The infant with a severe visual impairment is helped to reach directionally from tactile and proprioceptive cues. The caregiver attempts to gain possession of an object which pulls the infant's arm forward in resistance. If her action releases the object from the infant's grasp without upsetting him, the caregiver holds the object within reach in the same midline orientation. She makes a sound, and the in-

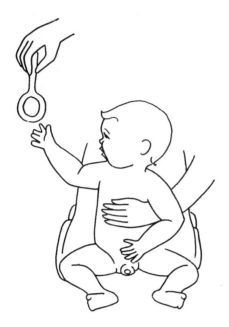

FIGURE 2-42. The hand is placed on the abdominal or thoracic area to facilitate a beginning rotational movement.

fant may reach in the trajectory his hand was pulled in. The caregiver gradually progresses to pulling his arm more to one side. At first the infant may reach toward the location where he last grasped the object. When the infant finally makes the tactual-auditory match, he can be encouraged to start reaching in midline and then directionally in response to a sound cue alone. He realizes there is a solid object out there.

The caregiver also facilitates moving from prone to sitting and later from sitting to quadruped with a rotation pattern versus the compensatory straight-line patterns that have been described. Specialized therapy approaches will have to be used if the infant has hypertonia or fluctuating tone. If the infant has hypotonia or an immature motor pattern, the caregiver can try the following approach. She lures the infant to raise up in a more adaptive way by progressive changes in the position of an enticing object. The caregiver will probably have to provide some help to give him the feel of the new pattern, which involves rolling from prone more to the side, resting on the elbow and forearm of one arm, and placing the other arm and hand in a propped position (Fig. 2-43A). The infant then pushes up with the propped arm, extending the leg on the same side as the propped arm, flexing the opposite leg, and pulling the pelvis back (Fig. 2-43B). The infant should be able to roll segmentally and reliably extend his arm laterally in the sitting position before expecting this adaptation. If the infant has hypotonia, he is encouraged to stay in the side sitting position for an interval before transferring weight to both buttocks. One side is elongated, which elicits the active involvement of the oblique muscles, and the legs are also closer together. This is another reason that specialized consultation is needed if the infant has hypertonia. There is often more involvement on one side, and the infant will prefer to sit on the better side, which can result in hip dislocation.

As the infant becomes more flexible in the sitting position, he needs to feel that he can prevent himself from falling backward with a protective extension response of the arms. This response may be initiated by an adaptation of the Catch the Baby game if enjoyable. The person behind the infant gradually allows him to fall farther backward before gently pushing him forward again, which may elicit a protective extension of the arms. Another approach can also be intertwined with a play period. The caregiver supports the infant's shoulders to provide an initial sense of security and rocks him backward in rhythm to la-la sung in two tones or another ditty (Fig. 2-44A). The modeling may elicit imitation of the sound or intonation. When the infant begins to extend his arms, the caregiver progresses to rocking him backward with no support to the shoulders but with her hand ready to catch the infant in a playful manner if necessary. He will gradually begin to use his abdominal muscles to help pull himself back to midline. Progression is then made to lifting both legs in an abducted, externally rotated position to pull off the shoes when undressing the infant, which tilts him back just a short distance. (Fig. 2-44B). This elicits a righting movement back to midline negating a need for protective extension.

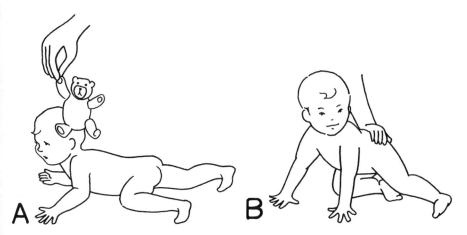

FIGURE 2-43. The infant gets the feel of moving from prone to sitting in a more adaptive way with the enticement of a toy and some assistance.

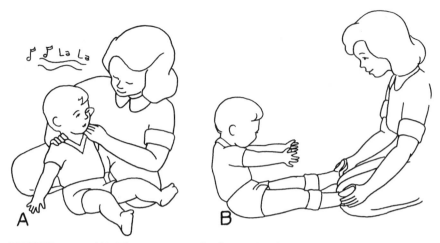

FIGURE 2-44. (A) The caregiver facilitates backward protective extension, providing more support initially. (B) She progresses to facilitating a righting movement back to midline.

As explained in the preceding stage, the effort of abdominal flexor muscles can relax the extensors if the infant has extensor hypertonicity. However, the infant may be able to overcome the extensor pattern only if he is tilted backward a certain distance and if he has enough strength in the abdominal muscles. This is just one example to illustrate that the above activities very possibly will elicit aberrant responses if the infant has hypertonia or fluctuating tone: stiffening and retraction of the head, shoulders, and arms, Moro reflex, excitability, or disorganized movement. Specialized therapy will have to be used to facilitate a more normal backward protective response if one is forthcoming.

Summary

When the infant can sit more stably, he feels free to differentiate body segments, rotating one part and holding with another part as a counterforce. This flexibility allows the infant to expand perceptual experiences across midline in a new position. The upper extremities can assume a more functional orientation: abduction, external rotation, and an upward orientation of the radial fingers. This paves the way for an adaptive radial-digital grasp and explorative examination schemas. The infant can also flexibly combine and recombine schemas in different ways to achieve a goal and to imitate unfamiliar actions.

A stable sitting position frees cognitive energy to interact with objects and environmental events, especially if the infant's breathing becomes more regular and slower as the result of increased thoracic volume. With a more stable platform, intercostal muscles become more mobile and active in respiratory adaptations, which has significance in terms of lengthening the babbling chain. The better sitting alignment may facilitate expansion of the vocal tract resulting in more flexible movements of the larynx and articulators. The infant can more flexibly vary the intonation of his vocalization, and affective expressions become more differentiated. He also adds new consonants and vowels, and the pitch quality of certain vowels becomes more stabilized.

Approaches to Foster Interaction and Movement Patterns in Quadruped Position

Approaches will be outlined in this section to facilitate the following habilitative outcomes if the infant has hypotonia or immature motor development.

- Develops increased proximal stability.
- Moves the extremities reciprocally with a rotational component.
- Adjusts to a gravitational shift with an equilibrium response.
- Develops increased stability in the arms as the background for explorative schemas.
- Strengthens the respiratory muscles and increases endurance.
- Practices distancing and proximity-seeking behaviors.
- Associates a label or gesture with familiar persons and objects.
- Displaces objects in different spatial orientations relative to the body.
- Searches for an object hidden in alternate locations.
- Forms means-end relationships from environmental regularities.
- Organizes experiences into a higher-order representation of body parts.

Simultaneous with the facilitation of a more stable sitting posture, the caregiver also helps the infant get the feel of the quadruped position. She does not prematurely encourage a position higher from the horizontal surface, if the infant does not bear weight on extended arms in prone position or sit in a more erect position with an abducted ringed position of the legs illustrated in the preceding stage. If the infant has hypertonia, the quadruped position should not be encouraged without consultation with a team member trained in specialized therapy, because this position may reinforce hip flexor tightness. Specialized approaches will also be necessary if the infant has fluctuating tone to inhibit disorganized movement and abnormal reflex patterns.

If the infant has hypotonia or immature motor development without apparent abnormal tone, the caregiver helps the infant test his

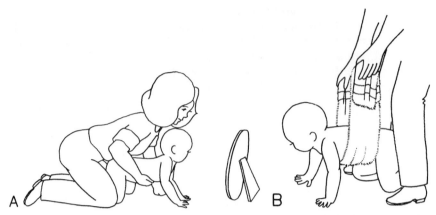

FIGURE 2-45. (*A*) The caregiver helps the infant get the feel of assuming the quadruped position and (*B*) progress to superimposing proximal mobility on distal stability.

readiness to assume this new position. She provides assurance and some support by placing her hand on the infant's abdomen, and she also corrals his legs if he has hypotonia to prevent an exaggerated abducted position and aberrant sensory feedback (Fig. 2-45A). The caregiver observes for signs of lack of readiness: retraction of the head, locking or hyperextension of the elbows, exaggerated abduction of the elbows with a hanging effect of the shoulders, collapse of one or both arms, collapse of the hips on the feet, or an exaggerated lordotic curve in the back. These responses signal a need to emphasize the development of proximal stability and mobility down lower in the prone, total support position.

If the infant can comfortably assume the quadruped position, the caregiver gradually withdraws her support. The imitative lure of a sibling down in the same position or a mirror will add enticement. If the infant does not gradually initiate proximal movement, the caregiver can again provide support under the abdomen with her hand or with a towel around the infant's chest and abdomen and help him get the feel of proximal mobility. Some developmentally disabled infants have to be introduced to the feel of a movement before they will initiate it on their own, even though they are ready. The caregiver helps the infant rock backward and then backward and forward, progressing to a side-to-side movement with a slight weight shift at first (Fig. 2-45B). If the infant has hypotonia, the rocking excursion should be shorter and brisker in a somewhat bouncing fashion to maintain joint compression and facilitate sufficient dynamic stability. If the proximal mobility elicits aberrant compensations or emotional stress, the infant is not ready. The caregiver must also monitor the effect of pressure from the towel on breathing. If the infant leans into the towel for support, he is not ready for proximal movement. This will restrict expansion of the rib cage for deeper respiration during heavier work patterns.

If the infant initiates proximal movements on his own in a pleasurable manner, flexibly uses locomotion as a means to an end in the combat crawl pattern, or reaches out to a sound cue if he has a severe visual impairment, he no doubt has the incentive to learn a new way to move forward in space. If these background components are missing, facilitative approaches are likely to elicit resistance or passive resignation. It may be that the infant needs only to have the caregiver help him get the feel of superimposing distal mobility on proximal stability in a creeping pattern. She can repeat an earlier approach and place her hand on the infant's abdomen or place a towel around his abdomen and chest, monitoring the pressure on the thoracic area. The caregiver helps the infant move forward toward an enticing visual or sound cue. She corrals the infant's legs if they exaggeratedly abduct. It is expected that the arms and knees will be more abducted at first, and the movement will thus involve a wider weight shift from side to side and lateral trunk flexion. If the new mobility pattern elicits aberrant compensations or stress, the infant is not encouraged to practice this new pattern. Sensory feedback will be distorted and physiologic benefits will be compromised. Locomotion will be an unpleasurable effort.

The infant is gradually encouraged to use the new form of mobility to venture farther away in his sensate world. The environment is adapted by having him practice in a smaller room initially and by adjusting the complexity and diversity of stimuli to either perk him up or tone him down. The most motivating impetus is the caregiver's loving and proud look and encouraging vocalization. She is also responsive to the infant's need to return to her for emotional refueling. The caregiver may have a tendency to decrease her emotional support, because she is worried about reinforcing dependency. The intervener helps the caregiver realize that premature withdrawal of herself as a safe anchor and guiding beacon will actually encourage dependency and timidity or disoriented exploration. A mediated environment should decrease the incidence of behaviors that elicit negative interaction and restrictiveness. Or the opposite may occur. The caregiver is reluctant to set any limits because of the vagueness of the infant's signals. She feels that he will not understand. The caregiver may very well be right. And this points to the need to consider readiness for a new mobility pattern in terms of all aspects of development.

If the infant feels free to explore, he uses what senses he has to map his environment and give meaning to events. The infant with a severe visual impairment searches for the sounds and smells in the kitchen and relates these to mealtime. He searches for the television which is making a sound and finds the knobs. The infant discovers the vent emanating warm air, which he begins to match with the sound of the furnace. The infant with a severe auditory impairment matches the feel and sight of the vent with the emanating warm air, the vibration of the piano with a bouncing movement, and the displacement of clothes in the dryer with vibration. The caregiver labels discoveries with a word, gesture, or another more effective mode relative to the nature of the infant's disability.

The infant may begin to creep after a moving object, especially if the object moves slowly, for example, a Jack LeLanne exercise ball. A ball with a bell inside provides an extra sensory cue that may help other infants as well as the infant with a severe visual impairment. The infant is encouraged to find the kitchen cupboards and practice displacement schemas. He is an undoer initially—takes objects out. A contrasting, easily grasped object can also be placed in a larger box for him to take out and eventually release back in. Hiding games are expanded to alternate displacements when the infant consistently searches for an object in one location even when the obstacle is more difficult, for example, imbedded in a cloth under a box. When the new search activity is introduced, a very enticing object (daddy's watch) and easily removed obstacles (diaper, undershirt) are used. If the infant resists parting with the object after he finds it so that it can be hidden under the second obstacle, he is allowed to explore the object for a while. Most important, hiding games should be fun. The infant may initially search in the location where he found the object the first time when an alternate displacement game is introduced.

The infant with a severe visual impairment is encouraged to search for a sound cue. A sound is made in one location on the rug— bell ringing. When the infant creeps to that location, the sound is activated in another location, which encourages him to creep and follow the displacement. He may progress to listening for the sound of a box sliding on the rug. The infant then progresses to searching for even a more subtle sound in this stage or the next stage—lifted box being placed back down on the rug in a new location. The caregiver gradually makes the search more difficult for the infant, regardless of his impairment, to challenge but not overchallenge his adaptability.

Practice in displacing the body and objects in space provides tactile, proprioceptive, vestibular, and auditory input that may play a role in the maturation of the sensory system. If receptors are modified and newer pathways transmit impulses to higher centers at a faster speed with less spread to other areas, the infant's sense of his own body movements and surface contact will be more localized and discriminative. Practice in creeping also strengthens the proximal muscles, which provide the background for rotation. In addition, there has been an emphasis on the refinement of reciprocal movements and the rotational component in the combat crawl pattern rather than hurrying the infant to assume a higher position. The caregiver strengthens the background components by engaging the infant in activities that facilitate equilibrium reactions. He may enjoy an adaptation of the Catch the Baby game. The infant is encouraged to assume the quadruped position, and a familiar person kneels on each side of him. The infant is tilted back and forth laterally in rhythm with a ditty. Less assistance is provided as he begins to make the adjustment back to midline. The caregiver can also place a hand on each of the infant's hips and tilt him back and forth when he is engrossed in an activity in the quadruped position or is creeping down the hall.

Summary

As the creeping movements become more refined, there is less wasted motion. Faster movements increase the need for air exchange, which strengthens the respiratory muscles and increases the vital capacity. Also, the evolvement of more differentiated bodily movements correlates with the evolvement of more dissociated oral movements. With these background components, the infant may become more vocal in a longer babbling chain, and the caregiver assumes the role of a responder more often. The infant can also more actively seek distance from or proximity to his caregiver, which fuels beginning autonomous function. As he moves about with more facility, unilateral weight bearing increases the muscle strength in the arms as the background for blending stability and mobility. More adaptive schemas evolve to explore the novel features of objects.

Other Approaches to Facilitate Vocalization

As discussed in the summaries, activities in the sitting and quadruped positions facilitate a more mature breathing pattern. Pleasurable movement during the above activities may also facilitate vocalization, and the caregiver can pick up on this and enter into vocal play, which encourages imitation. It may very well be that sessions in the rocking chair with the caregiver during a relaxed period in the day will be the most facilitative. Slow, rhythmic rocking may relax the infant with hypertonia to the point that he can vocalize and attempt imitation. Brisker or more arrhythmic rocking may perk up the infant with hypotonia. The infant should be in a comfortable position with his head, shoulders, and trunk aligned for more normal apposition of oral structures. He should also be positioned so there is face-to-face contact with the caregiver. The caregiver initially imitates the infant's babbling sounds. She then models a new combination of an old sound, such as consonant medially (ubu) or at the end (ub-ub). At times the caregiver models a new consonant sound that requires a movement similar to a sound already in the infant's repertoire. For example, if the infant can say da-da, the caregiver models la-la. If the infant begins to show signs of tension with increased muscle tone or a change in the vocal quality (weak and breathy or forced and grating), the caregiver should not continue to encourage vocalization. She may also have to attenuate her response and avoid attaching too much affective meaning to the infant's vocalization, until he has become comfortable forming the sound. Otherwise, the infant may become too excited, which interferes with oral coordination. It is also important to speak more slowly if the infant has a response latency.

When the infant is involved in the common round of daily events during the described activities and during mealtime and other care routines, the caregiver facilitates a visual-auditory association by tuning in to the infant's focused attention. When he is looking at or pointing to a person or object, actively exploring an object, or gesturing a need, the caregiver applies a label. Also, the caregiver just naturally says up when she reaches out her hands, and she likewise relates other words to meaningful gestures. In her eagerness for the infant to talk, the caregiver may label animate and inanimate objects in a programmed manner. She can be redirected to the value of her own spontaneous sociability. If the infant relates communication with pleasurable interaction, sounds and words will be associated with positive inner sensations. He will want to reproduce a sound and practice it to remind him of the pleasurable association. This has broader significance because sociable, friendly infants tend to score higher on cognitive tests.[51] It is difficult to continue talking to an infant who does not respond vocally. In one study[52] the mother was less verbal with a twin who had cerebral palsy. Yet, receptively the infant may be able to match words to a significant person or persons and objects if they are becoming separate entities.

If the infant is suspected of having a conductive hearing loss or a loss has been verified, the caregiver can speak more loudly. Also, tubes are inserted and hearing aids are being fitted during the first year in some diagnostic and treatment centers. The team members collaborate with the caregiver to decide whether to relate a simple gesture to persons and objects or use the T-K speech approach mentioned in the preceding stage, or a combination of the two approaches.

Approaches to Foster Interaction and Movement Patterns in Kneeling Position

Approaches will be outlined in this section to facilitate the following outcomes if the infant prematurely assumes this new position:

- Maintains a supported knee-standing position with less exaggerated compensations.
- Visually orients to other humans and inanimate objects from a new spatial orientation.
- Displaces objects in space from a vertical orientation.
- Displaces an obstacle from a completely hidden object.

Approaches will also be outlined to facilitate the following outcomes if the infant has hypotonia or immature motor development:

- Develops increased proximal stability in a more upright position.
- Superimposes mobility on stability to move laterally toward a stimulus.
- Superimposes rotation on stability to reach in different spatial orientations.
- Differentiates flexion and extension and leg movements to assume a half-kneel position.
- Exerts a downward and diagonal pull on the ribs.
- Displaces and retrieves objects in new spatial orientations.
- Imitates bodily movements.
- Moves in rhythm to music.

Movement higher up from the center of gravity in a knee-standing position is not prematurely encouraged. The infant needs to develop stability and flexibility in postures closer to the surface. However, there are always exceptions to any generalized statement. Knee-standing is sometimes facilitated with specialized therapy, if the infant with hypertonia has tightness in the hip flexors. Also, some infants use straight-line patterns to move up higher from the surface in an attempt to seek closer proximity to a stimulus before they have mastered readiness components.

When the infant signals a desire to view his world from a different angle, the caregiver helps him stabilize his body so that he can attend to her face and other interesting sights from this new vantage point. If the infant with hypotonia fixates with extension, the caregiver places her hand on the abdomen to facilitate the feel of holding with the flexors also. She pushes the buttocks inward if the pelvis is exaggeratedly tilted to give the infant a feel of more body weight on the knees (Fig. 2-46A). If the infant with hypertonia is cognitively impatient to move up to this position before he is ready and the caregiver and intervener

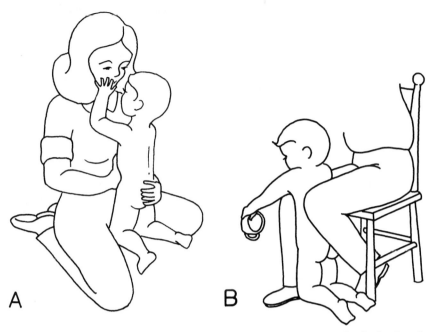

FIGURE 2-46. The caregiver provides support to compensate for lack of midline stability if the infant or child has (A) hypotonia or (B) hypertonia.

do not have access to a specialized therapy resource, they can try the following approach. The caregiver holds the infant against her body and slowly and rhythmically rocks him. The muscles may relax enough so that the infant can maintain the position without a lot of superficial static holding. This frees cognitive energy to attend to what lured him up higher in the first place. If the infant with hypertonia begins to pull down into flexion, he can be helped to place his arms on the caregiver's shoulders. Or the caregiver keeps the infant's arms extended to explore her face or gently swipe a cloth off a completely covered object in her mouth by rotating them outward at the shoulder level as illustrated in Figure 2-28B in the preceding stage.

When the infant with hypertonia feels more secure, he can stand on his knees between the caregiver's legs when she is sitting in a chair. His arms rest over the caregiver's knees, if necessary, to prevent him from thrusting backward or pulling down into flexion. The caregiver provides the necessary support with her legs to align his hips and maintain weight on both knees (Fig. 2-46B). The infant may lure his caregiver into the old game of him dropping and her retrieving. The infant can also kneel on a sturdy, upholstered chair using the back as a support to observe the common round of daily events and engage in the drop and retrieval game from a higher vertical orientation. The height of the back of the chair is important, if he has a tendency to pull into flexion. The infant, regardless of the nature of his motor impairment, may enjoy the above positions and support when he is adapting to this new position higher from the center of gravity.

When the infant with hypotonia or immature motor patterns feels more stable in the kneeling position, he can be engaged in an adaptation of the Catch the Baby game, with a person on each side helping him shift weight slightly from one knee to another in a playful way. If the infant enjoyed this game in lower positions, he may continue to relax and enjoy the game in a higher position. He is also encouraged to engage in imitative dancing that involves a swaying, lateral weight shift and an up and down bouncing action. The above approaches may elicit stress, increased tone, disorganized movement, or other aberrant compensations, if the infant has hypertonia or fluctuating tone, and should not be used.

The infant with hypotonia or immature motor development is gradually lured to adapt the weight shift and move laterally to grasp an object after the caregiver retrieves it. The infant is then encouraged to assume the role of retriever, which involves reaching down to the surface. Initially, the caregiver adjusts the position of the object so the infant is reaching down in more of a straight-line movement. She gradually adjusts the object to elicit a more diagonal reaching orientation. The caregiver places her hand on the abdomen if necessary to facilitate involvement of the flexor muscles in the rotation movement.

The above activities facilitate increased midline stability and trunk rotation and serve as precursors for the assumption of a half-kneel position. The differentiation of leg movements when sitting (flexing one leg and extending the other leg) and when creeping also serves as an important precursor. When the infant progresses to the point at which he can place weight on the knee of one leg and the foot of the other leg, he can practice grasping his caregiver or a piece of furniture and raising up to the bipedal position in a more adaptive way.

Approaches to Foster Interaction and Movement Patterns in the Standing Position

Approaches will be outlined in this section to facilitate the following outcomes if the infant has hypotonia or immature motor development:

- Develops increased proximal stability.
- Superimposes mobility on stability to cruise laterally.
- Differentiates body segments to rotate away from midline with counter-rotation.

- Develops increased awareness of the lower extremities.
- Develops increased control of movements in the legs and feet.
- Perceives the size and height of animate and inanimate objects from a new vantage point.
- Inserts the arm and hand in different spatial orientations in space.
- Imitates body movements and moves in rhythm to music.

Approaches will also be outlined to facilitate the following outcomes if the infant has hypertonia:

- Maintains a supported position with less exaggerated compensations.
- Develops some awareness of the lower extremities.
- Experiences less competing physiologic demands with the descension of abdominal contents.
- Expands perceptual experiences.
- Intentionally applies means to achieve a goal.

If the infant has hypotonia, he may signal a desire to assume the bipedal position even though he lacks the background components. The caregiver provides some assistance to help minimize the dysfunctional effect of compensations. She adjusts the angle of her body support to slightly flex the infant's knees if the legs hyperextend. Her body also provides some of the support to decrease the need for fixation. If there is an exaggerated anterior pelvic tilt, the caregiver places her hand on the infant's abdomen to elicit use of the flexors, and she presses the buttocks in with the other hand as illustrated in the kneeling position. The caregiver lifts one of the infant's legs a very short distance off the surface and then the other leg to give him the feel of weight bearing on the whole foot, if his weight is on the medial border with pronation of the ankles.

When the infant becomes comfortable standing in a less compensatory pattern, he is encouraged to imitate bouncing up and down and swaying back and forth in rhythm to a ditty. This will increase dynamic proximal stability as the background for distal mobility. When the infant feels more stable, he very probably will release one arm and hand from the support role. The caregiver gradually entices him to rotate his head and shoulders to orient to her voice, a little to the side at ear level and then above ear level. She also encourages him to reach sideways a short distance to grasp an enticing object. Both of these movements involve a weight shift. The caregiver progresses to placing an enticing object a little farther to the side. As the toddler reaches for the object, he may take a lateral step to realign the body and maintain his balance. When the infant begins to step laterally, the caregiver playfully lifts one of the infant's legs a very short distance and then the other in a musical game to give him the feel of weight over the lateral border of the foot if his own weight shift does not elicit this. More important, continued practice at rolling (especially uphill), creeping, and lateral knee walking will increase midline stability and balanced strength in hip and leg muscles. The legs will move more in line with the hips, and the weight shift will be more directly over the knee and foot. The more direct weight bearing over a limb increases the infant's awareness of his lower extremities and increases the control of leg and foot movements.

As the infant develops increased midline stability he is also encouraged to gradually open up surrounding space with trunk rotation. The caregiver encourages the infant to reach toward an enticing object or orient to a sound somewhat behind him. The position of the object or sound is gradually adjusted to facilitate increased rotation. The infant is also encouraged to reach down and retrieve an object from the surface that is gradually placed more to one side. Again, the caregiver places her hand on the infant's abdomen to facilitate flexor involvement if necessary. These rotational movements and the gravitational force in an upright position *may* continue to angle the ribs downward.

The above activities will be helpful if the infant does not have abnormal muscle tone but has a strong positive support reflex. This reflex is functional when the infant first attempts to stand in the preceding stage because of the protective increase in extensor tone. The reflexive response gradually decreases in strength with the evolvement of the following components: proximal stability, trunk rotation, and more reliable equilibrium responses in the sitting, quadruped, and supported standing positions. Touch-pressure input to the feet helps modify receptors just as in the hands. This form of input can facilitate a more adaptive, less protective response to the surface during weight bearing. The caregiver firmly massages the feet when washing and drying them during the bath, moving from the heel, up the lateral border of the sole to the ball of the foot. She also encourages the infant to kick against her body and other surfaces with the *whole* foot.

If the infant has hypertonia, his cognitive development may be disparately ahead of his motor development. He signals a desire to assume a standing position and expand perceptual experiences even though he lacks the background components. If there are no specialized therapy resources available, the caregiver can help the infant stand in a slanted position up against her legs with his arms over the legs to give support to the upper body (Fig. 2-47). She flexes one of the infant's legs if necessary to decrease a strong extensor pattern and static holding. He thereby senses less aberrant input in the leg and foot. The caregiver alternates and lifts the other leg. Now that the infant is finally up at eye level with his sibling, together they can listen to a record that is not too arrhythmic. The infant engages in goal-directed behavior by pressing an easy switch rigged up by one of his caregivers to turn the record

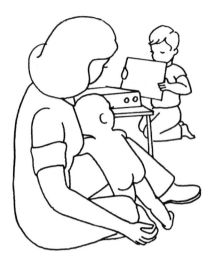

FIGURE 2-47. The caregiver provides support to help the infant with hypertonia interact with his environment in the upright position.

player on. The caregiver gradually adjusts her legs so the infant is more upright. She also gradually lets him bear weight on both legs simultaneously, if this does not elicit an extensor pattern. The upright position has physiologic benefits: facilitation of bone growth if the infant can assume a 60-degree or higher angle, less crowding of internal organs, including the lungs, which increases the thoracic volume, and possibly facilitation of a downward angle of the ribs. Specialized therapy will have to be used to superimpose movement on the standing position if this is a realistic goal.

Summary of the Effect of Approaches in the Different Positions

All the experiences in the different positions provide the infant with sensory input, which enhances his awareness of body parts and their relationship to one another. The internal referent of his body becomes more coherent, and he begins to sense what is me and not me. The experiences also enable the infant to view his caregiver and objects from different perspectives and experiment with their position and mobility in relation to his position and mobility. The infant's varied perceptual experiences challenge the central nervous system to become more adaptive in discriminating and integrating input. The infant singles out the parts of a new stimulus that relate to past experiences, leading to constancy. This ability to create order prevents the infant from perceiving a blur or continuous variation. He primitively begins to realize that each new ball shares properties with other balls that he has explored and that a ball can move from place to place. Thus, the infant can more adaptively deal with and enjoy novelty. Some infants' nervous systems will never evolve to this level of internal organization.

Adaptation of Equipment to Expand Experiences and Mobility

Some infants may never develop the necessary background components to independently assume positions and functionally move in the environment. Yet a particular infant may be cognitively ready for expanded experiences. The team collaborates with the parents to design adaptive equipment that will provide the necessary midline support when the infant is sitting, standing, and assuming other positions. If the infant is freed from postural stress, he can possibly prehend the world with his eyes and explore objects in different spatial orientations. The infant should be changed from one position to another at intervals in relation to his level of comfort, fatigue, and interest. He is then in control to the extent possible. A new position in a new location somewhat simulates the explorative movements of the normal infant and may increase the disabled infant's alertness and interest.

Equipment may have to be designed to provide a more effective mode of locomotion. If it takes too much energy to get somewhere, the infant will be discouraged from exploring his world. On the other hand, the appropriate degree of exertion can improve physiologic functions. He should be able to get on and off the device himself, if at all possible, to encourage budding autonomy. This implies that the form of mobility is as functional as his compensatory pattern. Technology is being applied to the need for an efficient means of locomotion during this stage of development, and new devices are becoming available. It is also important to adapt equipment to transport the infant on outings. This will ease the burden of expanding his social and stimulus world.

There is controversy over the use of a walker. This form of mobility can gear the infant for walking before he is ready and also reinforces compensatory patterns. In one study of normal infants[53] the walker facilitated a very different movement pattern with questionable transference value to bipedal locomotion. Walker training interfered with the development of strength in antigravity muscles, which support the body in more efficient alignment, and also interfered with the evolvement of equilibrium reactions. The lateral shift was wider in the walker, which placed less weight over the limb.

Adaptation of Objects and Experiences to Foster Exploratory Schemas

If the infant lacks the background components for the evolvement of more refined exploratory behavior, he will remain dependent on gross action schemas (mouthing, shaking, banging) to obtain sensory feedback from objects. The caregiver may need support to continue to provide a stimulus world that matches the infant's cognitive/perceptual level. The caregiver may become less discouraged or less apt to pressure the infant to perform schemas beyond his readiness, if she realizes that exploration of a variety of objects with the more gross schemas and stabilization of these schemas leads to an evolving interest in novel and more complex objects.[54]

More versatile and adaptive exploratory schemas may be facilitated by some of the following approaches. The infant is given an object with only one very obvious indentation or projection, which may facilitate exploration with the fingers or visual examination. A loosely grained sponge at bath-time or soft bread dough may elicit the poking schema for the first time, because the infant does not have to accommodate his finger spatially to a circumscribed area. When the infant with hypertonia is relaxed during his bath, he may begin to poke in body crevices and explore the genital area in new ways, for example, pull on his penis. If the motor-impaired infant's alertness and attention suggest that he is capable of visually exploring details, the caregiver can move an object closer in and farther away and at different angles. If the movement maintains the infant's interest, possibly he is obtaining meaningful input, although animal studies cited in the previous stage suggest that the infant has to move the object himself. So little is known at present about how the developmentally disabled child perceives and integrates input. If the infant has a visual deficit, the caregiver can turn the object so the infant feels a different tactual sensation. He may then begin to use his hand and fingers to turn the object and explore its surface; his hands become less blind. The infant who has fluctuating tone may be able to use his less involved lower extremities (feet) to explore objects in more functional ways.

Objects can be adapted in ways other than those already discussed to help the infant combine schemas in a means-end relationship. The infant may be able to pull a string if a dowel or cone is attached to the end. The dowel or cone should be larger if the infant has a strong grasp reflex. If he is attempting to pull the string, the caregiver can provide some assistance to let the infant link an end result with his approximated action. The infant's level of interest, alternate glances between the string and object, and repeated attempts will give some indication that he is processing the experience or obtaining meaningful feedback in ways that are not fully understood at this time. A sound-making object is attached to the string if the infant has a visual dysfunction. Some infants, especially if they have a low response level, are alerted and motivated by a light going on after they pull a cord. A light has to be used with caution if the infant has seizure activity. Technology is beginning to be applied humanistically to the development of switches that the motor-impaired infant can actuate to elicit an effect. An apparatus can be designed so that each schema elicits a different effect:

press a plate to make a bell ring, swipe a wand to make the clown pop up. The infant has his own surprise box, so to speak. The effect may have to be more attenuated if he is excitable.

Some adaptations have already been discussed to facilitate practice in restructuring the visible displacement of an object. If the infant with motor involvement looks at the obstacle intently or tries to remove it, the caregiver can completely remove the obstacle to give him an opportunity to visually verify the displacement. The infant may also become interested in hiding games that involve alternate displacements. The infant indicates that he remembers where the object was hidden by intently looking at the correct obstacle. The caregiver experiments with the type of obstacles, the type of object, and the distance between the two obstacles. A music box often elicits a very motivated search. An attachment with a significant person or persons is also important for the development of object permanence according to Bell's study reported by Ainsworth and associates.[55] The affective component adds that special predictability, meaning, and excitement to the stimulus world.

If the infant has motor involvement, the caregiver may have a tendency to use an intrusive approach during imitation games. She may need help choosing actions that interest the infant and do not require cognitive or motor adaptations beyond his capability. It is also important to wait for a response if the infant has a processing latency versus modeling the action again. If the caregiver becomes too focused on the infant's performance, she may manually help him imitate, even sitting behind him. Learning will then be negligible, and the infant will feel done unto and less in control of himself. In one study,[56] the infant had to participate actively in a game to elicit an affective expression. He did not smile or laugh if the caregiver placed his hand on her tongue or helped him stuff the diaper in her mouth.

Need for Alternate Caregiving Resources

The infant may never progress beyond this stage or may remain in this stage for a rather long period of time. It will be difficult for the caregiver to continue to provide the emotional refueling that the infant needs to support beginning autonomous function. It will also be difficult to continue to adapt the environment with just the right level of stimulation. The burden of care is relative to physical growth, because the infant may still be dependent in terms of his basic needs. He is only beginning to assume a more active role in feeding himself and making bodily adjustments when dressed. Budding independence in itself can be frustrating, especially over a protracted period. The family very possibly will feel a need for assistance with the infant's care at some point in time via resources outlined in the first stage.

The mother's attitude toward sharing her role may be very important based on the results of one study.[57] If the mother strongly feels that the infant should have one exclusive caregiver, she may experience role conflict if she shares the role with another caregiver or caregivers. The infant will sense his mother's anxiety when she separates from him each day, and the mother/infant relationship can be negatively affected.

The results of another study[58] suggest that the infant still needs a close relationship with a significant person, an organized physical and temporal environment, and an appropriate level of stimulating experiences. He had a blend of familiarity and novelty and a relationship with a caregiver or caregivers on whom he can depend to provide emotional refueling and to meet his basic needs. If the infant has to relate to too many caregivers, each one cannot possibly become closely acquainted with him. The caregiver will be less sensitive and responsive to his signals. There will also be less consistency if the infant is frequently moved from one caretaking environment to another. He may not form a secure attachment with anyone. The infant may wander aimlessly or hyperactively, as if the lighthouse beacon went out, or he may respond with some of the other behaviors described earlier. The evolving concept of the coherence of himself, other persons, and objects will be in jeopardy. It is a challenge for caregivers to plan an environment that meets the infant's needs to the extent realistically possible.

FOURTH STAGE: THIRTEEN THROUGH EIGHTEEN MONTHS

FRAMEWORK FOR ASSESSING NORMAL DEVELOPMENTAL PATTERNS

Description of Normal Motor Patterns

In the last stage the infant developed midline stability, more mature equilibrium responses, and flexible movement patterns in the sitting and quadruped positions. He also learned new ways of dealing with gravity as he gradually moved up to the supported bipedal position. The infant initially used both of the upper extremities to provide support in the kneeling and bipedal positions, just as he has all along. Likewise, he practiced proximal movement in the new positions. By the end of the preceding stage, the infant felt stable enough to superimpose distal mobility on proximal stability in the higher, supported, bipedal position. He released one arm to reach out in surrounding space and down on the surface, rotating the trunk. The infant also released one foot from a support role to cruise laterally. The muscles in the hips, legs, and feet became more stable with the increased demands of unilateral weight bearing: the hips adducted back in line with the shoulders, the feet pointed straight ahead, and the knees aligned over the feet: There was more direct weight bearing over the limb. The infant also adjusted to a gravitational shift when cruising with a more reliable equilibrium response. With the support of background components, the infant combined parts of motor programs into a more adaptive whole to cruise around a corner, which involves a diagonal movement and rotation.

The infant comes to this stage with increased stability in an extended position against gravity and an enhanced somatosensory awareness of the legs and feet. He feels daring enough to stand without upper extremity support, and the process repeats itself. The infant's legs abduct to widen the base of support, the arms go up in the old pivot prone position to help maintain his balance, and the toes may curl in an attempt to grasp the surface. When the infant feels wobbly, his arms return to the support position or he plops down on his buttocks bending at the knees.

The infant returns to a lower position to practice moving the lower extremities forward in a reciprocal pattern. He walks on the knees. As the infant develops increased midline stability and more mature equilibrium responses in the lower position, the knee-walking pattern becomes more refined with increased differentiation of the shoulder and pelvis. The infant also practices the reciprocal pattern up on his feet by walking forward a few steps when the caregiver holds both his hands and then just one hand.

One day the most heralded of all motor feats evolves. The infant leans toward his caregiver or a piece of furniture, and his feet follow in hopping steps to keep the body aligned with the head in a vertical righting response. The toddler has a strong drive to practice moving his upright body through space. He gets up to walk from point to point, gradually increasing the distance between the two sources of support, and he reverts to the creeping pattern less and less. The toddler walks for the joy of walking, seemingly unconcerned about the whereabouts of his caregiver and unruffled by the numerous falls and bumps. He rights himself and goes on his way to conquer the open space of the world.

The toddler's walking gait is very immature and inefficient because of the demands of this new form of mobility. He has to shift weight to one leg and foot and maintain dynamic stability and balance while moving the other leg and foot. The toddler slides down the spiral and falls back on old patterns. The legs are widely abducted and externally rotated with an out-toeing foot angle. There is a forward inclination of the trunk and a related anterior tilt of the pelvis (lordotic curve). The arms assume a high guard, pivot prone position. The toddler shifts his weight to one side, moves the opposite leg, and then shifts his weight to the other side to regain his balance. There is excessive hip flexion during the swing phase and limited hip extension at the end of the leg swing, which gives the appearance of high stepping when in fact there is minimal foot clearance. The steps are short with flat-footed contact and little ankle movement. Thus, the gait is relatively rigid and halting in nature, and the infant descriptively becomes a toddler.

In the course of practice, the toddler gains the courage to assume the bipedal position out in the middle of the floor without the help of a support. He goes through a lot of wasted motion because of immature equilibrium responses. The toddler rotates all the way over and assumes a quadruped position, straightens his legs in a plantigrade position, and pushes up to standing in a vertical righting response. The body follows the head in a straight-line plane at this point in development.

The toddler alternates walking with other motor patterns to maintain a balance between the flexor and extensor muscles and between stability and flexibility. He also has a drive to practice moving his body in different spatial orientations, which allows him to view the sensate world from different perspectives. The toddler creeps under the table to get an object and learns through experience not to stand up while still under the table. He adaptively adjusts to a smaller space by swim crawling under his crib to reach an object. The toddler creeps upstairs and crawls down backward or bumps down one step at a time on his buttocks. He climbs up on the couch or chair and turns around to sit down, which involves a lot of wasted motion. The toddler gets even more daring and climbs up onto the arm of the couch or over the back of the couch dropping his feet down to the floor. He may even climb over the rails of the crib. The toddler squats and rocks forward to reach an object, rocks back, stands up, and squats again to inspect another object. This series of movements strengthen the quadriceps, prevent tightness in the hamstrings, and increase the stability and flexibility of the knees and ankles. The toddler also adapts his movement patterns to use another object as a means of locomotion. He rides astride a wheeled toy pushing himself in a straight-line pattern down the hall. The toddler progresses to planning the movements of his arms and legs to make a turn and go into a room.

It is evident from the above descriptions that the toddler practices using his body in new ways as a means to achieve a goal. He approaches and moves away from his caregiver and an object, perceives them from different vantage points, and masters a new feat to further his budding autonomy. The toddler actively experiences being inside, outside, up, down, on, under, and over. These movements are an important aspect of the repertoire of experiences that help the toddler understand the relationship of his body to objects and the relationship of one object to another. As emphasized in the first part of this chapter, all the developmental patterns are intertwined.

Walking and the above activities increase the strength of muscles that keep the toddler upright with very limited surface support. The experiences also elicit an adjustment to gravitational shifts with an equilibrium response. Maturational changes are expressed by a rather amazing improvement in the walking pattern by the end of this stage compared with the initial fledgling steps. The base of support narrows until the feet are within the trunk width. There is a gradual decrease in hip flexion during the swing phase and an increase in hip extension at the end of the swing phase with a less high-stepping effect and a related increase in the stride, although minimal at this point. There is a less marked forward inclination of the trunk and anterior tilt of the pelvis, which decreases the exaggerated lordotic curve. The pelvis becomes somewhat less rigidly fixed with a slight forward rotation on the swing leg side and a slight backward rotation on the side of the support leg. The beginning rotational component directs the leg movement in a somewhat more anterior-posterior plane also reflected by the increased stride length. There is a beginning lateral pelvic shift toward the support leg, which transfers some of the forward inclination of the body sideways over the extended leg. The arms move down to a medium and then low guard position with a minimal synchronous arm swing. The upper extremities still have to fix somewhat to compensate for immature equilibrium reactions. The arms immediately move back to the high guard, pivot prone position in response to a stress situation such as walking on an uneven surface.

The toddler adapts the forward walking pattern to step sideways or backward to pull a wagon or other objects. He carries an object when he walks, even lugging a heavier pillow into another room. If the toddler comes upon an unstable surface, he may revert to creeping in order to carry an object and negotiate the obstacle simultaneously. By the end of this stage, the toddler adjusts the placement of his feet to walk up steps when holding onto his caregiver's hand or another support; he then creeps down.

The toddler also begins to hurry his gait in the form of a primitive running pattern. The stress of a new adaptation elicits regression, and the toddler slides down the spiral again. The base of support widens, the forward tilt of the trunk increases with an accompanying downward pelvic tilt, the arms move up to a high guard position, the legs move stiffly with minimal knee flexion compared with the mature

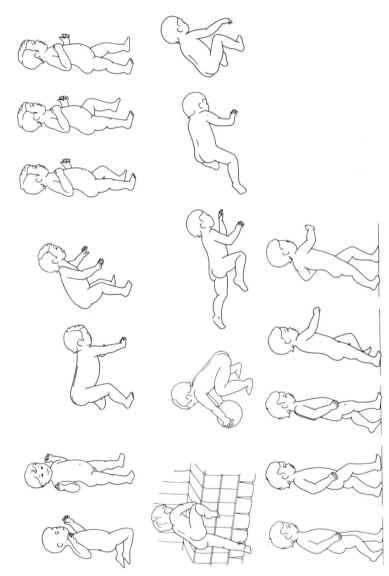

FIGURE 2-48. The first nine figures illustrate motor patterns that evolve at the beginning of this stage, and the remaining figures illustrate patterns that evolve by the end of the stage.

running gait, the steps shorten with minimal clearance off the surface, and the pace is slow.

As in the lower positions, the equilibrium response continues to mature over a period of time. Midway or at the end of this stage, the toddler adjusts to a weight shift in all directions. If he is held under the arms and moved to the side, forward, and backward, the toddler adapts by stepping in the direction of the weight transference to move the base of support under the center of gravity, realign his body, and maintain the position. The *beginning* rotational and lateral pelvic movements that become part of the walking pattern at the end of this stage also have a balancing effect. This effect will be discussed more fully in Stage V when the adaptations are more observable.

However, the toddler has a long way to travel in developing optimal midline stability and antigravity adjustments and integrating bodily movements. He still goes through a lot of wasted motion to change his position in space when rising from supine to standing. The toddler rotates to the prone position, assumes a quadruped position, and raises up to standing with less pushing assistance of the arms. There is enough leverage in lower extremity movements to eliminate the stiff, interim plantigrade position.

From a short-term perspective, the child has come a long way in this stage from tottering instability to using locomotion to get from place to place. The progression of motor patterns is illustrated in Figure 2-48 and qualitative changes are outlined in Table 2-16.

EVOLVEMENT OF PREHENSION SCHEMAS. In keeping with the cephalocaudal progression, upper extremity control is ahead of lower extremity control. The infant became aware of his arms and hands in previous stages through weight bearing, movement over the limb, and the myriad of sensory input from exploring objects. Also, the more heavily myelinated pathways that carry localized tactile and proprioceptive sensations become innervated in the arm and hand first.

The background components for more refined manipulative schemas continue to evolve in this stage. There is higher order integration of sensory input. The feedback mechanism becomes more effective with the faster transmission of impulses via the newer pathways. There is enhanced awareness of the relationship of the arm and hand in space from all the experiences reaching out in different orientations. There is increased awareness of body parts and the relationship of one part with the other, which improves bilateral coordination. The muscles in the arms become further developed as the toddler climbs, alternates between creeping and walking, and carries, pushes, and pulls heavier objects.

TABLE 2-16 Evolvement of motor patterns (Fourth Stage)

FUNCTIONAL ADAPTATION	QUALITATIVE DESCRIPTION
Stands unsupported	Widens base of support—abducts legs Curls toes to provide distal stability Moves arms to protective, pivot prone position Wobbles, returns arms to support position or sits down Maintains position with less reliance on arm support and less falling
Walks, fledgling compensatory gait	Abducts and externally rotates legs Moves arms to high guard, pivot prone position Inclines trunk forward, tilts pelvis anteriorly Flexes hip excessively during swing phase Extends hip minimally end of swing phase Moves foot in short step, whole foot contacts surface
Rises to standing without support	Rotates over to prone Assumes quadruped and then plantigrade position Pushes up to standing with arms
Walks with less compensatory movements	Narrows base of support—feet within trunk width Moves arms down to medium and then low guard position Decreases forward inclination of trunk and anterior tilt of pelvis Rotates pelvis and shifts pelvis laterally to slight degree Decreases hip flexion during swing phase Increases hip extension at end of swing phase Increases stride length slightly
Rises to standing, less wasted motion	Rotates over to prone Assumes quadruped position Raises up to standing with less pushing assistance of arms

TABLE 2-16 *(Continued)*

FUNCTIONAL ADAPTATION	QUALITATIVE DESCRIPTION
Adapts walking gait to primitively run	Widens base of support—abducts legs
	Moves arms to high guard position
	Inclines trunk forward, tilts pelvis anteriorly
	Moves legs stiffly, minimal knee flexion
	Moves feet in short steps, minimal clearance off surface
	Moves at slow pace

These maturational changes are reflected by further differentiation of arm, hand, and finger movements and more refined blending of stability and mobility. The toddler adaptively grasps bits of thread and flecks of dust with precise thumb-forefinger opposition, and he transfers a little bit from one hand to the other. The toddler can also move his hand to wave bye-bye without moving his elbow. He becomes both an undoer and a doer as his release becomes more adaptive. The toddler refines his movements to release one object in his hand, and then a second object, with successive extension of the fingers.

However, a new challenge elicits downward movement along the developmental spiral. If the toddler attempts to release a small object on top of another, there is regression to undifferentiated movements with a pronated orientation of the forearm and hand and an exaggerated extension of the fingers during the release. The tower of two blocks topples at first. Likewise, when the toddler begins to use an object as an extension of his arm (intermediary tool), this requires both grasping and manipulating the object in relation to another object and space (scribbling on the wall). There is regression back to a total, undifferentiated movement of the proximal and distal parts with a pronated palmar or even an ulnar-palmar grasp. The new movements become somewhat less awkward with practice during this stage.

The toddler coordinates bilateral movements to clap his hands and bang objects together more rhythmically. However, he cannot move his hands in different directions or use one hand as the stabilizer while manipulating with the other hand. The toddler pulls barrels apart versus using a twisting motion. Thus, there is a way to go to achieve manual dexterity. The progress in this stage and the qualitative nature of prehension schemas are outlined in Table 2-17.

TABLE 2-17 Evolvement of prehension schemas (Fourth Stage)

FUNCTIONAL ADAPTATION	QUALITATIVE DESCRIPTION
Refined differentiation of arm, hand & finger movements, lower level skills	Grasps very small object with precise pincer movement
	Releases one object in hand, then second object with successive extension of fingers
	Moves hand to wave bye-bye without moving elbow
More adaptive bilateral coordination	Transfers fleck of dust from one hand to other
	Claps hands and bangs objects together more rhythmically
Undifferentiated arm, hand, and finger movements, higher level skills	Releases one object on another with pronated hand, exaggerated extension of fingers
	Manipulates intermediary tool (crayon) with ulnar-palmar or palmar orientation of the hand
	Pulls barrels apart versus a twisting movement

Description of Normal Oral and Language Patterns

There is a continued intertwining of two forces to angle the ribs downward and enlarge the thoracic cavity: the enhanced gravitational pull of an upright, bipedal posture and rotational trunk movements in the various positions. The endless mobility involved with creeping, climbing, walking, and even a primitive runlike gait places an increased demand on ventilatory muscles, which enhances the strength and endurance of the muscles. Increased midline (axial) stability provides a platform for mobility of the thoracic muscles. The above influences and continued growth of lung tissue are reflected by a further decrease in the respiration rate and deeper breathing.

The toddler regulates the slower respiratory cycle and air pressure to expand his babbling to sentence length. He also has sufficient air volume to form a word that contains a fricative consonant—h.[1] The increased vital capacity and ability to meet higher ventilatory demands allow the toddler to selectively increase the loudness of his utterance. This requires an adaptation of the respiratory cycle which may be rudimentarily similar to that of adult research subjects[2] described in the following paragraph.

During a loud utterance in the upright position, the rib cage muscles become more active to effect a deeper inspiration, stretching the spring to a greater length, which enhances the recoil forces and increases the relaxation pressure. There is less forceful inspiratory braking of the recoil forces because a higher subglottal pressure is required for loud vocalization. As the relaxation pressure decreases, there is more forceful supplementary assistance by the expiratory muscles, including the abdominal group, to maintain the higher pressure level. The abdominal contraction also prevents the rib cage expiratory forces from driving the diaphragm footward with the aid of gravity in the upright position. This would place the flattened diaphragm at a mechanical disadvantage for the subsequent inspiration. Thus, the stiffer abdomen keeps the diaphragm tuned at the optimal length. The tauter abdomen also provides something for the rib cage muscles to develop pressure against. Otherwise, some of the effort and energy potential would be dissipated pushing out a relaxed abdominal wall— paradoxical movement.

There is also abdominal muscular activity during the inspiratory phase when the loudness of the utterance is increased, reflected by a progressive inward movement of the abdomen as the inspiration increases in depth. As described above, the rib cage muscles become more active in the upright position during a deeper inspiration. However, these muscles cannot act alone or the diaphragm would be pulled upward (headward) during the rib cage elevation, decreasing the change in thoracic volume. There has to be resistance either by a contributing contraction of the diaphragm or by a hydraulic pull of the liquid-filled abdomen on the undersurface of the diaphragm, which achieves the same effect. The rib cage muscles have something to pull against, which prevents wasting inspiratory effort pulling the base of the thorax upward. If one tries to inspire more deeply with the abdomen in an outward, relaxed position, one gets an idea of the need for balanced resistance. It is apparent that the different muscle groups enter into a teamwork relationship during certain aspects of speech breathing.

Structural changes are still in progress. There is further elongation of the pharyngeal and oral cavities with continued descension of the larynx and posterior one third of the tongue in the neck. A rather marked decrease in the frequency (pitch) of the voice begins in this stage as the vocal tract lengthens and the folds become longer and broader.[3,4] The articulators continue to become more mobile, which is necessary for further dissociation and refinement of oral movements.

Increased control is also the outgrowth of a higher-order cortical representation of oral structures and movements, higher-order sensory integration and discrimination, and a more effective feedback mechanism. The toddler continues to develop competence planning and modifying movements of the tongue, lips, and jaw; these experiences increase the stability and flexibility of the muscles in an intertwined relationship.

The chewing action becomes less effortful, and the tongue is guided away from approximating first molars by sensory cues. The toddler begins to inhibit the pumping action of the jaw when drinking from a cup, and he can keep the jaw more stable while moving the tongue to lick an ice cream cone and make the la-la sound. The toddler can also move his tongue in a circular motion and in and out without moving the lips. He moves his tongue in a more directional and refined way to lick in bits of food from the chin and corner of the mouth. With increased control, the forward movement of the tongue is inhibited during swallowing.

Dissociation of oral movements and increased breath control are important background components for the very complex synergistic pattern involved in blending sounds to form a word. The toddler also has a new capacity for trial-and-error experimentation discussed more fully in the subsequent section on cognitive patterns. He therefore begins to imitate more words in this stage. The toddler also practices blending sounds in a random babbling jargon with recognizable question or statement contours. He is recapturing the sentence-length utterance he has heard while interacting with the caregiver and other significant humans. The toddler has a primitive sense of turn-taking in speech, and he will stop and listen to the caregiver's response. He then answers with another babble sentence. The toddler may throw in a word as if it somehow belongs in the context, and his vocalization is accompanied by gestures and body activity.

The toddler's vocalization is still very repetitive, and the expressive vocabulary increases slowly. From the myriad of words he has heard, the toddler may utter no more than a dozen or so or possibly only three or four during this stage. There is a lot of variation among children and between the sexes. There is controversy over the class representation of the initial one-word utterances—nouns, prepositions, verbs, and relational words (more, all gone).[5,6,7,8] Nelson[9] reported that the initial words represent several classes. However, once a body of words is acquired in the expressive vocabulary, object words (nouns) dominate. The toddler overextends the meaning of some words; for example, daddy refers to all men, up to all vertical movements, back to any reversible movement. A certain sound may be used for a loosely assorted number of objects—quah for duck, water, and milk. Some words are ritualistically tied to a frequently occurring, single situation or context. For example, the toddler says more only to request another serving of cereal at breakfast; he says flower only at grandmother's house. Relational words may become less context bound earlier than object words—more cereal, more tickling, more cookie.[10] With expanded experiences, a word begins to carry more than one meaning in what is termed a holophrase. Bye-bye can express a departure or delightful anticipation.

Most of the single word utterances occur while the toddler is performing an action involving a present object. He is more apt to encode changes that carry the greatest amount of information to himself and others. If the toddler transfers an action schema from an old to a new object, he verbalizes the new object. He is developing the ability to signal a novel event with a word as well as with visual alertness and sensory-motor exploration.[11]

The toddler begins to coordinate person and object when expressing a need at times. He vocalizes, reaches or points, and looks at the adult. This emergence of a more intentional gestural and vocal signal correlates with the new cognitive ability to use a novel means to achieve a goal; this will be discussed in the subsequent section on cognitive patterns.[12,13]

There is controversy over whether comprehension of linguistic form takes precedence over expression of this form and whether receptive and expressive language represent different underlying processes. There is also disagreement over what cues the toddler uses to respond to language and whether he responds better to one word, two words, or a sentence in this stage.[14,15,16] The results of two studies[17,18] suggest that it is the semantic information rather than the syntactic word order that has communicative value. The toddlers responded as well to a mixed-up word order as they did to a sentence with the usual agent/action/object sequence, even after they could express this syntactic form in a two- or three-word utterance in the next stage. However, the results of another study[19] suggest that the toddler can perceive and categorize the role of agent and recipient of an action or event before he can express these concepts in a two-word utterance. In line with this finding, some investigators[20,21] hypothesize that the toddler reduces the caregiver's utterance down to the most regular parts in a sentence: agent/action/object. The toddler cannot apprehend all three parts at one time in this stage; he relies on the situation, gestures, and other nonverbal cues to fill in the gaps. Benedict[22] observed that the toddler understands more action words than object words, whereas he more frequently verbalizes object words. In contrast, Gleitman, Shipley, and Smith[23] reported better discrimination of nouns than verbs.

All the investigators recognized the toddler's reliance on environmental cues in this stage. He is more apt to understand a request in a context involving a certain time, place, and person.[24,25] The toddler very quickly responds to the utterance, "Go get Mommy's shoes," if she is dressing in the usual place at the usual time. There may be a beginning expansion of comprehension to referents out of sight and to unusual instructions by the end of this stage. The toddler will go look for a person or an object[26] and tickle a book.[27] Comprehension may also be related to the nature of exploratory behavior. If the toddler does not adapt his schemas to the unique properties of an object in a functional way (brings spoon to his mouth) or in a representational way (places spoon in doll's mouth), he does not follow verbal requests to perform these actions.[28] The toddler often feeds himself instead of a doll in response to a request. He gets the idea but applies the idea to the wrong object. His actions only gradually become other-centered toward the end of this stage and on into the next stage. The toddler may initially have an internal movement image of an object, but he has not related the object to a word. He will bring the cup to his mouth to drink but will not hand the cup to his caregiver or say cup upon request.

The toddler's receptive language expands in other ways as he interacts with his caregivers. He fetches an increasing number of objects which fuels the toting schema more fully described in the next section. He points to some labeled body parts and a two-dimensional representation of very familiar animate or inanimate objects in a book. The toddler may label one or more of the pictures himself toward the end of this stage. He may relate a spatial orientation to a word without a gestural cue—up, down, and possibly in. The toddler also understands and more consistently responds to regulatory words (no, stop, hot) if the environment has been contingent.

The toddler's speech is primarily directed to adults, and the content is structurally egocentric, which has functional significance.[29,30] His communicative attempts foster the attachment process by initiating proximity and interaction in both a social way and to gratify his needs. The caregiver's contingent responsiveness to the toddler's gestures and vocalization gives him the feeling that language is a very effective means to attain a desired result.

The toddler is building on the substrate acquired during the first year to intertwine components into more complex patterns. This allows him to blend sounds and form a fledgling vocabulary of words, simulate adult conversation with turn-taking babbling sentences, and adapt oral movements to alter the texture of foods. The toddler links sensory input to associate some words with recurring concrete events and thus attaches a meaning to symbols. The evolving patterns further outlined in Table 2-18 serve as a springboard for rather phenomenal advances in the next stage.

Description of Normal Cognitive Patterns

During the first year, the infant organized his experiences into progressively higher order and more complex internal structures. This process

TABLE 2-18 Evolvement of oral and language patterns (Fourth Stage)

Coordinates respiratory movements in more adaptive teamwork ways
    Maintains a steady flow of air to babble in a sentence-length utterance
    Increases the air volume to produce the "h" fricative consonant
    Selectively regulates the subglottal pressure to increase the loudness of the utterance
Moves elongated oral and laryngeal parts with increased flexibility relative to structural changes
    Vocalizes with a rather marked decrease in the pitch quality
    Moves tongue directionally to lick bits of food from chin and corner of mouth
    Inhibits forward movement of the tongue during swallowing
Develops increased ability to dissociate oral movements
    Begins to inhibit pumping action of jaw when drinking, more adaptive lip accommodation
    Keeps the jaw more stable when moving the tongue to form la-la sound
    Moves the tongue in different directions without moving the lips
    Blends stability and mobility of articulatory movements to form three or more words by end of stage
Associates visual input with an internal referent of vocal movements and past sensory-motor experiences
    Uses a word to refer to a number of objects with a common characteristic—labels all men daddy
    Uses a word to express more than one meaning (holophrase)
    Coordinates vocalization and a gesture with visual orientation toward an adult to express a need
Links receptive and expressive language with the immediate context and a particular situation
    Ritualistically ties certain words with a frequently occurring single situation
    Primarily vocalizes when performing an action involving a present object
    Relies on a familiar context and nonverbal cues to comprehend an utterance
    May progress to understanding utterances about familiar persons or objects not present in the immediate environment.

was reflected by an expanding repertoire of schemas to interact with other humans and inanimate objects. Initially, the infant was more inwardly directed which was adaptive in view of his immature nervous system. During brief, awake, alert states he used rudimentary behaviors to seek and maintain interaction with his caregiver. He also focused on bodily activity and came upon interesting sensations, which he repeated in what Piaget termed primary circular reactions. As competing physiologic demands decreased and periods of sustained attention increased, the infant became more outwardly oriented. He adapted old schemas and came upon new schemas to explore external events but still in a relatively primitive way. The infant repeated an action over and over in what Piaget termed a secondary circular reaction to recapture an interesting effect that he stumbled upon. Variations of the effect came about just as unexpectedly. The infant solidified the secondary schemas through practice, which paved the way for more flexible coordination of schemas to achieve a goal. Thus, the infant's exploratory behavior became more intentional and object-centered. The novel features of an object began to capture the infant's interest more so than the object's potential to nourish his habitual schemas.

The infant graduates to toddlerhood in this stage with the ability to actively confront and test reality in the role of a curious experimenter. He explores an object with one of the schemas in his repertoire and elicits an interesting, unexpected response. A circular reaction occurs to repeat the novel effect but in a more advanced way than in primary and secondary circular reactions in Stage I and II. The toddler draws upon the flexibility and intentionality acquired in Stage III to deliberately vary repetitions and produce different effects through what Piaget termed tertiary circular reactions. For example, the toddler releases two blocks in his hand and focuses attention on the trajectory of the blocks. He is intrigued by the new spatial/temporal effect, and the toddler repeats the spectacle in a new way to pursue novelty more actively. He releases one of the blocks and pauses before releasing the second block. The toddler may vary the novel effect in subsequent repetitions by increasing the pause between the two release actions and by changing the angle when he releases the second block. Thus, tertiary circular reactions are a more advanced expression of the explorative behavior that evolved in the preceding stage. The toddler even more intently accommodates his actions to the unique properties and potentiality of the object.

Through an active process of trial-and-error experimentation, the toddler begins to discover new and unfamiliar means that are not already in his repertoire. In the preceding stage the means-end schemas were coordinated or combined in new ways, but the schemas themselves were not new. This increased adaptiveness fosters a more persistent problem-solving approach, and the toddler becomes more reliant on his own resources as the stage progresses. He sees a favorite toy in the neighbor's yard, but he finds that the toy is out of reach on the other side of the picket fence. When the toddler's use of familiar ways to retrieve the toy are unsuccessful, it becomes a matter of innovation. The caregiver fuels the problem-solving by unobtrusively placing a toy rake in view. The toddler draws upon past experiences integrated in internal structures and a more effective feedback mechanism to reorganize schemas and devise a new means. The toddler discovers that if he places a certain end of the rake in a certain position relative to the object, he can accommodate for a gap in space and move the toy within reach. He has added an intermediary means by using an object as a tool to obtain another object. All the props must be in the toddler's immediate perceptual field, and he has to be a part of the action. He cannot mentally develop a plan to attain his goal and go find a rake or another tool. The toddler still has to act to think, and the new means evolves from trial-and-error groping. The addition of an intermediary enhances the toddler's awareness of a spatial-temporal series. He senses that the action of his hand and the tool are in front of the goal and that one action must occur before the other.

As the toddler practices tertiary circular reactions, he becomes more aware that there are causal forces outside of himself. The illusion of his own magical powerfulness begins to wane, demonstrated by a change in his behavior during ball play. The toddler no longer gestures in a magical way or places the caregiver's hand on the ball as though he has to remain a part of the throwing action. He now places himself in the spatial-temporal series by standing in a certain place. The toddler then expects that his caregiver will throw the ball to him on her own. He also begins to realize that outside causal forces affect him as an object among other objects. If the caregiver raises her watch above the placemat which is within reach, the toddler realizes that the pulling schema will no longer achieve his goal; he cannot obtain the enticing no-no. The toddler has to submit to an intruding causal action which affects his relationship with the object as well as the relationship of the object to the support. Thus, there is a beginning transference of power as the toddler tests reality.

The toddler comes upon new ways to relate one object to another through tertiary circular reactions. In Stage III, the infant focused on the relationship between his actions and an object and only primitively began to discover the relationship of one object to another through displacement schemas. In this stage the toddler actively builds upon this rudimentary awareness. He spends a lot of time toting objects from one point to another and displacing them in different ways. Arrangements are mapped and modified through trial-and-error experimentation, which places objects in different perspectives: near, farther away, close to one another, far apart, above, below, beside, in, out, tilted, reversed. The toddler more actively experiments with putting objects together and taking them apart in a contents-container relationship, and he recognizes that some objects are too large to fit in the container and no amount of stuffing will work. He begins to recognize that flexible objects will fit through a small opening if their shape is altered. The toddler also learns that objects have to share a common boundary to a certain degree for one to be placed on the other. A round can has to be placed so the flat surface is resting on the block. He begins to match the shape of forms as they become more constant through trial-and-error groping. For example, he fits a round shape in an indentation or through a hole with some heavy pressing and turning.

The toddler does not always explore his environment in a very active, motor way. His beginning recognition that the actions of others are independent from his own emphasizes his role as an observer. There are periods of stillness when the toddler is absorbed in watching his caregiver put on her makeup, the man load the garbage, or the play of other children. This very focused attention was related to later competence in a longitudinal study conducted by White and associates.[31]

Although the toddler is realizing that other persons and objects exist apart from him and his behavior, he cannot reproduce an image of a person or object without the support of concrete, external perceptual cues. Animate and inanimate objects have not become sufficiently coherent in time and space. The toddler's short-term memory gradually increases, evidenced by resuming his search of an object after becoming distracted by another event for approximately five minutes or maybe even longer. He can also seriate events to follow sequential, *visible* displacements. If an object is displaced under cloth A, brought into view, and then placed under cloth B, the toddler may initially regress and search where the object was first displaced (A). He more flexibly unlocks his internal image from one particular position, reconstructs the series, and searches under B to find the object. The toddler progresses to searching directly under the last place where the object visibly disappeared (B). His ability to arrange events serially gradually becomes more flexible, and the toddler searches under the last place the object disappeared in either direction: $A \rightarrow B, A \leftarrow B$. By the end of this stage, a third displacement can be added to the sequential series: $A \rightarrow B \rightarrow C$. The toddler may again revert and look under A or B first. He then progresses to searching directly under C. He also progresses to looking under the last place the object disappeared in either direction: $A \rightarrow B \rightarrow C; A \leftarrow B \leftarrow C$.[32,33] The toddler cannot make an inference about what took place out of sight and follow an invisible displacement. This requires a mental representation independent of a perceptual cue, an ability that evolves in the next stage. Some toddlers may begin to engage in this higher level of search behavior toward the end of this stage. As discussed in the preceding section, the toddler may look for his caregiver or an object in another room outside his visual field.

The toddler continues to order experiences into primitive subschemas or groupings that are the forerunners of classification schemas that evolve later. With an increased focus on the inter-relationship of objects, he categorizes objects that fit in a container and objects that do not fit in absolute terms. Other categories of object-to-object relationships also evolve, for example, objects that stack, objects that nest. The toddler may start gathering objects in a pile in this stage. There is no consistency in his selection; an object may be included one time and excluded another time. Proximity is an influential factor but not always. The toddler's rudimentary functional classes also gradually expand and become more flexible. In the preceding stage, the object had to be very similar to objects the toddler had explored to be included in the grouping. By the end of this stage, he places a miniature cup in the category of objects used for eating.[34] The round of daily events continues to provide the context for grouping certain objects or events together: bath, quiet time on mommy's lap, and pajamas belong with bedtime. The coffee pot and stove go together and mean hot! The toddler may say hot, and the word then becomes a part of the grouping. Whereas perceptual matches initially evolved exclusively around body modes, the actions of other humans and objects are having an increasing influence on the categories.

The toddler's imitative skills reflect a higher-order internal representation of body parts and an increased ability to motor plan movements. The toddler very systematically attempts to reorganize his schemas to imitate the actions of others, and he gradually attends to more details in an attempt to make his movements correspond to those of the model. There is progressively less trial-and-error groping as his ability to motor plan improves. He also begins to imitate novel movements that he cannot see himself perform (facial gestures). Of course there has to be a certain degree of congruence between the modeled visible and invisible actions and the toddler's level of competence.

The functional exploration of objects continues to be a precursor to symbolic play. The toddler acts on objects in ways that he has experienced himself or in ways that have been frequently modeled by other persons. The action centers on himself initially in this stage—brings the spoon to his mouth. Midway or toward the end of the stage, there are signs of decentralization. The toddler directs the action to another object—places the spoon in the doll's mouth. There is a ritualistic quality to the toddler's behavior, because he cannot mentally order two or more actions in a multi-schema combination with an element of make believe. He does not scrape the spoon across the dish and place it in the doll's mouth or feed the doll and put her to bed. This flexibility evolves in the next stage.[35]

Play in the more true sense is still lighthearted in this stage. The toddler comes upon a new discovery, and he may immediately repeat it in a playful rather than a more serious experimental way. For example, he places his face in the bath water and accidentally blows bubbles. The toddler laughs and repeats the action, varying it somewhat but only to entertain himself. The toddler may insist on going through this play ritual at the beginning of his bath for a month, which can be exasperating to the caregiver.

Referring to the outline of cognitive patterns that evolve in this stage in Table 2-19, it is evident that the toddler assumes the role of experimenter with gusto. He makes many new discoveries including the beginning realization that objects exist apart from him and interact with each other. He also realizes that outside causal forces impinge on his actions.

Description of Normal Affective Patterns

If the toddler has had a predominantly positive relationship with other humans and inanimate objects, he takes off on his own two feet after the initial period of unsteadiness with an elated mood and a heightened responsiveness to the sensate world. Mahler, Pine, and Bergman[36] emphasize that an upsurge of exhilaration characterizes the practicing subphase of the separation/individuation process. Thus, the emotional tone of mobility and exploration is the important element rather than the development of motor skills per se.

The toddler becomes almost totally engrossed in the mastery of his own body and the physical realities of the world to the near exclusion of interest in his caregiver's whereabouts at times. He can give full reign to his urge to explore because of a sense of power derived from a predictable, contingent environment and a trust in the accessibility of his caregiver. The toddler achieves a delicate balance between a beginning sense of autonomy and a sense of oneness with the world and perceives no contradiction between the two.

To maintain this delicate balance, the toddler occasionally looks around and locates his caregiver. He also comes to her at times for a brief emotional refueling or for gratification of other needs. This dependency almost gets buried by his new demeanor as a grandiose conquerer. Ainsworth and associates[37] emphasize that the context determines the intensity of attachment behaviors, which is vividly demonstrated when the caregiver chooses to leave the toddler rather than he choosing to leave her. He may protest her departure, especially if he is left with a person who is not involved in his care everyday. The toddler usually calms down when he realizes that his caregiver has in fact gone, and he tries to console himself with his usual activity. However, he senses the loss of his caregiver's beacon which lights up the contours of the outer world and "sculpts them into a circle of safety."[38] The toddler may become low keyed, focusing on inner sensations which remind him of his caregiver's presence. Or he may seek comfort from a cuddly blanket or favorite toy that has a symbolic link with his care-

**TABLE 2-19 Evolvement of cognitive patterns
(Fourth Stage)**

Intentionally varies repetitions of schema to produce different effects (tertiary circular reactions)
- Releases an object with arm in different positions to vary trajectory
- Focuses on motion of object rather than release action

Subordinates action schema to object
- Actively explores novel potentiality of object
- Adapts schema to unique properties of object

Applies experimental orientation of tertiary circular reactions to problem situation
- Discovers new means through trial-and-error experimentation
- Invents intermediary means (tool) to achieve a goal
- Increases intentionality of action with novel adaptation and addition of intermediary means

Begins to discover relationship of one object to another
- Places objects in different spatial arrangements—in and out of container, stacked on top
- Studies relationship of objects rather than their relation to self and its actions

Clearly views object as separate from his actions, places in spatial/temporal series
- Resumes search of object after longer interruption (five minutes or more)
- Follows sequential visible displacements, initially searching in order of displacement (A then B)
- Seriates events to search in last place object disappeared in either direction

Becomes increasingly aware of independent causal sources outside self
- Recognizes another person acts on their own without his involvement
- Begins to recognize the necessity of spatial contact between two objects to effect a cause
- Submits to an outside causal force—does not pull support if object is raised above it

Adapts self to reality in more systematic and flexible ways
- Corresponds movements to those of model more precisely
- Imitates novel actions cannot see himself perform
- Begins to direct actions to another object—spoon in doll's mouth

Adapts reality to self in expanded ways
- Varies action schemas to entertain himself rather than to seriously experiment
- Ritualizes the playful repetition of an action schema

Orders reality within context of own actions and rudimentarily within context of actions of other persons and objects
- Categorizes objects in interrelationships—objects that stack, objects that nest.
- Categorizes objects as a group of things—pile
- Expands functional class to include more and less familiar objects—miniature cup with eating
- Categorizes certain objects or events as belonging together—bath, pajamas, story with bedtime
- Includes word with grouping—coffeepot, stove, "Hot!"

giver. As mentioned in a previous section, his internal representation is not coherent enough in time and space to reconstruct a picture of his caregiver in her absence. His subdued mood demonstrates strength. The toddler longs for the person he has become attached to, but he can maintain his emotional equilibrium when she is away by using inner forces to conjure a state of well-being and rhythm related to her presence. The length of time the toddler can maintain this continence depends on individual characteristics and situational variables.

When the caregiver returns, her greeting may be sufficient. The toddler does not feel a need to establish proximal contact with her. Or the toddler may run to his caregiver and remain in close proximity for a longer period than in the preceding stage. Or the toddler may start to run toward his caregiver and then turn away, or he may burst into tears. Possibly, he feels safe enough to express some of his anger and disappointment when she left him. Or it may be that the bona fide caregiver does not immediately match up with the perfect mothering sensations he conjured in her absence. After the toddler has integrated his caregiver as the all-good mothering object again, or after he has released some of the tension of maintaining his equilibrium while she was away, he is more accepting of her overtures. After a period of emotional refueling, the toddler is off to explore the world again, and it is difficult to believe the babysitter's report that he was so quiet and good.

The toddler's exuberant, explorative spirit often makes it seem as though he is getting into everything. Some of his reality testing invades another person's possessions, and the toddler's longer short-term memory and more persistent search behavior diminish the effectiveness of the distractive approach. If another object is substituted or he is taken to another part of the house, the toddler may persistently come back to explore the novel properties of the enticing object. Also, in his urgency to master his own body and the world, the toddler appears oblivious to danger. His caregiver may find him teetering on the arm of the sofa or attempting to climb on a high object. It is no wonder that the budding experimenter and conquerer elicits more interaction of a limit-setting nature. If the caregiver has been nurturing, a close attachment no doubt is evolving, and the toddler will have a desire to please. This will increase compliance but not without repeated testing.

The toddler's saving grace is his repertoire of behaviors, which tilt the scales in a positive direction. His appealing babbling jargon and other communicative skills functionally foster the attachment process with a significant person or persons. The toddler continues to assume a more active role in initiating interaction, and he also becomes a more active participant during spontaneous play, which is more rambunctious in nature at times. He loves to assume a center stage position and ham it up, which elicits a lot of positive social attention and reinforcement.

The toddler experiences an array of sensations as he creeps, walks, squats, climbs, and bumps into unyielding objects. His feedback mechanism becomes increasingly more discriminative as the sensory system matures, and the toddler becomes more aware of subtle bodily movements. He also becomes more aware of the behind or back surface of his body as rotational movements become more flexible in the lower positions. When he is up walking, the male toddler may bend over to look at his penis and scrotum from a new vantage point. The female toddler may lean over from a sitting or squatting position and visually inspect the vulva and vagina, which her hands have already discovered in previous stages. Many toddlers also fondle their genitals and playfully tense and release perineal muscles at nap and bedtime. All the above experiences enhance the toddler's inner representation of his body/self. As he becomes more aware of his own boundary, the toddler becomes progressively less dependent on his caregiver as a reference point or beacon to orient his interaction with the sensate world. The caregiver gradually takes on the role of a very important auxiliary helper who predictably provides support from the wings. Mahler, Pine, and Bergman postulate that this beginning differentiation of self, coupled with a history of a positive attachment with a significant person, is an important component in the development of autonomous function. Thus, attachment and separation continue to evolve simultaneously in an interrelated way at higher levels.

The sense of power that the toddler invests in his own budding autonomy and adaptive skills is asserted during daily care routines. Even more so than in the preceding stage, the toddler wants to do and not be done to. Thus, he is usurping his caregiver's center focal position in another way. The toddler may impatiently squirm during diaper changes and dressing, and he draws upon his increased bodily awareness and motor planning capabilities to practice removing easier garments, albeit not always at appropriate times. The toddler may insist on feeding himself the entire meal at some point during this stage, and he uses an old means (his fingers) with facility. However, the use of a new intermediary means or tool requires trial-and-error experimentation. The toddler must construct new spatial relationships when using an extension of his hand. He regresses and grasps the spoon with a palmar orientation, and he may use his other hand to help fill the spoon. The toddler initially misses his mouth or turns the spoon before or when it enters the mouth because of the awkward pronated orientation of the forearm and hand. He falls back on finger feeding, progressing to alternately using his fingers and the spoon. Although there is progressive improvement with practice as evidenced by less spillage, the toddler must continue to refine his use of the spoon in the next stage and beyond.

He also uses his adaptive experimental focus when drinking from a cup. The toddler has to figure out the relationship between the liquid level, gravity, the edge of the cup, and his mouth. Initially in this stage, the toddler may tilt the cup too quickly when bringing it to his mouth, and the liquid spills down the front of him. Through trial-and-error groping he learns how to adjust the tilt of his familiar cup if he looks at the level of liquid; but the toddler still has a lot to learn about the relationship between container and contained. If he is given a narrower or wider cup, he tilts it at the same familiar angle, and the liquid either spills or nothing comes out. By the end of this stage, the toddler begins to realize that the liquid level is not absolutely fixed, and he can adapt to different cups. He holds the cup with both hands and adjusts the tilt without visually monitoring the level of the liquid. The messiness of the toddler's trial-and-error experimentation is compounded by his interest in displacement—transferring food to the cup, attempting to pour milk from the cup into the bowl.

As the toddler becomes more aware that other humans and objects exist apart from him toward the end of this stage, he definitely begins to sense his own separateness. The toddler may attempt to stave off the full reality that he is alone in the world as a separate person by entering into what Mahler, Pine, and Bergman term the rapprochement subphase. Anxiety enhances the expression of attachment behaviors, and the toddler more actively elicits the caregiver's attention and involvement in his exploration. Bye-bye is now supplanted by Hi as the predominant expression. Mommy is more often vocalized in an attention-getting tone, and other directive words may be added to the toddler's vocabulary—Look! The toddler loads the caregiver's lap with toys from his shelf and shows her a new schema he has applied to one of them. A little later he comes back to share a discovery or to elicit her help with an experimental problem. There is something of a role shift; the toddler is the introducer and mediator of stimuli more frequently. He is also beginning to acquire communicative and cognitive skills that need to be rehearsed and perfected via interaction with another person.

The toddler becomes more socially engaging with other familiar persons, sharing his toys and discoveries with them. He interacts with another toddler in a rudimentary way: distant visual monitoring, smiling, vocalizing, and exploring objects in a parallel orientation. This side-by-side relationship may elicit aggressive behavior when both toddlers want the same object. In one study[39] it was found that there is a higher level of physical contact and proximal behavior if the toddlers have very frequent contact with each other and if the caregivers are attentive and actively involved in fostering interaction. There is very little proximal contact with strange toddlers. If the toddler meets an unfamiliar adult, he continues to express conflict between wariness and friendly curiosity by averting his gaze, lowering his head, and smiling with a shy, coy affect.

The toddler's sociability is egocentric in nature. He is just beginning to perceive his separateness, and the toddler is incapable of putting himself in another person's place to understand the other person's feelings. He can only rudimentarily sense that other persons have separate drives that may conflict with his and that other persons have rights of possession. The toddler's needs always occupy the center stage position, which creates conflict in his relationship with other humans at times.

Although the toddler's egocentric nature is annoying at times, this centering of attention on his needs perpetuates the attachment process. The evolvement of affective patterns in this stage outlined in Table 2-20 reflects the toddler's intertwined focus on practicing his budding autonomy with a grandiose sense of power and maintaining his bond with other humans. There is an increased need to verify this bond at the end of this stage when the toddler begins to realize that he is a small, vulnerable person.

GROWTH-FOSTERING ENVIRONMENT

The infant's graduation into toddlerhood signals a need for another menu change. The Master Chef prepares a smorgasbord in keeping with the diner's increased interest in novelty and experimentation. The assortment of food represents the right blend of free choices and nutritional precautions. Once the meal is laid out, the Chef moves from a central focal position to the wings. However, she provides assistance and support upon request.

Translating the symbolism, the caregiver expands the sensate world by baby-proofing the home environment even more stringently than in the preceding stage. She places dangerous substances inside a locked enclosure, because the toddler will learn to climb to who knows where during this stage. Special locks are placed on certain doors, hazardous tools are immediately put away after their use, precious possessions are stored away, and the backyard fence is checked for weak areas. The toddler is then free to cross over more and more thresholds.

The parents and other family members allow the toddler to practice creeping and cruising until he feels ready to take off on his own two feet. They avoid the temptation of hurrying this developmental pinnacle to increase the likelihood of congruence between emotional,

**TABLE 2-20 Evolvement of affective patterns
(Fourth Stage)**

Achieves delicate balance between a sense of oneness with the world and a
  sense of autonomy
  Practices the mastery of locomotion skills and physical realities with an
    elated mood and heightened sensorium
  Verifies caregiver's presence as an emotional anchor and spatial referent
    less frequently
More actively asserts his budding autonomy in the daily round of events
  Becomes more resistive and impatient during passive handling—diapering
  Removes easier garments albeit not always at the appropriate time
  Uses the fingers to feed himself with facility
  Uses an intermediary tool (spoon and cup) with progressively less groping
    and spillage
Balances autonomous function with a perpetuation of the attachment process
  Egocentrically assumes the center stage, hamming it up to attract and
    maintain attention
  More actively expresses needs and elicits interaction with gestures and a
    word
  Continues to react to strangers with wariness
Interacts with peers in an egocentric, rudimentary manner
  Visually monitors a peer at a distance, smiles and vocalizes
  Sits beside a peer to explore an object
  Does not understand needs, feelings, or possessive rights from the peer's
    perspective
Organizes experiences into a more coherent inner referent of his body
  Senses more subtle body movements with increased discrimination
  Orients to the back side of body during flexible rotation movements
  Senses body edges as he bumps into more unyielding objects
  Becomes more visually and tactually aware of the genital area
Attempts to stave off the awareness of his separate existence toward end of
    stage with increased attachment and proximity-seeking behaviors
  More actively elicits the caregiver's attention and involvement in his ex-
    ploration of the expanded world
  More actively elicits interaction with other familiar persons

cognitive, and motor readiness. The toddler will then more fully sense
the elation of this new expression of autonomy. When the exciting day
comes, everyone celebrates the toddler's masterful feat. When he feels
steady, the family members give the new conquerer their blessings as
he sets out to explore from a new spatial perspective.

The caregiver responds to the toddler's need to verify her availability, his need for a quick battery recharge, and his need for a lunch or
nap break. Her contingent responsiveness facilitates pleasurable forays
out in the sensate world. Mahler, Pine, and Bergman postulate that the

initial pleasurable experiences help the toddler approach new situations in a positive and confident manner, more so than any other variable.

Of course, the caregiver's eyes and ears are constantly attentive to such things as toilet swishing and too venturesome climbing. Certain limits are consistently established to protect the toddler, maintain the workability of interesting objects (dishwasher), and protect the rights of other members of the family. The caregiver intervenes with as little fanfare as possible, distracting the toddler with another interesting event if possible. However, she avoids the temptation to use food, which can upset his hunger-satiety rhythm. If the toddler is persistent, a short spontaneous play period may be the most effective distractive approach when time permits. The toddler may have to be physically removed from a situation at times and possibly placed in his playpen for a short interval when the caregiver realizes that she is losing her cool. A breaking point is a reality that the toddler gradually has to learn to deal with. However, the caregiver avoids the frequent use of restrictions that limit the flexibility of movement and expansion of the sensate world, for example, confinement in a playpen, crib, or in one room. The overall emotional tone is such that the exhilarated mood characteristic of this stage predominates. Overall, the toddler has a good feeling about the mastery of his body and the world out there.

As the toddler moves about the house and fenced yard, he is exposed to a myriad of experiences whereby he can practice tertiary circular reactions. The toddler pushes his car one way and then another way on the furnace grill. He pulls the lever and produces an interesting effect in the toilet, which he repeats. The toddler further exploits the novelty by swishing his hand in the toilet just as the caregiver appears.

The toddler also comes upon many problem-solving situations during his daily exploration, for example, a ball rolls under the couch. The caregiver facilitates the use of a tool by placing a yardstick in view. She also gets down on the toddler's level to support problem solving efforts if necessary. When the toddler drops pieces of food on the floor during lunch, the caregiver encourages him to help clean up the mess with a miniature broom and dust pan, which involves both imitation and the use of intermediary tools.

The caregiver facilitates the toddler's interest in displacing his body and objects in space and experimenting with the interrelationship between objects. He is free to move and climb within safe limits. The toddler is also allowed to explore some of the kitchen cupboards again in this stage. The caregiver makes available objects that can be combined in different arrangements—stacked, nested, piled. She collects shoe boxes, old books, large spools, and different sized caps, cans, boxes, and bowls. Assorted objects are also placed in a kitchen drawer. The caregiver rotates all the objects to provide variety. The toddler will no doubt displace objects from the drawer into a container and then back. On one day, the caregiver selects objects from the drawer that are too large for the container, if the toddler does not come upon this problem on his own. On another day, she gives him a container with a narrower opening and one or more chains which he may learn to adapt to the opening. The caregiver provides the toddler with a box that has an attached rope, a small wagon, or other object which he can load and push or pull from point to point. All the above activities raise different questions versus a more closed, set response.

The suggestions illustrate that it is not necessary to purchase a lot of expensive commercial toys. However, the toddler will enjoy receiving one or more novel toys on special occasions. He is likely to be interested in toys that involve applying a schema to one part which produces an effect on another part, for example, a surprise box. Toys that involve displacement in a number of ways also have an appeal— shape cash register, mailbox with basic form holes, a slot, and a drawer. The pounding board with balls that sink through the hole, pop out in view through another hole, and roll along a slot intrigues the toddler because of the multiple displacements. There is a variety of commercial toys that involve a contents-container relationship (animals in the barn, peg people in a bus); stacking (rings on a dowel); nesting (graded boxes); and form matching (puzzle with circular shapes).

The engrossment in locomotion and exploration does not diminish the toddler's enjoyment of spontaneous play periods. Imitation games expand to include more actions in pat-a-cake and other similar games that involve a series of gestures, correspondent identification of additional facial and body parts, and more movements to music. The caregiver also encourages imitation when the toddler is intently observing her actions at intervals during the day. She gives him a turn stirring the cake and a comb and roller for his hair. Ball play is a favorite with the toddler chasing versus catching the ball.

The caregiver still captures the toddler's interest in hiding games. He now enjoys hide-and-seek with his caregiver disappearing behind a door or couch. The toddler may initially regress and search in a privileged position; he looks where he found his caregiver the first time. She has to call or partially appear from the new position. The toddler also enjoys following visible displacements. During dressing, an object is placed in one shoe, out where he can see it, and then placed under his shirt where it is left. When the toddler can follow the sequential displacement, the direction is reversed: shoe ← shirt. A third displacement is gradually added to the sequential series: shoe → shirt → diaper. The caregiver again progresses to reversing the displacement direction: shoe ← shirt ← diaper. The toddler's delight in novelty can be exploited by successively displacing the object in the caregiver's pockets following the above progression. The game can be varied in another way by placing the object under the toddler's diaper and piling his shirt and plastic pants on top of the diaper. The object can also be placed inside a sack or easily opened box inside another sack or box. The toddler might initially become engrossed in the displacement of the obstacles in the latter two variations. An object is hidden in the toddler's shoe and dropped behind him to facilitate awareness of the back portion of his body.

Movement input is still an enjoyable part of spontaneous play. Many toddlers now enjoy being swayed up in the air faster or higher, being turned upside down to walk on their hands wheelbarrow fashion, and being placed astride the foot or back of a less secure human horse. The toddler may also enjoy being pushed in a chair swing and being placed part way up the slide on his stomach with his caregiver ready to catch him at the end. He enjoys rides in the wagon, wheelbarrow, and possibly strapped in a carrier on his caregiver's bike. He likes to push himself astride a wheeled toy and activate a rocking horse. In all the movement activities, the caregiver lets the toddler's responses determine the intensity and duration of the input.

When interacting with the toddler throughout the day, the caregiver assumes the role of responder more frequently. Contingent responsiveness to the toddler's overtures supports his budding autonomous function and helps him associate words with an immediate interest. The caregiver also adapts her verbalization to the toddler's developmental levels. She speaks more slowly, uses fewer words, and a simpler syntax which emphasizes the regular agent-action-object sequence. This highlighting facilitates the understanding of roles (initiator and recipient of actions) and word meanings.[40] The caregiver does not overdo labeling or the encouragement of word imitation. This approach can discourage the toddler's practice of spontaneous, inflective babbling in sentence units. The caregiver responds to the babbling jargon in a turn-taking sequence with a short sentence related to what she and the toddler are experiencing at the moment. She responds very positively to all the toddler's spontaneous communicative attempts via words or gestures; and she listens with a sincere desire to understand him, using all available cues. The toddler continues to get the feeling that language is powerful in causing something to happen.

During the course of daily events, the caregiver also takes advantage of opportunities to place the toddler in the role of responder so that he can practice decoding language. She sends him on simple fetching errands which feed into his toting schema. The caregiver's verbal request emphasizes key words accompanied by gestures, if necessary. She also encourages the toddler to point to labeled pictures of familiar persons in a plastic cube or album and familiar objects in a magazine or story book.

As in the previous stages, the environment has a sense of rhythm and organization. In one study[41] there were certain environmental parameters that consistently related to optimal development: temporal, regularity, low noise and confusion level, lack of overcrowding, adequate space for exploration, and environmental responsiveness to the child's actions and cues. Thus, the novelty of the toddler's exploration is balanced with a common round of daily events. The caregiver attempts for the most part to allow enough time for daily routines; this decreases episodes of frustration and irritation when the toddler asserts a desire to practice his autonomous function or insists on performing a play ritual.

The caregiver has had a lot of practice shifting gears, which helps her respond to the toddler's increased interactive overtures toward the end of this stage. She avoids re-engulfing the toddler or detaching herself in the role of a dominating teacher. Instead, the caregiver sensitively shares the toddler's discoveries and achievements, which encourages his rehearsal of evolving social, intellectual, and language skills. She also encourages his overtures with other familiar persons.

The caregiver simultaneously gives the toddler an opportunity to practice using his inner strengths to cope with separation. The caregiver braves the possible protests when she leaves and temporary rejection when she returns. She also helps the surrogate caregiver understand that if the toddler becomes subdued, efforts to cheer him will probably be of no avail or will actually interfere with his adaptive coping mechanisms. The caregiver avoids straining the toddler's coping capacities too much by just dropping him off in a strange situation, except in an emergency situation. She also adjusts the length of her absence to his tolerance level if at all possible. Some toddlers can only tolerate a few hours away from their caregiver without beginning to fall apart, whereas others can tolerate a weekend provided they are with someone they know and trust. The toddler may have a surrogate caregiver during the day. He no doubt will become accustomed to the routine as long as the parent reappears at the usual time and the surrogate caregiver is responsive to his needs.

FRAMEWORK FOR ASSESSING ABERRANT DEVELOPMENTAL AND INTERACTIVE PATTERNS

The infant with a disability is making an important developmental transition from infancy to toddlerhood, although he may be older chronologically. In keeping with the preceding stages, the assessment framework has a functional focus. In what ways does an identified impairment affect the toddler's ability to take off on his own two feet with an elated mood and a heightened responsiveness to the sensate world. What effect does an impairment have on the attachment and separation/individuation process.

The developmental transition may be imbedded in a very supportive matrix. Family members are emotionally attached to the toddler, and the parents have a nurturing and yet realistic caregiving perspective. Although they are inclined to view two key milestones (walking and talking) as the most salient measures of the child's developmental progress and functional potential, the parents are able to maintain a balanced emphasis with the support of consultation resources. Their child senses that the world will hold him just as his parents have held and nurtured him, and he ventures out in the role of an experimenter when *he* feels ready.

Effect of an Aberrant Response Threshold and a Disturbed Relationship

On the other hand, there may continue to be a disturbance in human relationships or the toddler's response pattern that prevents him from experiencing the true measure of exhilaration and omnipotence characteristic of this stage of development. The toddler with a very permeable stimulus barrier may continue to have a low frustration level, which interferes with the evolvement of more focused exploratory and problem-solving behaviors. If the toddler learns to walk, he is easily overloaded by all the novel experiences, expressed by escalated disorganization, motor disinhibition, and receptor fatigue. The toddler may quickly move from one stimulus to another in a reckless manner, and he may experience anxiety about running away with himself if he has not been helped to control volatile state changes and escalating behavior in a very effective manner. The disorganized movement increases the risk of mishaps, and the toddler may overreact to injuries. The caregiver may respond to mishaps with negativism, physical punishment, and mobility restrictions.

It may be that restless, albeit less reckless, movement is evoked by confusing internal stimuli. The toddler does not receive accurate feedback from his own movements, and he never quite knows where his body is in space or if he or the world is moving. His energy is always divided between trying to make sense of internal and external stimuli.

The toddler with a low response threshold is dependent on his caregiver as a stimulus barrier. A disturbed relationship may compound the dependency because the toddler is very unsure about the caregiver's accessibility. He frequently seeks proximity, and distress reactions quickly escalate to a crying state. The toddler may strongly resist separation and any attempts to console him during the caregiver's absence. He may also resist his caregiver's attempts at consolation when she returns, or he may insist on remaining in close proximity for a long interval. The toddler may express a disturbed relationship in another way. He gives up attempts to seek pleasurable proximity, and his behavior becomes resistive or ignoring in nature. The toddler may indiscriminately accept care from anyone albeit in his temperamental way.[42]

At the other end of the continuum is the toddler with a relatively impermeable stimulus barrier. If he learns to walk, he may confront a minimal number of stimulus events which elevate his arousal level. The toddler wanders around rather aimlessly, too unwary of strangeness and novelty. He may have a very minimal awareness of danger, which increases accident proneness. However, he under-reacts to an injury because of a high threshold to pain. The toddler's explorative behavior may still be characterized by more gross actions because of a lack of emotional support and encouragement, slow processing of novel features, or low muscle tone, which interferes with the evolvement of more differentiated arm, hand, and finger movements.

The toddler with a high threshold is also very dependent on his caregiver for environmental mediation but in a different way. The stimulation level needs to be revved up. The toddler may be most alert when his father is in the role of caregiver and engages him in excitable play. His father provides the stronger, arrhythmic, intermittent stimuli that the toddler needs to alert his nervous system and increase his responsiveness to the environment.

The toddler's reaction to being left by his caregiver may still be attenuated in this stage. He immediately responds to the friendly overtures of a stranger, and the return of his caregiver elicits minimal proximity-seeking behavior.[43] Or the toddler may begin to respond to a strange situation with signs of stress and attachment behaviors.[44] His timetable was delayed compared with the so-called norm.

A weak affective component can affect the separation/individuation process and other areas of development, irrespective of whether the toddler has a low or high stimulus threshold. He may continue to be preoccupied with the caregiver's whereabouts rather than mastery of motor skills and physical realities in the sensate world. The toddler may have a sense of powerlessness and a lack of confidence that he has any control over what happens to him. Or he may sense the lack of a beacon to light the way and sculpt the world in a safe circle. The toddler's vocalization may be limited and out of synchrony with his caregiver's activity and other environmental events, because communicative signals have minimal interactive meaning. He is not motivated to imitate words, nor does he view a word as an effective means to an end.

There is the other extreme in a disturbed relationship as discussed in the preceding stage. The toddler may be smothered with nurturing attention, which also interferes with the practice of autonomous function. Upright mobility signifies an end of the caregiver's possessiveness of her infant. She may hover over the toddler and intrude on his attempts to practice the role of explorer instead of providing encouragement from the wings. The toddler becomes cautious and reluctant to venture out, and he may over-react to falls and other obstacles when he musters the courage to take off on a short foray.

The caregiver may have difficulty shifting gears if the toddler, irrespective of the nature of his disability, evolves to the rapprochement subphase and attempts to woo her back into his circle. The results of one study[45] suggest that the disabled toddler demonstrates this behavior as much as or more than the normal toddler. The caregiver may not allow the toddler to be the introducer and mediator of stimuli, because she is too entrenched in this role, or she may view the wooing behavior as regressive. There is the danger of two contrasting responses: pushing the toddler back out on his own or re-engulfing him to reinstate the bliss of oneness.[46]

Effect of Sensory Impairments

Some of the ways sensory impairments affect the toddler's interaction with his caregiver and objects have been discussed in the above paragraphs. Also, many of the impairments described in Stage III continue to affect the toddler's development and can be reviewed by the reader to avoid repetition of content. The following discussion will further delineate the effect of a loss of sensory function or an impairment of sensory function on developmental patterns in this stage.

VISUAL IMPAIRMENT. If the child has a total loss of vision or very minimal vision, mobility patterns will very probably continue to evolve via a different timetable. If the child forms a match between sound and touch toward the end of the preceding stage or the beginning of this stage, he may soon thereafter begin to creep toward a sound cue which now signifies the presence of a substantive animate or inanimate object out there. The impetus of a sound cue may shorten the interval between the assumption of the standing position and mobility. Even so, walking is generally delayed. If the child takes off on his own two feet toward the end of this stage and becomes a toddler, he has to go through a tedious process of remapping space one step at a time in the new upright orientation. The toddler lacks the most efficient receptor for filling spatial gaps and monitoring the flux in the environment which requires an adaptation—chair moved in a different place. It is no wonder that the toddler with a severe visual impairment is a more cautious explorer.

A more coherent representation of animate and inanimate objects also comes about in a more laborious way through tactual, auditory, and kinesthetic exploration of unique features. The toddler has to rely solely on his own movement to learn that objects undergo various displacements in space independent of his actions, since he cannot see movement; and experimentation with bodily displacement is more limited with the delayed emergence of mobility skills. Thus, an elementary concept of the permanence of animate and inanimate objects and the relationship of one object to another may continue to emerge more slowly.

Labeling is likewise delayed because of the inability to coordinate input from the two most efficient distance receptors—visual and auditory. The toddler also continues to assume the more passive role of responder during most of this stage rather than the initiator of communication. He has no visual cue of the presence of an object or a person. He uses auditory cues to belatedly practice distancing and proximity seeking when he begins to recognize the caregiver's objective existence. He listens for his caregiver's voice to verify her presence, and he intermittently comes back to home base. He also belatedly expresses separation anxiety. The toddler may exhibit a high level of distress, because he cannot visually latch onto reminders of his caregiver's presence in a familiar environment nor can he readily map the new space in a strange environment.

Dysfunctions of the visual system described in the preceding stage continue to interfere with the evolvement of more elaborate schemas. A peripheral or central impairment may become more observable in this stage when the toddler attempts to engage in more focused exploration. He may hold objects up close or farther away or tilt his head to one side. The toddler may turn his head when a moving object approaches him. His behavior may become disorganized when he begins walking and is confronted with a new array of visual stimuli. If there is an imbalance of eye muscles (strabismus), it is impossible for both eyes to focus on the object at the same time; and the toddler has to learn to compensate by focusing with one eye, which negates three-dimensional vision. He does not realize that he has a problem at this early age, because he senses that everyone sees the way he does. The toddler compensates for the strabismus and other dysfunctions at a price that may be expressed by eye itching, eye blurring, dizziness, headache, and even nausea.

AUDITORY IMPAIRMENT. A permanent or fluctuating hearing loss continues to deprive the toddler of the important auditory link in the feedback loop. If the toddler has a fluctuating loss, he may receive enough auditory input to derive the meaning of certain words with the help of contextual cues. However, the lack of constancy of auditory cues may cause confusion regarding the meaning of some words. The toddler also misses stress patterns that highlight certain words; he therefore has more difficulty conceptualizing the role of agent and recipient of an action in this stage and the subsequent stage. The toddler does not hear linguistic boundaries that serve as the basis for practicing babbling sentence units and rudimentary turn taking. He is also deprived of the deluge of auditory information, even if he has a fluctuating loss, which is initially needed to produce words effectively. The toddler may only hear part of a word, since there is a 30 decibel difference between some vowel and consonant sounds.[47] The toddler continues to miss and confuse emotional cues in the speech of others; thus, he has a limited ability to express affect in appropriate ways. His voice has a monotone quality and may be too loud or too soft.

The toddler has a more limited awareness of temporal series, which interferes with an emerging concept of the coherence of objects in time and the formation of certain means-end relationships and expectancies. For example, the toddler does not hear his caregiver's voice, her footsteps, and the turn of a doorknob that signal her impending arrival when he is involved in a no-no.

If the toddler with a hearing loss also has a vestibular dysfunction, he has a more vague sense of where he is in space. Walking may be delayed, or his gait may remain very unstable. A superimposed impairment increases the likelihood that the caregiver will describe the toddler's behavior with adjectives frequently associated with a child who is deaf: overpossessive, restless, and disobedient. A more negative perception may especially coincide with the evolvement of bipedal locomotion if the toddler also has a vestibular impairment. He is confronted with new internal and external input which he cannot make sense of or cope with in an organized way. There is the risk of a stressed relationship with the caregiver and frequent restrictive intrusion.

As discussed in the previous stage, the toddler may have normal hearing acuity, but he has difficulty making sense of input. Sound may continue to be a noiselike wave of confusion that causes a sensory overload and disorganized behavior. Or the toddler may act as though he is deaf at times and respond at other times because of his poor ability to localize sound in space or his difficulty in processing auditory stimuli. The toddler may not have the capacity to coordinate what he is seeing or feeling with a particular auditory stimulus; he cannot form cross-modal associations. He may have difficulty processing rapidly changing, dynamic sounds and sequencing rapid auditory events. Words spoken at the normal pace may therefore be incomprehensible. Or the words may sound like Donald Duck talk, and some toddlers speak with this tempo no doubt reflecting what they hear. The toddler may be able to understand speech presented at a slower pace.[48,49]

VESTIBULAR IMPAIRMENT. The importance of antigravity adjustments becomes even more apparent in this stage when the toddler learns to walk. If he has a vestibular dysfunction, he may have difficulty mastering this feat which was briefly discussed in the above section. The toddler may not adjust to gravitational shifts with a more mature equilibrium response in the lower positions; he either goes with the force of gravity or quickly changes to another position. He therefore lacks the armamentarium to cope with the stress of shifting weight to one foot and maintaining dynamic balance while moving the other leg forward. However, the drive to develop is strong, and the toddler may learn to walk by relying more heavily on the visual and proprioceptive senses to monitor where he is in space. The toddler keeps his eyes on the floor and fixes the proximal muscles. The walking pattern reflects the stress superimposed by the vestibular impairment: very rigid trunk and pelvis, very wide base of support, and an exaggerated pivot prone position of the arms. The toddler falls frequently, possibly in a splattered way, because he does not realize that he is falling until he hits or almost hits the surface. Protective responses are either delayed or absent. The toddler may veer to one side, and he may also bump into objects because of a distorted sense of movement in space. His face may look battered most of the time. The toddler has difficulty walking in the dark and on uneven surfaces because of a decreased ability to substitute vestibular cues for visual and proprioceptive cues. He may avoid climbing and other movements that involve gravitational shifts.

At the other end of the continuum, the toddler may sense only more intense vestibular input, and he seeks movement. The toddler spins himself around in a sitting position, walks around in a circle, and enjoys motor play involving fast movements. He also wants to swing or stay on the merry-go-round for a longer interval than other toddlers.

TACTILE AND PROPRIOCEPTIVE IMPAIRMENTS. If the tactile and proprioceptive systems are dysfunctional, the toddler lacks the higher-order sensory processing capabilities necessary to refine his motor performance. He is more vaguely aware of the position of his fingers, feet, tongue, and other body parts at a particular point in time. The toddler's movements remain poorly planned and clumsy, and he may assume rather strange positions. The delay in the evolvement of more differentiated movements interferes with the toddler's ability to explore objects in more elaborate and experimental ways, form words, walk, and climb to new heights.

If the protective withdrawal response has not become more selective, the toddler's overall behavior will no doubt continue to be protective in nature. He may maintain a wide personal space, prefer to touch rather than be touched, walk on his toes, over-react when he falls or bumps into an obstacle, become very upset during his first haircut, and resist foods that do not have a bland texture.

If the toddler has a high receptor threshold, he is more responsive to intense tactual input as discussed in the preceding stage. He enjoys having his hair cut, feeling the fuzzy pet, and other forms of input that the toddler with a low threshold avoids. He may have a low sensitivity to pain, responding to falls and injurious mishaps in a very attenuated manner.

Summary

It is evident that especially if the toddler has more than one sensory impairment, he will not assume the role of conquerer with an exhilarated mood and a heightened sensorium comparable with that of a nondisabled toddler. He has to map alternate, slower routes; and it takes longer to learn about the unique properties of objects and realities in the sensate world. If the toddler has difficulty coordinating input and movements, this affects his ability to create varied effects and devise new means to achieve a goal via trial-and-error experimentation. A weaker conceptualization of means-end relationships and outside causal sources may impede language development. The toddler has more difficulty recognizing relationships that exist between words and the context. He may also have a more limited ability to generalize a word to other objects that share common features, if he cannot explore the unique properties of objects in more focused and elaborate ways. Sensory impairments may intertwine with other organic impairments to limit the toddler's ability to refine movements and coordinate a number of dimensions or functions at one time. He cannot begin to reach or point, vocalize, and look at an adult to express a need. The toddler continues to rely more heavily on gestural communication.[50,51] A world of relationships is evolving more slowly because of an interruption in the network of sensory systems.

Effect of Motor Impairments

The infant may lack the background components for the transition to toddlerhood because of motor impairments that cannot in reality be separated from sensory impairments. There is the broader issue of a balance between areas of development. Ideally, the toddler's beginning awareness that other persons and objects exist apart from him and his behavior parallels the evolvement of upright mobility (walking). However, there is the risk of an imbalance between the toddler's social/emotional, cognitive, language, and motor development when he has a disability with all the ramifications discussed earlier.

Looking more narrowly at the motor skill itself, the toddler may lack some or all of the following background components that signify a readiness for walking: (1) pelvic mobility in all three planes; (2) proximal stability in the sitting position (hips aligned with the shoulders and the extended legs aligned with the hips); (3) mature equilibrium reactions in the sitting position; (4) rotational dissociation of the pelvis from the shoulder in the sitting position and when creeping and changing from one position to another; (5) dissociation of the legs from the pelvis and one leg from another when creeping and pulling to a standing position; (6) proximal stability in the supported standing position (hips aligned with the shoulders and direct weight bearing down over the knee and foot); and (7) a flexible cruising pattern with a weight shift to the lateral border of the foot. Thus, there is a lot of preparation that leads to the pinnacle of motor functions when the toddler lets go with his arms and only feels a source of support with the bottom of his small feet. He must then shift weight to one small foot and step forward to walk.

COMPENSATORY WALKING PATTERNS. If the infant has hypertonia, he may never become a toddler. He cannot develop sufficient normal muscle strength and balance to maintain his body in an upright position. Or the infant may not be able to assume a standing position because of contractures that developed from sitting in a W position with the knees very flexed and the ankles extended. The child may adapt the W-sit position to walk on his knees.

If there is less abnormal tone in the arms and trunk than in the legs, the child with hypertonia may learn to walk. He compensates for the more involved parts by excessive use of the less involved parts— head, upper trunk, and arms. The toddler flexes the lateral surface of the trunk to raise one leg and bring it forward. He leans his head and trunk forward to transfer his weight, and the internally rotated, stiff legs are carried along by the mobility of the upper body. The legs are adducted, and the toddler walks on his toes with the body weight on the inside of the feet, which narrows the base of support. The steps are short and tripping in nature with a forward momentum as the toddler seems to fall from one leg to the other (Figs. 2-49A and B). Toe walking is an adaptive means of maintaining extension in the legs to stay upright. If the toddler dorsiflexed the foot, this may elicit flexor tone in the whole leg, and he would collapse. The toddler may be able to stop walking only by falling down, because he cannot stand still without holding on to a support. The stress of walking may increase abnormal tone to the point that the legs and feet cross. The stress may also elicit an ATNR response with the head turned to one side. The arm on the face side is extended, and the arm on the occipital side is flexed.

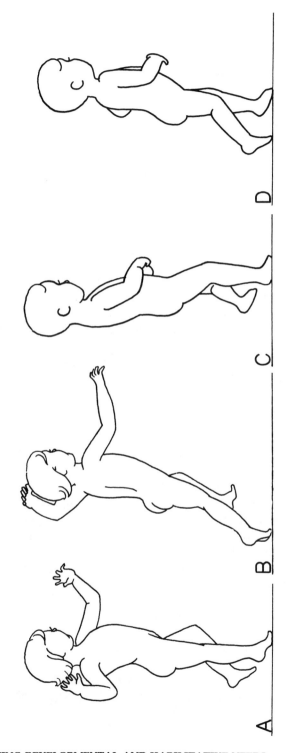

FIGURE 2-49. (A and B) The child with more involvement in the lower extremities learns to walk primarily by using less hypertonic upper body parts to move forward. (C and D). The child with more active flexor muscles uses a pigeonlike backward and forward bodily lean to lift the foot and step forward.

The toddler with more active flexor muscles may compensate in a different way. He walks with the upper trunk, arms, hips, and legs in a more flexed position. The toddler has to lean backward with his trunk to raise the leg and step forward, which tilts the pelvis posteriorly. He then moves his body forward to transfer the weight at the end of the swing phase (Fig. 2-49C and D). The pattern resembles the movements of a pigeon.

If the child has fluctuating tone (athetosis) and the lower extremities become more involved, he may not make the motor transition to toddlerhood. When the feet touch the surface, the input elicits a total extensor pattern with neck and shoulder retraction, stiff extension of the legs with weight on the toes, and possibly even scissoring as illustrated in Figure 2-37A, Stage III. However, if the lower extremities remain mobile and less involved than the upper extremities, the toddler may learn to walk in a compensatory way. He hyperextends the hips and knees and leans the trunk and shoulders backward to reinforce the extensor tone, which keeps him upright and prevents a collapse into flexion. The toddler controls the tendency to thrust backward in an exaggerated fashion by internally rotating the arms and extending them in front of the body. He may also internally rotate the legs. The toddler steps with wooden-soldierlike shuffling movements that involve only a slight weight shift to maintain the extensor pattern. The toes may contact the surface first because of the continued influence of the positive support reflex. The toddler is then able to dorsiflex his foot and contact the floor with the sole surface. He may fix with the medial border of one or both feet to provide added distal stability. The arms may move somewhat more to one side and then the other side in a pendulum effect as the toddler walks. The head moves from flexion to extension during the swing phase with the chin pointed upward (Fig. 2-50A and B).

If hypotonicity predominates in the tonal fluctuation pattern, the toddler may also learn to walk but with a different compensatory pattern that resembles the initial normal gait. There is exaggerated hip flexion and dorsiflexion of the ankle, which creates a high-stepping effect. The arm on the swing leg side extends backward to counteract the exaggerated flexion. The toddler hyperextends and throws back the support leg to compensate for the lack of stability. The upper back is rounded, and the chin juts forward. The weight is transferred forward with a lurching body movement that increases the anterior pelvic tilt (Fig. 2-50C and D).

If the infant has marked hypotonia, he may also not learn to walk. He lacks sufficient muscular strength to support himself in an upright position and to shift stability demands to one foot and leg. The infant with less marked hypotonia may toddle in an exaggerated way if

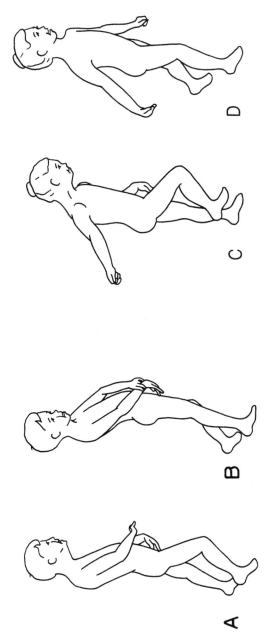

FIGURE 2-50. (*A* and *B*) The child with fluctuating tone adapts an extensor pattern to walk with a shuffling gait. (*C* and *D*) If there is a predominance of hypotonicity as the tone fluctuates, the child walks with a high-stepping effect.

he has lax ligaments and very hyperflexible joints. The legs widely abduct and externally rotate, the knees hyperextend, and the toes may curl in an attempt to increase distal stability. The ankles pronate, which shifts the center of gravity inward. The gait resembles a duck waddle because of the wide weight shift from side to side and excessive pelvic mobility. The weak hip musculature does not provide sufficient proximal stability. The shoulders are shrugged because of the tendency to fixate in the midline as a compensation for weak muscles. The arms may assume a rather aberrant high-guard position (Fig. 2-51). The toddler may have to rely on a support to pull up to standing for a longer period because of weak musculature in the trunk, hips, and legs and immature equilibrium reactions. He may also have difficulty standing back up after squatting.

The toddler with hypertonia or fluctuating tone may not be able to lift his head and trunk into an extended standing position out in the middle of the floor, or he may be very delayed in mastering this skill. Likewise, the toddler cannot grade movements to assume a flexed squat position and raise back up to an extended position. The toddler with hypertonia may experience muscular resistance and discomfort when he tries to flex his hips, knees, and ankles simultaneously to squat.

The infant may not have abnormal muscle tone, but he precociously begins walking with very little preliminary practice in creeping and cruising. Or he primarily practiced mobility in a walker. The tod-

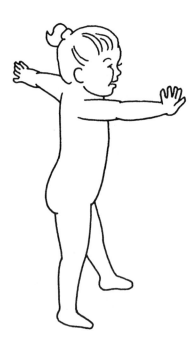

FIGURE 2-51. The child with hypotonia begins walking with a wide-based, exaggerated, toddling gait.

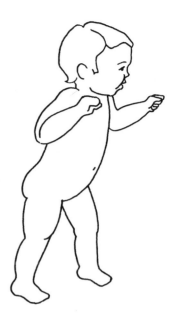

FIGURE 2-52. The early walking pattern is qualitatively different from the norm if the toddler without abnormal tone walks before he is ready.

dler's initial gait may differ from the norm in a number of ways. He compensates for inadequate midline stability and immature equilibrium reactions with a stronger positive support response of the legs and possibly toe curling in an attempt to increase distal stability. There is a more forward inclination of the trunk and more flexion at the hip joints. The legs are more abducted with a greater degree of out-toeing, and the arms are in a more fixated, pivot prone position. The toddler walks with more superfluous weight shifting because of the wider base of support, and leg movements are stiffer with less flexion of the knee during the swing phase (Fig. 2-52).

Summary

It is evident from the above descriptions that the disabled toddler's adaptiveness is rather incredible. He uses all the resources that he has, including primitive reflex patterns, to master the feat of walking. The compensations reinforce abnormal patterns that can cause deformities: scoliosis, flexor contracture of the hips, knees, elbows, wrists, and fingers; equinovarus or equinovalgus deformity of the ankle and foot from toe-walking and turning the sole inward or outward, and subluxation or dislocation of one or both hips. If the toddler with athetosis has low postural tone, he is not likely to develop contractures. However, there is the risk of subluxation or dislocation of the mandible, finger, shoulder, and hip joints because of the excess mobility. Although walking with a crude gait poses problems, confinement in a wheelchair or the use of braces and crutches may also cause complications, and the adaptive mobility aids increase the child's dependency. This again is a habilitative dilemma. It is felt that early specialized therapy facilitates a less compensatory pattern, especially if the emphasis is on preparation for walking versus hurrying the acquisition of this skill.

A toddler who walks with a compensatory gait does not experience the same sensations as the toddler who does not have a disability. The center of gravity is more deviant, which gives him a different sense of his anatomic midline as a reference point for movement. He does not have the same awareness of his lower extremities, because he does not sense weight bearing and movement over the limb to the same degree. The disabled toddler may not view his genital area from a new vantage point. The male lacks the steadiness to lean over and examine his penis when standing and walking, and the female lacks the flexibility to lean over and visually examine her genital area when squatting or sitting. The disabled toddler's sense of body/self is therefore different and very possibly less coherent. A comparison of some of the above described compensatory patterns with even the fledgling initial walking gait of the nondisabled toddler (Fig. 2-53) illustrates some of the differences in terms of the orientation of body parts, the degree of fixation, and the walking movement.

The compensations represent a wasteful expenditure of energy because of excess movement or an inability to inhibit some of the cocontraction and thus reduce the overactivity of muscles. The toddler may fatigue very fast, because he runs out of aerobic fuel after walking a short distance. His oxidative capacities are limited if there is an inadequacy of one or more of the following transport links: capacity of the heart and respiratory muscles to work, capacity of the blood to carry oxygen including the circulatory hemoglobin level and blood volume, and the extraction capacity of active muscles.[52]

The tolerance for activity is further decreased when other conditions are superimposed on the compensatory walking pattern. Chronic respiratory infections interfere with the air flow, and certain cardiac diseases limit the ability to adapt to increased energy demands. Excess fat in and around the chest wall provides resistance, which decreases the efficiency of the respiratory muscles. Thus, the overweight toddler walks with a higher physiologic cost.

EFFECT OF MOTOR IMPAIRMENT ON EXPLORATIVE SCHEMAS.
Competing physiologic demands affect the toddler's ability to take on the role of a conqueror and experimenter with gusto. He has difficulty remaining in an alert, attentive state to explore the potential of an object more fully and devise a new means through trial-and-error experimen-

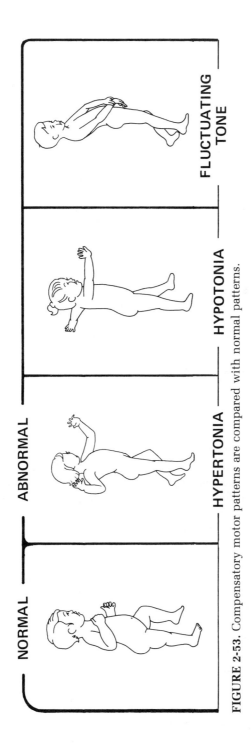

FIGURE 2-53. Compensatory motor patterns are compared with normal patterns.

NORMAL

ABNORMAL

HYPERTONIA

HYPOTONIA

FLUCTUATING TONE

tation. The effortful and awkward mobility patterns also limit displacement of the body and objects in different spatial-temporal series. The toddler may have to keep his arms in a high guard protective position. Or he may have to use his arms and hands to operate crutches or another assistive device. The toddler therefore cannot tote an object from A to B and then back to A. Clumsy upper extremity movements limit his ability to map different arrangements and study how objects relate to each other in space (stack, nest, place in and out, rotate, and reverse). If the toddler lacks a framework of spatial experiences, he may not seriate events to follow multiple, visible displacements of an object and his caregiver.

If the toddler cannot explore his world in more elaborate ways and derive new intermediary means, he may have a more vague awareness of external causal sources. He does not find out that the stick must touch the object to move it, which dilutes the notion of efficacy phenomenalism. The toddler also misses experiences that help him realize that he can be the recipient of a cause as well as the cause. In fact, the toddler may not even view himself as a causal agent because of his limited ability to elicit environmental results all along the continuum of development and feel a sense of power. An illusion of omnipotence precedes the beginning transference of power to other animate and inanimate objects.

EFFECT OF MOTOR IMPAIRMENTS ON ORAL AND RESPIRATORY PATTERNS. As discussed earlier, the toddler may have weak respiratory muscles and a limited vital capacity. He may also lack the necessary neuromuscular control to coordinate the activity of respiratory muscles. The toddler cannot regulate the level of airway pressure and the air flow to expand his utterance to a jargon sentence or assert himself with a louder tone. He may not form the fricative h consonant sound, which requires increased intercostal activity and an air flow four to five times the value of b, d, g.[53]

The lack of coordination interferes with the emerging force and counterforce interplay of muscles with one group pulling or pushing against the resistance provided by another group to increase efficiency. If there is an imbalance of rib cage and abdominal forces, effort is dissipated pushing out the lax abdominal wall or pulling up the thoracic floor. If there is a weak interplay, the rib cage and abdominal muscles cannot begin to adjust the geometry of the respiration system to offset the forces of gravity in the upright position and keep the muscle fibers of the diaphragm optimally tuned. The thorax cannot take over more of the workload to execute a deeper inspiration and prevent the diaphragm from descending too much. A very lax abdomen cannot prevent the diaphragm from being driven footward by rib cage expiratory forces. Thus, the complex mechanisms are lacking to prevent excess flattening of the diaphragm, and the muscle fibers are at a mechanical disadvantage. The inspiratory phase is therefore longer, which impedes the trend toward a longer expiratory phase during vocalization.[54,55]

Anxiety and tension from a feeling of unsteadiness or from pressure to walk before the toddler is ready may tighten pectoral and neck muscles. The tension shrugs the shoulders and juts the head and chin forward, which distorts the airflow and oral movements, especially at the front of the mouth. Anxiety or tension also affect the regularity of respirations.

If the toddler has difficulty dissociating larger movements, he very probably will also continue to have difficulty dissociating oral movements. The toddler may attempt to use the jaw as the main articulator rather than the tongue, which results in sound distortions. There may still be a lot of movement in the jaw when he drinks from a cup and licks an ice cream cone. The toddler may have difficulty moving his tongue in all directions and moving the tongue without moving the lips. There may still be a forward movement of the tongue when the toddler makes certain sounds, chews, and swallows.

With the lack of important components, the toddler's vocalization may not take on the form of early language that initiates interaction with the caregiver and fosters the attachment process. His babbling utterance is shorter, and the vowel and consonant sounds are more distorted. The voice quality may be breathy, too soft, or arrhythmic. The toddler has a limited ability to enhance the meaning of his vocalization by varying the loudness and the pitch.

FRAMEWORK FOR HABILITATIVE APPROACHES

This may be a rather stressful period for the family. The parents and siblings may become anxious about the evolvement of walking and talking. Yet, the parents may have mixed feelings. It is difficult for them to visualize their fragile infant or their rather passive infant making the transition to toddlerhood and becoming more independent. Or they may be concerned about their very restless, reactive infant's increased potential of creating chaos in the home and severely injuring himself. Or the parents may wonder if their motor impaired infant will ever learn to walk and become more independent. They may wonder if their disabled infant will ever be able to communicate with them in a more functional way.

There may be a need for more support from extended family members, friends, and professional interveners. In a longitudinal study which extended over the first one-and-a-half years,[56] the father's relationship with his parents was the most important variable. If the father felt that his parents were very supportive, he had more positive feelings toward his disabled child, interacted with the child more frequently, and felt good about the changes in himself. The mother's positive feelings were related to a broader social support network that included her husband's parents. A more formal professional support system did not have a significant impact on the adjustment of either the father or mother. The findings also suggest that there may be a trade-off. When the parents relate to their developmentally disabled child in positive ways, they internalize some of the stress of the parenting demands evidenced by physical symptoms and more negative feelings about their marital relationship. The father has more symptoms of stress, and he perceives the child as having a disruptive influence on the marriage.

These findings emphasize the importance of placing the professional relationship with the family in the proper perspective as just one aspect of a network of supportive resources. The intervener must sensitively recognize priority shifts in terms of the needs of the disabled child, his parents, and other family members, and use these shifts as the basis for dynamically adjusting the intervention focus. Thus, the intervener makes every attempt to avoid placing an imbalanced emphasis on the developmentally disabled child, which can disrupt his status as an integrated member of the family unit.

Although the parents may feel a need for more support during this transitional stage, they probably are becoming more independent in some ways if there has been a collaborative relationship with the primary intervener. The parents feel more confident in their own common sense and intuition, and they are less dependent on the intervener to help them read their child's signals and cues. Nor do they interpret or use information they hear or read in an unquestioning or generalized way. The needs of their individual child provide the framework for determining the appropriateness and relevance of information and suggestions.

The intervener more clearly senses the lifestyle of the family and the types of activities that are enjoyable. She uses this familiarity to create a better match between habilitative suggestions and the individual qualities of the child and his family. Thus, the activities in the following pages provide a framework for individual adaptations that have a unique character.

Approaches to Facilitate Evolvement of Bipedal Locomotion and More Elaborate Explorative Schemas

Approaches will be outlined in this section to facilitate the following habilitative outcomes if the toddler has hypotonia or immature motor development.

- Develops increased proximal stability.
- Walks on the knees with a more refined reciprocal movement.
- Coordinates lower extremity and rotational trunk movements to cruise around a corner.
- Develops increased strength in the lower extremities and somatosensory awareness of the legs and feet.
- Stands without support.
- Superimposes mobility on dynamic stability to begin walking.
- Develops increased endurance.
- Experiences pleasurable forays in a mediated environment.
- Organizes his movements in a series of spatial displacements.
- Develops a beginning understanding of object interrelationships.
- Intentionally creates varied effects through tertiary circular reactions.
- Devises new means to achieve a goal, including an intermediary means.
- Begins to transfer power to external causal forces.
- Groups objects and actions together in the natural environment.
- Imitates novel visible and invisible actions, words, and intonations.

Since walking may have a high priority habilitative status during this stage, the intervener helps the parents understand all the developmental parameters involved in readiness. I have found that parents are very responsive to this approach. Quality is a meaningful criterion, because parents want their child to walk with a gait that corresponds to the norm to the extent possible. They see this as an asset in view of integrative, mainstreaming trends.

If the child has hypertonia or fluctuating tone, specialized therapy will no doubt be required to foster a less compensatory gait. Facilitation and inhibition have to be applied in the right places at the right time. If there is a distance problem in terms of available resources, the primary intervener can work very closely with a specialized team in a regional center to help the parents implement a habilitative program. Mobility patterns are becoming too complex to provide interim suggestions that may be helpful.

If the child has hypotonia or an immature motor pattern without evidence of abnormal tone, the caregiver can experiment with a number of activities to help the child develop readiness for walking. This focus will increase the likelihood that the child will experience an elated mood when he takes off on his own two feet. The caregiver involves the child in activities described in this section in preceding stages if the quality of background components is still marginal. The activities may have to be varied some because of the child's increased size and developmental level. For example, there may still be a need to strengthen proximal muscles in the shoulders, trunk, and hips. The pivot prone response can now be facilitated by placing the child on his stomach over a large bolster or beach ball and rocking him forward as rapidly as he can tolerate (Fig. 2-54A). This response is not facilitated if it is aberrant in ways described in Stage II. This may be a sign of undiagnosed pathology.

If the child has a rather slow protective response and weakness in the shoulder, arm, and back muscles, he may enjoy another activity. The child is held by the caregiver and tipped downward to elicit protective arm extension. Or the child can be placed in a prone position on a small bolster or ball and rocked forward. He may develop enough strength to hand-walk toward an object, shift weight to one arm, and place the ring on a low dowel (Fig. 2-54B). If the child is on the bolster or ball, the caregiver rolls it forward as the child hand-walks forward. He may initially have to rely on a ball or bolster for support to hand-walk if his shoulder girdle and arm muscles are weaker.

The child is spontaneously engaged in other activities during the day to increase his endurance and the strength of proximal and upper extremity muscles. He may imitatively assume a forearm support position on his stomach to look at pictures of familiar persons in an album with another family member. He is also encouraged to creep imitatively a longer distance with a sibling or his caregiver to take socks to a drawer or tote other objects. An increased creeping speed is encouraged at times by a catch game, which exercises ventilatory muscles. The child's fatigue level is closely monitored as a gauge for the intensity and duration of the game.

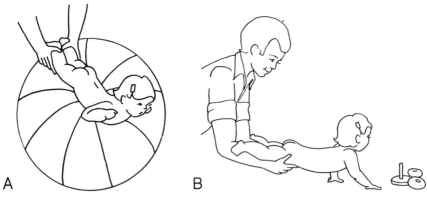

FIGURE 2-54. (A) The pivot prone response is elicited with a forward movement of the ball. (B) After the child is tipped downward to elicit protective extension of the arms, he is helped to hand-walk toward an object.

Readiness for bipedal locomotion is further facilitated by encouraging the child to practice reciprocal leg movements on his knees down closer to the center of gravity. Knee-walking is intertwined with an activity that fosters a tertiary circular reaction if the child has a tendency to habitually focus on one action when exploring objects— push a car in a certain way. An incline is formed by placing a board, foam wedge, or firm sofa pillow at the end of a coffee table or other low piece of furniture; and a container is placed at the end of the incline (Fig. 2-55). Various objects (big ball, small ball, big wheeled pull toy, small car) are placed on the other end of the table. The caregiver encourages the child to knee-walk over to obtain an object and walk back to roll the object down the incline if he does not do so on his own. The child may experiment with the way he rolls the one object even trying to roll it up the incline, or he may try all the objects and find that each of them creates a different effect in terms of the sound, speed, and other characteristics. The activity can be varied by placing an upturned box at the end of the runway with a hole in it so that the object can roll inside the box. The child has to see the object disappear in the box to search and retrieve it, because he very probably can only follow visible displacements in this stage. As the child moves between the table, ramp, and container, he practices assuming different positions and moving in different ways (knee-walking, creeping, sitting), which is a desirable outcome. The toddler who is not disabled frequently changes his position when exploring objects.

The activity is adapted somewhat if the child has a visual impairment. He is lured to knee-walk toward an object at the end of the table with a sound cue. The caregiver then moves over to the incline and vocally encourages the child to knee-walk toward her, and she helps

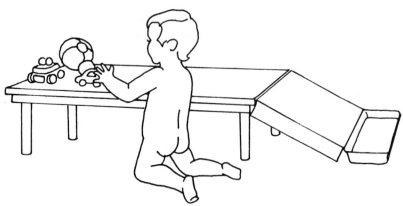

FIGURE 2-55. The child is engaged in an activity to facilitate knee-walking and tertiary circular reactions.

him roll the object down the incline. The child is encouraged to knee-walk back to the first location with a sound cue from a different object. He may move back on his own to roll the second object down and create a new auditory effect. The caregiver gradually includes objects that have a more subtle sound trajectory.

There may be a tendency to help too much or take over, which gives the child the idea that there are certain acceptable ways to experiment with an object. He will subordinate his actions to the caregiver's wishes rather than subordinating his actions to explore the potential of the object. If the child's frustration or fatigue level is low, he may give up very easily. The caregiver unobtrusively provides some supportive assistance by moving the objects on the other end of the table over closer to the ramp or even by retrieving an object for the child to roll down again. A longer period of sustained attention is an important goal and justifies the added support.

As the child practices knee-walking, he develops increased midline stability, which serves as the background for more reliable equilibrium reactions and a more refined reciprocal movement. An adaptation of the catch the baby game provides an enjoyable way for the child to practice adjusting to a gravitational shift. He is nudged from side to side and forward and backward by trusted family members. Elements of the game can also be incorporated in the bath routine. The caregiver taps the child's shoulders or hips from side to side when she is drying him after the bath (Fig. 2-56). She also progresses to tapping him backward and forward, preventing him from falling either way. The child will gradually become less reliant on the alternate tapping as he begins to make the adjustment back to midline in the kneeling position.

The child is also engaged in activities that facilitate refinement of the cruising pattern, expansion of perceptual experiences, and awareness of the spatial relations among objects. When the child is cruising, he is encouraged to raise up on his toes to reach an object on a higher piece of furniture. The object is positioned on a placemat at times to facilitate devising an intermediary means—pulling one object to obtain another object. The caregiver progresses to moving the object to the side of the mat or above the mat to help the child more fully recognize the placed upon relationship of the object to the support. He also begins to recognize that he has to submit to outside causal forces. The pulling schema will no longer fetch the object to him. The caregiver places the object back on the support or within reach, and she also places a container on the floor to one side, which encourages the child to release the object in the container with a rotational movement. He is then lured to cruise around a corner to reach more objects and place them in the container. The child may be receptive to changing his spatial orientation in another way. He stands with his back against a wall, rocking

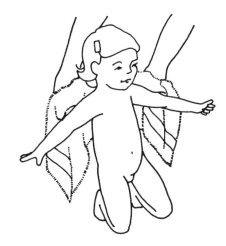

FIGURE 2-56. The child is nudged from side to side to elicit an equilibrium response in the kneeling position.

back and forth in rhythm to music. He gets the feel of weight shifting from a new vantage point, and he may cruise laterally with his back to the wall.

The activities increase muscular strength in the shoulders, trunk, hips, legs, and feet. The child will no doubt feel ready to practice standing by himself with just slight support from his caregiver (her hand and then her finger) when she is down at his level changing his diaper or dressing him. He gradually feels brave enough to stand on his two feet with no support at all.

An imitation game just naturally evolves when the dyadic pair are at eye level. The caregiver sniffs her nose and then sniffs her nose on the diaper. The modeling may encourage the child to sniff his nose in different ways to vary the effect, and the movement also strengthens facial muscles. The game may set off a play ritual that continues for a month during dressing. The child will no doubt enjoy modeling other novel actions—placing a hat on and off his head. He must actively reorganize his schemas to copy reality. If the caregiver has to manually help him imitate, the action is too novel or difficult. The child should also not be pressured to direct an action to his caregiver or another object—place the hat on her head or a doll's head—until he signals a readiness to do this on his own.

The caregiver emphasizes other senses to facilitate imitation and increased awareness of body parts if the child has a severe visual impairment. She sniffs her nose on his hand or another body part, if tolerated, to provide both a tactual and auditory cue. The caregiver can also rub her nose against the child's nose. He may tactually explore the caregiver's face to find her nose and initiate the rubbing action. The child may imitate placement of a hat on and off his head if there is a visor, which is easier to find, handle, and adjust.

When the child begins to stand alone, the caregiver gives him the feel of a lateral weight shift out and away from a support. She initially provides a sense of security by supporting him under the arms. The caregiver tilts the child to one side to elicit abduction of the weight-free leg and the arm on that same side and lateral flexion of the head in an attempt to adjust back to midline (Fig. 2-57). The child is then tilted in the opposite direction, which elicits placement of the foot back on the surface and a weight shift to that leg. The activity is connected to a song that repeats a word and a melody, and the child may attempt to imitate the intonation or word. The caregiver progresses to placing a towel around the child's chest after the bath and moving him from side to side monitoring the amount of thoracic pressure. He may also enjoy a Catch the Child game in the standing position, with one family member nudging him a short distance sideways to be nudged back by the other family member.

When the child feels more sure standing alone, he may begin to practice the forward reciprocal stepping movement of the legs by pushing a weighted doll buggy, box, or wagon. He may also enjoy practicing when holding onto his caregiver's hands, then one hand, and then a finger. One day the child makes the transition to toddlerhood by independently walking forward a few steps. His courage is fueled by the confident look in the eyes of family members, their en-

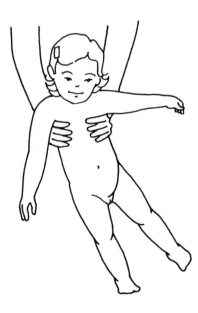

FIGURE 2-57. The child practices adjusting to a lateral weight shift in the standing position.

couraging voices, and their mirroring admiration. However, there is always the delicate balance between a need for just a little more encouragement and a sense of being pushed to do something too soon, before the child is ready.

The toddler bolsters his confidence for later forays by walking a short distance between two pieces of furniture. The caregiver encourages practice mapping different object relationships by stacking two blocks on one of the chairs and placing two additional blocks adjacent to the tower. The toddler may enjoyably knock the tower over, or he may imitate the arrangement by stacking the other two blocks. When the toddler walks over to the other chair, he finds objects nested inside each other. As he experiments with taking the objects apart and nesting them again, the caregiver places an assortment of objects on the first chair, and she places a container on the floor. When the child returns to the first chair, he may drop the objects in the container observing the effect each one creates. He sits down and puts them in and out of the container, gathers them in a pile, or carries one or more objects to another point as he creeps. The frequent change of positions and the varied displacement of objects is a positive outcome versus a more habitual explorative repertoire. The distance between the two chairs is gradually increased, which necessitates a readjustment of the child's spatial relationship with the chair.

The toddler is also involved in activities that increase the strength in the lower extremity muscles and enhance the somatosensory awareness of the legs and feet. The caregiver encourages the toddler to walk sideways over a lumpy surface (pillow or mattress) and then off onto a smooth surface while holding on to her hands or a dowel. With the security of a support, the toddler may progress to walking forward on these surfaces and on the pavement, dirt, and grass outdoors and even up a small incline. If the child resists all of these sources of tactual input, the caregiver experiments to determine what type of input he can tolerate. He may accept a firm massage of the heel, lateral border, and ball of the foot. A foot massage is very calming at bedtime for some children.

Facilitative approaches are adapted to help the toddler who has a severe visual impairment make the transition to bipedal locomotion. The caregiver holds both of the toddler's hands and walks backward. She then progresses to leading the way while the toddler holds onto her skirt. The caregiver gradually decreases her support by walking beside the toddler, holding onto one of his hands. She encourages the toddler to use the other hand to touch landmarks as a way of orienting himself to the upright vertical space. The caregiver also helps him learn to place his hand up for protection when he comes to a new area and when he bends down. If the toddler experiences a lot of discouraging bumps, he may feel more secure if he temporarily wears a helmet. However, the excessive bumps may be a sign of lack of readiness for walking. The caregiver helps prevent mishaps during the unstable phase by moving displaced objects and by keeping the furniture in the same arrangement.

The caregiver attempts to increase the pleasure of the toddler's mastery of his body and the physical realities in the world by using her sensitive observations and suggestions in Chapter 3 to mediate the environment. There is no universal cookbook answer. The toddler with a low response level will be perked up by a short, physically stimulating play period. He then takes off at his best, further revved up by the usual activity and objects in the home and the addition of objects with a high stimulus intensity. The reactive infant may be overwhelmed by the usual stimulation level reflected by escalated excitement and disorganization. He takes off at his best in an area where there is less activity and objects. A short period of slow rhythmic rocking may also help him become more organized. The caregiver learns to sensitively time a buffering activity that prevents some mishaps and keeps the scale tilted in the positive direction as much as possible. However, this may not be humanly possible if the toddler is very reactive.

If the toddler has a severe visual impairment or another type of disability, he may feel more secure if he can return to his playpen with the side rolled down when he cannot always track his caregiver's whereabouts. This is not to imply that the caregiver substitutes environmental props for her own emotional sustenance—a loving look, encouraging vocalization, contact when approached. However, there are realistic limitations in terms of the caregiver's accessibility and the time that can be spent engineering the environment for one family member. There will be intervals when the toddler will have to draw upon his own resources and fall back on something that reminds him of the supportive presence of his caregiver.

With the support of a beacon light and a mediated environment, the toddler gradually expands his spatial/temporal field. He witnesses activities that relate to a certain family member or room, which he categorizes in a relationship—Daddy shaves in the bathroom. He also gets into more things, witnesses new effects, and devises new means—turns the water on. Unobtrusive monitoring continues to be important.

Approaches to Foster Language Development

Interaction throughout the day provides the opportunity for spontaneous, meaningful communication. Although certain prerequisites for language have been reported by researchers, there are still insufficient data to define specifically the necessary background cognitive components. It is harmless to assume that the child makes sense of language, even if he cannot form words. His level of attention, manifested by facial expressions and other body language, provides the caregiver with a gross measure of his receptive competency. Electronic communication systems are being developed that allow the motor impaired child to demonstrate his receptive level.

The caregiver often naturally adapts her speech to the child's level just as she would if he did not have a disability. She correlates the length of her utterance and the grammatical simplicity with the child's cognitive capacities as she perceives them, emphasizing essential words. She also talks about the here and now, which the child is actively experiencing. The caregiver talks more slowly, which may be very important if the child has a processing problem. The utterance should also not be repeated within a short interval, as this can interfere with comprehension. The caregiver may have a tendency to use more nonverbal cues—pointing, reaching toward, tapping. In fact, the child may figure out what she is saying from the perceptual cues without understanding any of the words.[57] The caregiver can possibly prevent over-reliance on nonverbal cues by gradually decreasing her gestures. She can encourage refinement or expansion of the child's gestural or verbal request via a successive guidance system, "What do you want?" However, the sensitive caregiver avoids frustrating the child. Gratification of the request is not contingent on a certain response or standard.

The caregiver avoids using a programmed approach with an emphasis on labeling and expanding the vocabulary at too fast a pace. A symbol is only as good as the knowledge or meaning behind it. Also, motivation can become almost entirely extrinsic in nature. The child is very hesitant to name an object until he is absolutely sure of the mirroring admiration of the adult. This hesitancy interferes with spontaneity and the enjoyment of language. The child loses the inner desire to label for labeling's sake and to practice babbling sentence units over and over.

There is one approach that may be effective in energizing language directed from within rather than always from external verbal stimulation. The approach stems from the orienting response to novelty—selective attention to a change. If the child is releasing blocks in a container, the caregiver hands him a doll instead at one point. He may expressively make note of the change. However, the developmentally delayed child may be more apt to signal the new element at the gestural level rather than with a word.[58]

The caregiver can also try another approach to elicit gestural or verbal interaction. She gives the child a container and keeps the blocks, or she gives him a plate and keeps the sandwich, which is apt to facilitate some form of communication to get the object. There should not be a set condition for a response; the activity is only to be used as a catalyst. The caregiver must also keep in mind that there is controversy regarding just what types of words the child understands and verbalizes first and whether he uses a word for a label before he uses the word to acquire something.

The trend toward early diagnosis and treatment of hearing impairments is just as significant in this stage. The team collaborates with the parents to determine the best habilitative approach: insertion of tubes, hearing aid, T-K speech, signing. There is controversy over signing, which can confuse parents. Downs[59] pointed to one advantage of learning both words and signs. The toddler has a bimodal system to draw upon. Signing is also being used with disabled children who do not have a diagnosed hearing loss. Many signs are more concrete, because they look like the action that they represent, whereas a word is a more abstract representation of an action or object. The child may also be able to process a sign more easily, because it is slower than an auditory signal.

Readiness is a factor, and a good indication is the child's invention of his own gestural signs. This suggests that he is beginning to recognize that persons and objects are separate from his actions and that a sign is a means to an end. He is also developing a beginning notion of outside causal agents. There is the risk of programmed signs as well as programmed speech. If the caregiver freely uses gestures with her speech, this helps the child attach meaning to communication. However, gestures can be less natural if the caregiver has a more shy and inhibited demeanor or is depressed.

Regardless of the nature of the child's disability, the caregiver must be reminded of the importance of a mundane function, breathing, that has a pervasive influence on all aspects of development including language. Some of the suggested activities in earlier paragraphs strengthen muscles in the shoulder girdle, thoracic area, and abdomen and increase the need for air exchange. Some of the activities may also be instrumental in angling the ribs. There is an increase in the vital capacity and an increase in the ability to coordinate muscles and regulate the air pressure in more adaptive ways.

Water play is also an enjoyable way to foster more mature breathing patterns. The child practices breathing in with a more rapid and deep inspiration and breathing out in the water with a slower expiration. The water also facilitates increased mobility, especially if the child has hypertonia, because of less gravitational resistance. There is not as much danger of an overload. In one program that had a well planned swimming curriculum, I observed a decrease in the children's breathing rate and an increase in their vocalization by the end of a summer session. Slower, deeper breathing improves the blood-gas exchange for oxygen and carbon dioxide.[60] Thus, there are both physiologic and developmental benefits.

The child with hypertonia, and also some children with other disabilities, may become more tense when he attempts to speak, which impedes breathing and the movement of articulators. A short interval in an inverted posture with the head lower than the body as illustrated in Figure 2-11, Stage I, fosters relaxation and increases the lung volume. If the toddler has lax abdominal muscles, manual support to the abdomen has been effective in shortening the inspiration and lengthening the expiration in the upright position.[61] The support no doubt prevents excessive flattening of the diaphragm.

If the parents and other family members are very anxious for the child to talk, they may also lose sight of two primary facilitative forces: an intimate relationship with a significant person or persons and a predictable, contingent environment. The toddler senses that language causes things to happen, and he has a strong desire to elicit interaction with significant persons and imitate them. The social interaction is also very instrumental in helping the toddler attach meaning to his experiences and link words with objects and actions.

Approaches to Foster a Less Compensatory Walking Gait

The toddler with hypotonia or immature motor development may spontaneously engage in activities that facilitate a very observable improvement in the walking gait by the end of this stage as is the case with the toddler who does not have a disability. However, progress may be dependent on facilitative assistance to decrease some of the excessive movement or postural tension. More energy can then be channeled to exploratory behavior. Swimming helps develop muscular strength and flexibility and endurance. The caregiver also encourages squatting to increase strength in the quadricep muscles and reciprocally decrease tone in the hamstrings. The hamstrings may be overactive even if the toddler does not have abnormal tone because of postural insecurity and tension. The squatting also increases strength and flexibility in the knees and ankles. The caregiver has the toddler sit on the side of her lap with his feet on the floor during the dressing routine. He is encouraged to rock forward to reach one of his garments and rock back to give it to the caregiver. He is encouraged to rock forward two more times to reach additional pieces of clothing (Fig. 2-58A). He is then encouraged to raise up to put his shirt on or as a Jack-in-the-box popping up (Fig. 2-58B). The caregiver elicits repetition of the series of movements (rock forward and back a number of times and stand up) in accordance with

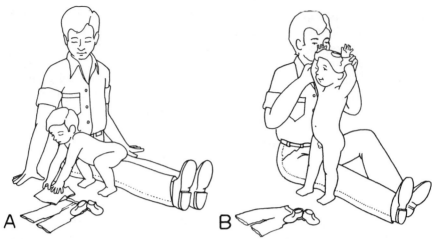

FIGURE 2-58. Movement between the squatting and standing positions is facilitated to increase stability and flexibility in the knees and ankles.

the toddler's tolerance level. The movements can be correlated with other activities to maintain interest and involvement—a song, imitative actions with rhythm instruments, placement of rings on a dowel.

Climbing also facilitates increased muscle strength and flexibility. The toddler may initially be more apt to climb on and off a low table or in and out of a low box, especially if the caregiver admires his feat. He is gradually encouraged to take on more difficult challenges—climb up on the couch to look at a book. However, the scattered, overactive toddler may climb recklessly because of a distorted awareness of spatial relationships and movement. He has to be closely monitored to prevent injury.

The toddler with hypotonia is engaged in activities to strengthen the shoulder, trunk, and hip muscles and the lower extremity adductors. The increased midline stability and more balanced muscular strength in the legs helps decrease the exaggerated, wide based gait. The toddler practices pushing and pulling a heavier wooden box or weighted wagon and pulling a heavier object on a blanket. The resistance increases muscular work and enhances proprioceptive feedback, which no doubt fosters the organization of a more coherent representation of body parts and their relationship to one another. The toddler is encouraged to roll up an incline again in this stage, which strengthens adductor muscles. He is also engaged in another activity while he is in a box that is small enough to prevent abnormal abduction of the legs. The toddler is encouraged to pop up and down like a Jack-in-the box.

Movement input helps facilitate more reliable equilibrium reactions in the bipedal position. The caregiver engages the toddler in activities that allow him to experience bobbing around in the upright position just as he has done in lower positions to find his anatomic center. He also practices realigning his body to maintain the position. The toddler may enjoy a catch the child game per an earlier suggestion. He is nudged off balance, but he is not allowed to fall by the surrounding family members. He may now enjoy being tilted in all directions: to each side and forward and backward. This activity may especially be helpful if the toddler does not have abnormal muscle tone but tenses his muscles in a fearful reaction to unsteadiness. The tension restricts breathing and more normal compensatory movements and increases the chance of falling. The toddler may relax in response to the enjoyable game and begin to more freely adjust with head, extremity, and trunk movements. The caregiver also helps the toddler practice adapting to a gravitational shift by holding his upper arms and moving him to one side, then the other side, forward, and backward in rhythm to a song, encouraging him to sing also. This facilitates stepping in the direction of the weight transference to move the base of support back under the center of gravity (Fig. 2-59A). The caregiver adapts the activity to let the toddler practice making an antigravity adjustment with the upper body. She grasps the toddler's knees, providing support above and below the knees to prevent flexion and to keep the feet on the

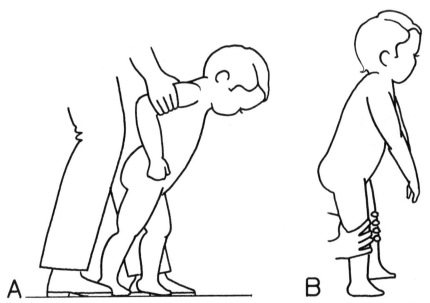

FIGURE 2-59. The child practices adapting to a gravitational shift in the standing position with the (A) lower part of the body and (B) the upper part of the body.

surface (Fig. 2-59B). The caregiver gently tilts the toddler forward, backward, and sideways in rhythm to a simple ditty that he can imitate or when he is engrossed in an activity that will not be disrupted in an annoying way by the movement. He has to adjust his head, trunk, and arms adaptively to counter the gravitational force, and the movement also fosters increased stability and flexibility in the ankles.

The toddler should not be involved in an activity if the movement input is not enjoyable or if the input elicits increased tenseness, disorganization, a Moro response, or other aberrant compensations that may reflect undiagnosed pathology. As emphasized earlier, the toddler with hypertonia or fluctuating tone should not be involved in the habilitative motor activities without specialized consultation. Suggestions provided in the section, Growth Fostering Environment, also have to be used with caution. The type and intensity of vestibular and other forms of stimulation have to be individually determined.

Summary of the Effect of Habilitative Activities

As the developmentally disabled toddler practices walking and other activities, his movements gradually become less wasteful, which decreases physiologic demands. He can direct more energy to active exploration, which increases his endurance. Thus a cycle evolves. With a background of increased motor and physiologic stability, the toddler can focus his attention on an object versus his own actions and exploit novelty via tertiary circular reactions. He also discovers new means via trial-and-error experimentation. The toddler displaces his own body in space in varied ways, and he also arranges and rearranges objects to study how they relate to each other. He observes the common round of daily events as he moves about, which serves as the basis for expanding functional meanings, recognizing events that belong together, and associating labels with actions and objects. At times, the toddler interacts with other persons and objects in a very lighthearted way simply to celebrate what he has learned as an explorer.

As tension in the neck, shoulder girdle, and thoracic muscles decreases and control of respiratory muscles increases, the toddler expands his communicative repertoire. He assumes the role of initiator more frequently to validate and perpetuate the attachment process. The toddler also asserts his budding autonomy more actively.

Adaptation of Equipment to Foster Mobility and Expand Experiences

Some children with a developmental disability may only be able to walk with some form of assistive device. Again, the team collaborates with the parents to determine readiness and the most appropriate mode of assistance. There are a number of important factors to consider. The premature use of crutches or the wrong type may encourage adduction and internal rotation of the upper and lower extremities and a flexed, more quadrupedlike posture. This has significance in terms of physiologic functions including breathing. There is also the problem of decreased explorative experiences when both hands have to operate crutches. The combination of a parallel walker and parapodium is a desirable option from this standpoint for the child with myelomeningocele, because he can at least stand with both hands free.

The energy demand is also a key consideration. Mobility is an unpleasant experience if the child feels as if he has run a marathon to get from place to place. Electronic carts and wheelchairs are becoming a more viable option with the development of adaptive inserts and electronic controls. Some children as young as 18 months learn to operate the controls and guide the cart or wheelchair. From a developmental perspective, it does not seem in the best interest of the child to make him struggle with a manual wheelchair or other form of mobility, if he can operate the more efficient electronic model. The effort can dampen the child's spirit, which is antithetical to the typical elated mood in this stage. The child may be less enthusiastic about practicing autonomous function when an electric wheelchair is finally considered. There is an ever-present dilemma in terms of humanistic needs and economic factors.

Adaptation of Objects to Foster Exploratory Schemas

Increased demands are placed on the caregiver if objects or the environment have to be adapted to facilitate more advanced explorative behavior and a variety of experiences. Some modifications have already been described in the activity suggestions. Bath time can be used to facilitate tertiary circular reactions, especially if the child is hypertonic. He may relax in the water if a special support has been devised by the professional team. The caregiver gives him a pliable squeeze bottle or another type of bottle or cup, a funnel, colander, and sponge, which create different novel effects when placed in an out of the water.

The caregiver can engineer different effects when a child with a motor impairment or another disability is swiping or releasing objects in a container in a repetitive way. The caregiver places an inverted pie plate in the bottom of the container, which elicits one auditory effect when the child swipes or releases an object. She exposes him to additional auditory effects by placing a rubber pad and other objects in the pan. Another novel effect can be added if the child does not have a visual impairment. A net or cloth is stretched over the pan in a hammock shape, which creates a swinging visual effect. It is hoped that the surface adaptations will direct the child's attention to the trajectory of the object and thus facilitate a *deliberate* variation of his actions, which is the essence of tertiary circular reactions. He may vary the angle, force, or tempo of his release.

Special electronic devices make it possible for the motor involved child to practice tertiary circular reactions and also to devise new means through trial-and-error experimentation. The system can be set up so the child elicits one effect if he activates the switch a certain way—strikes the wand laterally, another effect if he strikes the wand forward, and another effect if he strikes the wand backward. The ways the switch can be activated are adapted to the individual child's movement and cognitive potential. The system is then changed to provide more of a problem-solving challenge. The child has to experiment to determine which means schema elicits an effect or which of two or three switches activates an effect. As discussed earlier, there can be a tendency to solve the problem for the child rather than allowing him to experiment with trial-and-error groping within his fatigue and frustration threshold.

Displacement of objects and the body in space may be especially limited if the child has motor involvement. The child with hypertonia will no doubt be able to practice the contents-container relationship longer and with more enjoyment if the container is shallow and the objects are lightweight and easy to grasp—plastic bottles which fit his hand, pliable bean bags, balls with clutchlike projection. Magnetic shapes are easily moved around on the refrigerator with little effort, and they do not get away from him. If the child has weak muscles in the upper extremities and a low endurance, lightweight blocks may be more easily stacked, gathered in a pile, and displaced in other ways. The plastic cubes used to display photographs come in varied sizes, and pictures of very familiar persons and objects can be placed on each side if the child is not reactive to increased visual stimulation. Blocks can also be made by placing the lower half of two milk cartons together; the cartons come in two sizes. Somewhat heavier blocks may be easier to stack if the child has difficulty releasing an object or overextends his fingers when releasing an object.

There is somewhat of a dilemma in terms of habilitative activities. If the child has hypotonia and a low endurance, lightweight objects may be more facilitative in terms of focused exploration. However, the resistance provided by displacing heavier objects, pulling objects off a stronger magnet, and other activities, strengthens the muscles in the arm, hand, and fingers. There has to be a balance in terms of fostering increased stability and fostering increased periods of sustained attention.

If the child has a disorganized movement pattern (athetosis or hyperkinesis), heavier objects provide a stabilizing effect, which increases the child's functionalism. He is given heavier bean bags, bottles with a quiet safe ingredient inside to add weight, oranges, heavier cars, and other objects to displace in different ways. The child may experiment with placed upon (stacking), if the plastic or milk carton cubes are weighted with a safe, quiet ingredient, or if he is given grocery cans with the contents still sealed inside. He may push magnetic shapes around on the refrigerator easier if they provide more resistance. The child with athetosis may be able to control disorganized movements if he holds onto a short dowel secured by a plunger with one hand while manipulating with the other hand. Or his hands can be corraled inside a large ring as illustrated in the book by Finnie.[62]

Other adaptations may also facilitate an awareness of the relationship between objects. A child with motor involvement may be able to place circular shapes in a formboard if a knob is placed on the shape. The knob should be the same color as the circle and should not be too large to prevent distorting the shape. The child may also fit larger bracelets or other rings on a shortened dowel attached to a plunger if the dowel is securely vacuum sealed to the floor. The child who has a severe visual impairment is initially helped to displace objects in different ways by providing tactual cues. If he resists the assistance or does not experiment on his own after a number of guided trials, the activity is not right for him.

Hiding games involving successive, visible displacements can be adapted. The child may be able to follow the displacements if there is a distinct contrast between the obstacles and the object. The caregiver experiments with the nature of the sound and the distance between the displacements if the child has a severe visual impairment. If the child has a severe motor impairment, eye movements can express that he knows where the object is; and the caregiver uncovers the object to let him verify his visual search. His face brightens and his eyes light up. An electronic device can be developed whereby a switch activates each screen, or each screen is activated by a certain movement of the switch. The child can more actively search via trial-and-error.

Need for Alternate Caregiving Resources

The developmentally disabled child may always remain in this stage of development or remain in this stage for a rather long period of time. The impact is very apparent at the end of some days when it seems that the child has been into everything and the house is in disarray. This may especially be true if the child is dependent on buffering influences to prevent disorganization and utter chaos. As discussed in previous stages, there will no doubt be a need for resources to relieve some of the burden of caregiving. There are still many unanswered questions regarding the nature of the child's attachment to those involved in the caregiving role and the effect on his development. Does he form an equal attachment to persons in a surrogate caregiving role and how does this affect the attachment with his parents?

As discussed in other stages, some findings emphasize the importance of the child's relationship with an adult. In one study,[63] normal children 12 to 24 months had elaborate interchanges with adults in a day care center. The adult had the adaptive capacity to read the child's cues and mediate her repertoire of behaviors to pace and maintain the interaction, whereas interaction with a peer was much less elaborate because each child's limited social and communicative repertoire was quickly exhausted without the adaptive, adult influence. In another study,[64] the interaction of 12-month-old normal infants was dependent on the support of an attentive caregiver, even if the infants were in frequent contact with each other.

The results of a study by Piper and Ramsay[65] suggest that environmental parameters identified by Wachs[66] have a significant effect on all children whether they have normal or delayed development: temporal organization, predictability, adequate personal space, lack of a lot of noise and confusion, and a relationship with a limited number of adults. Some developmentally disabled children are very protective of their space and aggressively react to intrusion. Male children appear more vulnerable to stresses from a noisy, unordered environment.[67]

The above discussion raises questions about the staff/child ratio and the program model in infant programs, special education classes, and in respite and permanent care facilities. How many children can an adult relate to and still provide the emotional sustenance and mediation that the toddler needs to invest in the elated mastery of his body and the realities of the world? What should be the prime consideration in changing a child from one program to another: social/emotional development or other areas of development? What is the risk of a modular program overtaxing the child's adaptive capacities in this stage of development in view of the above identified parameters? What is the nature of the child's relationship with his caregiver? If he is becoming very attached to his caregiver, he will miss her stabilizing influence; and she should be encouraged to remain with him as long as is necessary for him to feel comfortable in a new environment. What has been the nature of the child's separation experiences? If these experiences have been positive, he no doubt is learning coping skills and will adapt to a new environment more quickly. If he has had unhappy experiences from being abruptly dropped off or being lured away with a toy only to later find out that he cannot return to his caregiver when he wants to, he will no doubt experience a lot of separation anxiety. Or it may be that he has repeatedly been admitted to the hospital, and the treatment program involved painful procedures. Or it may be that discretion has not been used when talking in the child's presence, which may negatively affect his budding sense of self.

Most of the questions cannot be fully answered because of the paucity of evaluation models to measure the relative effectiveness of various strategies. As I emphasized in another publication,[68] early intervention is still an experiment. The caregiver is still faced with the challenge of determining the best way to meet the toddler's needs in whatever environmental context he is in.

FIFTH STAGE: NINETEEN THROUGH TWENTY-FOUR MONTHS

FRAMEWORK FOR ASSESSING NORMAL DEVELOPMENTAL PATTERNS

Description of Normal Motor Patterns

When the toddler felt more steady on his feet in the preceding stage, he set out to master his own body and conquer the open spaces of the world. The investment of time and energy in this new endeavor was reflected by a gradual improvement in the walking pattern. The base of support narrowed, the arms moved down to a less fixated, low guard position, the forward sway of the body decreased, and the pelvis became somewhat less rigid. There was less flexion at the hip joint during the swing phase reflected by a diminution of the high stepping effect. Thus, bipedal locomotion was characterized by less overactivity of muscles and wasted motion by the end of the stage. However, features of the initial walking pattern resurfaced when the toddler hurried his gait to run rudimentarily. There was regression back to a wide base of support, an increased forward inclination of the trunk, a high guard position of the arms, stiff leg movements, and short steps with minimal clearance off the surface.

The toddler also falls back on old patterns when he attempts to perform more difficult feats at the beginning of this stage. Since jumping involves a more effortful movement than running, the toddler can only roughly approximate an upward thrust of the body. He either minimally crouches and his feet remain on the surface, or he raises one foot in the old steplike action. The toddler holds onto an adult's hand to step down versus jumping off a step. He also does not have the wherewithal to kick. The toddler is still learning to shift weight to one leg and foot and maintain dynamic stability and balance while moving his other leg and foot, and he is dependent on the longer double support phase in walking to maintain his equilibrium. He cannot narrow the base of support and shift weight completely to one leg and stand on one foot while he simultaneously plans the movements of the other foot and leg to kick a ball. The toddler has not constructed the relationship of his lower extremities in space to the same extent that he has with the upper extremities. He just moves against a large ball, pushing it forward with whatever part of his leg comes in contact with it. The toddler may step on a smaller ball in an attempt to kick it, or he may squat and push the ball with his hand or pick it up and throw it.

A strong drive to master the body and the physical realities of the world serves as a built-in impetus to practice motor skills again in this stage, and history repeats itself. There is a gradual improvement in the walking gait that rudimentarily resembles the adult pattern by the end of this stage. The heel strike begins to evolve, because there is enough control in the lower extremities to blend stability and mobility and primitively simulate the series of ankle and knee movements in the mature gait. The knee extends and the ankle flexes (dorsiflexes) in readiness to contact the surface with the heel. The knee then begins to flex and the ankle extends (plantarflexes) to bring the whole foot in contact with the surface. The stance phase involves a reversal of the movements with extension of the knee and flexion of the ankle to the neutral position. After the body has moved ahead of the support base, the ankle extends to shift contact to the forefoot in a beginning push-off motion. The knee then flexes in preparation for the swing phase, and the ankle begins to flex to clear the foot from the surface and in readiness to repeat the cycle and contact the floor with the heel.[1] Thus, there is beginning dissociation of the movement of the ankle and knee joints.

There is also less proximal fixation because of increased midline stability and more reliable equilibrium reactions. The pelvis rotates forward, albeit to a limited degree, on the swing leg side and backward on the side of the support leg. The pelvic rotation directs the leg movement in a more anterior-posterior plane, which decreases the external rotation of the swing leg and out-toeing. The more medialward movement increases the length of the stride approximately one-and-a-half inches compared with the first fledgling steps in the preceding stage.[2] There is a related decrease in the vertical shift of the center of gravity during each step. There is also a beginning lateral movement of the head, thorax, and pelvis toward the extended leg to realign the body's center of gravity more over the base of support, which increases stability. This beginning lateral shift decreases the forward tilt of the trunk and anterior tilt of the pelvis, and the lordotic curve continues to become less pronounced. The arms assume a less fixed position at the sides of the body, and there is a rudimentary reciprocal arm swing with only flexion of the elbow when the opposite leg swings forward. Thus, a counterbalancing effect is evolving with the shoulder and flexed elbow more forward and the pelvis on the same side backward. The thorax rotates in a direction opposite that of the pelvis.[3,4]

Although the neophyte characteristics of the toddler's walking gait are disappearing at the end of this stage with a related decrease in the energy cost, there is still wasted motion and inconsistent timing. The heel-toe pattern and pelvic and thoracic rotation become more refined and observable at the end of the third year. However, it is not until approximately the seventh year that the child's gait is almost similar to the adult's pattern.[5]

With increased midline stability and improved equilibrium reactions, there is a gradual decrease in wasted motion when the toddler moves from the supine to the standing position. At the end of this stage, the toddler rotates to the side, leans on one arm, and pushes himself to the sitting position. He then rotates over to the quadruped position and pushes up to standing in a straight-line plane, or he moves from the quadruped position to a half-kneel position, and then up to standing. The pattern therefore involves two steps: partial rotation and complete rotation, whereas at the beginning of this stage, the pattern involved a one-step complete rotation of the body over to the prone position. The toddler then assumed a quadruped position and pushed up to standing.

The running gait also gradually improves with practice. By the end of this stage the support leg is more extended, and the swing leg is more flexed, which propels the body upward and forward into a longer, albeit relatively short, nonsupport phase when neither foot is in contact with the surface. The base of support narrows some, but there is still wasted motion. The knee of the swing leg circumvents outward, around, and then forward, and the movement limits foot clearance off the surface and the length of the stride. The entire foot simultaneously comes in contact with the surface versus the heel, which reflects regression to an old pattern. The upper extremities move to a medium guard position with the arm opposite the swing leg flexed in close toward the midline of the trunk, and the palm is also facing more inward. The other arm is extended, abducted, and backward in a counter pattern to the forward, swinging leg.[6] The arms may go up in a high guard position when the toddler attempts to increase his speed. However, the running pace is relatively slow and effortful because of the wasted motion and the limited range and leverage of leg and arm movements. The gait has to be refined on into the preschool years before the child can change directions quickly and stop abruptly. The toddler runs in a straight-line plane.

The initial abortive kicking attempts are transformed into a primitive simulation of the adult pattern as the toddler develops increased midline stability, more reliable equilibrium reactions, and increased awareness of the position of the leg and foot in space. There is very little preparatory lifting of the lower leg backward and upward. Thus, the leg remains almost straight and moves in a restricted arc with minimal leverage. The ankle remains locked at a right angle, and the part of the foot that contacts the ball is determined mostly by chance. The toddler retracts the leg after the kick versus the more mature kick-through movement and compensatory backward lean of the trunk. The flight of the ball remains low because of the stiff leg and ankle movement.

A primitive jumping movement also evolves toward the end of this stage. The toddler adapts his walking pattern to jump off a step, lifting off with the support leg and landing on the foot of the forward leg, which involves a brief nonsupport phase. There is minimal flexion of either leg resulting in a rigid movement, and the arms raise up to a high guard position. The toddler may jump vertically off the floor, albeit in a very immature pattern. He minimally crouches and incompletely extends the legs at takeoff, and there is quick flexion of the hips and knees after the feet leave the surface. The upward movement is therefore minimal because of the lack of thrusting extension during the takeoff and in flight. It is difficult for the toddler to synchronize the actions of both feet during all aspects of the jump, and he may lead with one foot or land with one foot. He regresses back to the stepping movement he is mastering in walking and running. His arms also move to the old medium or high guard position, and the trunk inclines forward.

All the mobility experiences improve the toddler's movement patterns in other ways. He backs up and sits directly in the chair, whereas he initially climbed in the chair and turned around, which involved a lot of wasted motion. He ascends and descends stairs with both feet on each step, holding onto the rail for support. The toddler also climbs up the ladder and goes down the slide, and the caregiver may find him on a higher piece of furniture not quite sure how he got there. He frequently squats to interact with an object and flexibly squats to pick up an object. The toddler has come a long way in this stage in using his body as a means to an end. The progression and qualitative changes are outlined in Table 2-21.

EVOLVEMENT OF PREHENSION SCHEMAS. Although the lower extremity movements are becoming more flexible evidenced by the beginning heel-toe walking gait, the toddler still performs higher level skill functions with the upper extremities in keeping with the cephalocaudal continuum. As he becomes more stable while standing and walking, the upper extremities no longer have to be held in readiness to extend protectively if he falls. As the arms become freed from postural functions, there is related progress in the development of more

**TABLE 2-21 Evolvement of motor patterns
(Fifth Stage)**

FUNCTIONAL ADAPTATION	QUALITATIVE DESCRIPTION
Attempts to jump	Minimally flexes hips in preliminary crouch Raises one foot in steplike action Or extends the hips with weak thrust, both feet remain on the surface
Attempts to kick ball	Walks against ball pushing it forward Moves ball with whatever part of foot happens to contact it
Walks with rudimentary heel-toe gait	Begins to dissociate knee and ankle movement with extension of one joint, flexion of other joint Moves body weight across foot from heel to toe Begins to dissociate thorax and pelvis with a rotational movement Brings swing leg forward with a more medialward movement, lengthening the stride Decreases time spent in double support phase Begins to laterally shift the head, thorax, and pelvis toward the support leg Decreases forward tilt of trunk and anterior tilt of pelvis Begins to move arms in reciprocal pattern—elbow flexion opposite swing leg
Runs in simulated adult pattern	Narrows base of support somewhat, less abduction of legs Propels body upward and forward in short, nonsupport phase with increased extension of support leg and increased flexion of swing leg Circumvents knee of swing leg outward, around, and forward in wasted motion Contacts surface with whole foot Moves arms to medium guard position Begins to move upper extremities in counter-pattern—flexed leg forward, extended arm backward Runs at relatively slow, effortful pace
Adapts running pattern to jump	Flexes hips more during preliminary crouch compared with initial attempts

Table continues on next page

TABLE 2-21 *(Continued)*

FUNCTIONAL ADAPTATION	QUALITATIVE DESCRIPTION
	Incompletely extends legs and hips during the takeoff
	Quickly flexes hips and knees after feet clear surface
	Leads with one foot or lands with one foot
	Moves arms to medium or high guard position
	Inclines trunk forward
Adapts weight shift in walking pattern to kick ball	Minimally lifts lower leg backward and upward, or omits preparatory movement
	Moves leg in minimal arc and with minimal leverage
	Moves leg and foot as undifferentiated unit
	Retracts leg after kick versus a kick-through motion
	Minimally adjusts rest of body
	Propels ball in a low flight
Rises to standing with less wasted motion	Rotates to side, pushes up to sitting position (partial rotation)
	Rotates from sitting position over to quadruped, moves up to standing (complete rotation)
	Or rotates to quadruped, half-kneeling, then up to standing

complex manipulative skills. The progress is also related to other motor and explorative experiences—climbing, creeping at times, pushing, pulling, placing the body and upper extremities in different spatial orientations, and varying action schemas to accommodate to the unique properties of an object. The experiences facilitate increased stability in the shoulder, elbow, wrist, and fingers and a more coherent sense of the relationship of the two arms to each other, to other parts of the body, and to other objects in space. The varied input no doubt facilitates the maturation of the sensory system reflected by higher-order integration of tactile, proprioceptive, vestibular, and visual stimuli and a higher-order feedback mechanism, which improves motor planning.

There is progressive dissociation of arm and hand movements in higher skill functions just as there was in manipulative skills in Stage III. At the beginning of this stage, the toddler manipulates an intermediary tool (crayon) with an ulnar-palmar orientation that limits the range of movement to a scribble and vertical stroke. By the end of this stage, he manipulates the crayon with a beginning radial-palmar orientation that increases his range of movement and adaptability. The toddler can copy a vertical and horizontal stroke and possibly a circular stroke. He can also align objects in a horizontal orientation. There is a beginning radial orientation when the toddler releases one object on top of another, and the height of his tower increases to six or more blocks. With increased bilateral and reciprocal integration, the toddler learns to use one hand in a stabilizing role and one hand in a mobilizing role. He holds the handle of a grinder with one hand and turns the knob with the other hand. He dissociates movements to unscrew barrels with the two hands moving in opposite directions, which involves forearm rotation.

In keeping with the cephalocaudal continuum, the toddler can throw a ball and strike a ball with his hand or a tool (paddle) before he can kick the ball. He uses the same overhand pattern for both throwing and striking. The flexed arm is brought back in either an upward and backward or somewhat sideward and backward movement with an accompanying slight backward tilt of the body. The short movement arc places the hand above the shoulder. The toddler throws or strikes with a forward and downward movement of the arm and early extension of the elbow. Thus, there is a stiff whole arm movement with no differentiation between proximal and distal parts. The feet do not change positions because there is only a slight forward tilt of the body during the throwing action. There is no rotation of the shoulder or trunk except maybe slightly at the end of this stage when the ball is released. The toddler may be able to catch a larger ball by the end of this stage if the thrower does most of the adapting. The caregiver has to help him extend his arms with the palms facing upward. The ball is gently tossed from a close distance into the arms, and the toddler flexes his elbows and traps the ball against his chest just as he trapped a rolling ball against his legs in Stage III. There is no differentiation of the arm and hand movements. The throwing and catching patterns are illustrated in Figure 2-60 along with other motor patterns that evolve in this stage.

The toddler continues to refine prehension skills throughout the preschool and early school years as the most distal and rostral parts

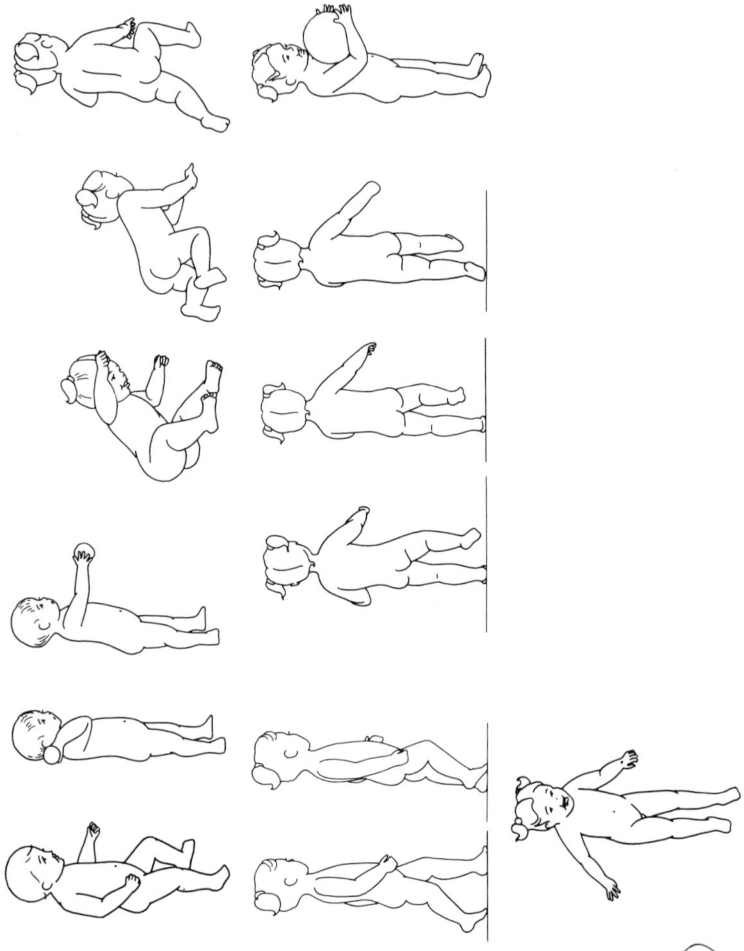

FIGURE 2-60. The first four figures illustrate motor patterns that evolve at the beginning of this stage, and the remaining figures illustrate patterns that evolve by the end of the stage.

DEVELOPMENTALLY DISABLED INFANTS AND TODDLERS

TABLE 2-22 Evolvement of prehension schemas (End of Fifth Stage)

FUNCTIONAL ADAPTATION	QUALITATIVE DESCRIPTION
Beginning dissociation of arm and hand movements, familiar higher level skills	Manipulates intermediary tool (crayon) with beginning radial-palmar orientation Releases an object on another (stacks) with beginning radial-palmar orientation Aligns objects in horizontal orientation with beginning radial-palmar orientation
Refined bilateral coordination and reciprocation	Holds handle of grinder with one hand (stabilizer) and turns knob with other hand (mobilizer) Unscrews barrels with two hands moving in opposite directions
Association of arm and hand movements, new skill	Throws and releases ball with no differentiation of arm and hand movements Catches ball by trapping it against chest with flexed elbows, palms face upward

become more mobile. The primitive avoidance response described in Stage I also becomes completely adapted. There are still remnants of the response in this stage reflected by overextension of the fingers and dorsiflexion of the hand as the toddler approaches to grasp an object, and overextension of the fingers when the toddler releases an object. A look in the future and remnants of the past should not detract from the progress that occurs in this stage in terms of coordinating forearm, wrist, and finger movements in different ways. The progress is summarized in Table 2-22.

Description of Normal Oral and Language Patterns

An ongoing process allows the toddler to intermesh phonation and breathing in more adaptive ways in this stage. There is continued lowering of the lateral aspect of the thorax as the ribs angle downward. The expansion of the thoracic cavity and the ventilatory demands of mobility and work patterns increase the vital capacity, and the respiration rate gradually decreases and stabilizes in the low 20s at the end of this stage. The slower rate coupled with increased neuromuscular control allows the toddler to lengthen the expiratory phase and regulate the air pressure to expand his babbling jargon. He also expands the number of words in his utterance to a two or three word phrase or telegraphic sentence by the end of this stage. The toddler develops the capacity to coordinate the movements of the smaller and faster acting thoracic muscles with laryngeal movements to adjust the subglottal pressure momentarily and stress a word or syllable. Thus, he can enhance the meaning of an utterance.[7] The increased air volume and thoracic control are also reflected by a more frequent and accurate h sound. Refinement of the respiratory pattern continues on into subsequent stages, and breathing does not become predominantly thoracic in the adultlike sense until the third[8] or seventh year.[9] The angulation of the rib cage is also not complete until the third or fourth year[10] or even later.[11]

Structural changes are also still in progress and continue to correlate with increased postural stabilization. It may not be until the third or fourth year that the rear portion of the tongue has descended in the neck to become the anterior wall of the pharynx, and the larynx has descended to form an adultlike supralaryngeal vocal tract. In-progress changes are reflected by a continued decrease in the frequency (pitch) of the voice, increased stabilization of vowel sounds, increased resonance, and increased flexibility of articulatory movements.[12,13]

The increased ability to dissociate the articulators also coincides with the evolving differentiations of the upper body from the lower body, the head and neck from the thorax, and the articulators from the head and neck. This ability to move body parts in more refined and flexible ways is dependent on more complex associations between sensory input, cortical perception, and motor performance.[14] Thus, an interplay of maturational processes continues to pave the way for more adaptive oral patterns. The toddler chews with his lips closed and a more refined and less effortful rotary jaw movement by the end of this stage. The buccinator muscle becomes actively involved in the chewing action.[15] Lip movements continue to supplant the more gross pumping jaw movements when the toddler drinks from a cup.

The maturational process is also reflected by a rather dramatic expansion of the vocabulary (150 – 200 words)[16] and the structure of the toddler's expressive language as he begins to combine words. However, he still has a way to go to master the complex synergistic pattern in fluent speech. The timing and precisional adjustment of oral movements is still relatively immature, and the toddler omits some consonant sounds. Or he may form a consonant sound at the beginning of a word but not at the end of the word. The toddler also substitutes a familiar sound for a sound that he has not acquired. The more refined grading of articulatory movements involved with the formation of some individual consonants and continuants (th) requires perception of subtle tactual and proprioceptive cues, and there is also a very subtle difference in the acoustic features of some sounds—r and l. The infant and toddler masters consonants with a maximal degree of difference first.[17] There is an exaggerated movement of the articulators and an overflow of movement in the eyes and head when the toddler attempts to vocalize some words and phrases. There may be concomitant movement in other parts of the body but to a lesser degree than in the preceding stage. The vocal quality is also inconsistently modulated with regression to a higher pitch and straining, especially at the end of a phrase.

In a broader sense, there is still controversy concerning the relationship between the evolvement of symbolic language skills and the evolvement of cognitive representational thought processes whereby the toddler can conjure an image of a person, object, or action when they are not visible. In view of the conflicting data, Leonard[18] purported that at this point in time the only conclusion that can be drawn is that the development of nonlinguistic representational skills parallels the development of linguistic skills. There is a structural similarity between the two functions. The results of two studies[19,20] suggest that the ability to internally devise a means to an end is the representational skill most closely tied to verbal language development. This new way of thinking will be more fully described in the subsequent section on cognitive patterns.

Although there is still unanswered questions regarding the essential background components for language development, research findings reflect the rapid expansion of the toddler's functional communicative repertoire in this stage. A word becomes chock-full of meaning with a sentence intonation reinforced by facial expressions and other body language (holophrase). The toddler then progresses to the two-word stage, and he experiments with semantic-syntactic relationships. The following examples illustrate the different combinations he may use to express an array of meanings: agent/action (mommy sleep), agent/object (daddy ball), action/object (eat cookie), action/indirect object (give daddy), action/instrument (up mommy), relational (more cookie), negativism (no sleep), agent/location (daddy *chair*), possessive (*daddy* chair). As with single words, the toddler uses vocal inflection and intonation to get the message across. He adds contrastable stress later in this stage to express possession and location or destination illustrated by the underline in the above two examples. He also orders a vertical sequence of words or two-word phrases to communicate a message that the adult expresses in a horizontal, multiword sentence: "Paul go." "Go bye-bye." "Go car."[21]

There are variations in style during this early language acquisition period that may be influenced by the parental style of interaction with the child.[22] The toddler may primarily use nominals, "push car," or he may primarily use pronominals, "push it," and only later begin to use nominals. He may use a pivot word in a constant position to try out new combinations—"eat cookie," "eat meat."[23]

Echolalia also characterizes this stage, with the toddler repeating what his caregiver or another person says. Although some investigators downplay the role of echolalia, Rodgon[24] postulates that imitation is an active reconstruction versus passive matching. The toddler preserves the word order and central idea and acquires rules that govern the semantic-syntactic structure of language. He may defer the imitation to a later time or creatively include some words that were not in the adult model. The more stilted repetition is gradually interwoven with spontaneous utterances in this stage and on into the subsequent year.[25]

The toddler may expand his utterance to three words at the end of this stage, and the third word usually fills in a word that was implied in the two-word utterance—"Paul eat cookie" instead of "eat cookie." If the toddler adds an adjective, one of the parts of the subject-verb-object sequence must go. The toddler says, "Eat good cookie" rather than "Paul eat good cookie."[26] His rudimentary sentence is telegraphic, consisting of essential words with a predominance of nouns and a lesser number of verbs. As discussed, a few adjectives are added but rarely adverbs or other parts of speech.[27,28]

The above descriptions exemplify that the toddler's speech is predominantly context-bound, particularistic, and concrete. His utterances are still primarily directed to adults, and the content centers on expressing his needs, labeling persons and objects, reporting his actions and concrete events, eliciting actions from others, and repeating what others say.[29] The toddler's speech is still structurally egocentric, because he has a limited ability to address or adapt his utterance to the listener nor can he perceive the other person's viewpoint. Thus, many of his utterances have a monologue quality. However, this does not imply that his speech is not socially functional. The content serves to validate and perpetuate the attachment process and to assert a beginning sense of separateness. This aspect will be further discussed in the section describing affective patterns.

There are some signs that language is becoming freed from the immediate context. An object may elicit an internal representation of a person or experience no longer perceptually present. For example, when the toddler sees a bottle, he mentions the name of a child whom he has observed sucking on a bottle in the past versus just labeling the bottle.[30] He begins to use verbs that refer to an internal state that is less conspicuous—"Johnny want." The toddler is also beginning to use speech in a rudimentary heuristic way to elicit information with an infrequent, elementary question, such as "Where ball?"

The controversy spills over into this stage in terms of the relative development of receptive and expressive language. Investigators argue whether comprehension precedes production during just the telegraphic stage or during the earlier holophasic (one-word) period and the telegraphic stage. There is also continued disagreement whether the toddler comprehends syntactic form (word order) and conceptualizes the role of the agent and recipient of an action in the adult sense before or after he combines words.[31,32] Golinkoff's findings[33] suggest that the toddler categorizes roles in a manner similar to the adult. However, he very possibly places more importance on the agent and action than the object when interpreting an event. Miller and associates[34] report that the two-year-old child typically assigns himself the role of agent when responding to a request, ignoring word order that places a toy in the role of an agent. It may be that the toddler realizes that certain classes of inanimate objects cannot move on their own by the end of this stage.[35]

Although the underlying process is still not fully understood, there is considerable improvement in the toddler's comprehension capacities. He receptively associates a label with many three-dimensional objects, and it becomes more of a challenge to associate labels with two-dimensional representations. The toddler enjoys pointing to pictures of familiar persons and objects, and he expressively labels some of them. With all the displacement experiences, he understands the meaning of the preposition in and possibly on.[36]

Just as with expressive language, the toddler is receptively becoming freed from the context. He comprehends an increasing number of utterances related to a person or object that is not in his perceptual field. The evolvement of a more mature concept of the object allows the toddler to evoke an image of the person or object and search for them in locations where he has frequently experienced their presence.[37] He shows signs of beginning decentralization by following a command to direct an action to another object—comb the doll's hair. At the end of this stage, the toddler can decode and maintain a mental image of a two-part command long enough to perform the task. He is beginning to use language to help him think and to direct his actions, which will be further discussed in the following two sections.

The oral and language patterns that evolve in this stage are outlined in Table 2-23. It is evident that the toddler is well on his way in acquiring the most significant mechanism whereby he can interact with other humans. He is beginning to symbolically represent reoccurring relationships between objects and events in his world, and he functionally expresses his internal representation with words, phrases, and intonations. The rather phenomenal progress in this stage catapults the toddler into the talkative preschool years.

**TABLE 2-23 Evolvement of oral and language patterns
(Fifth Stage)**

Develops increased ability to coordinate disparate neuromuscular systems and
    intermesh phonation with breathing
    Adapts slower respiration cycle to babble in longer jargon sentence, pro-
        gressing to two or three word utterance
    Momentarily adjusts the subglottal pressure to stress a word or syllable
    Produces vowels with a more demarcated pitch quality
    Vocalizes with an overall lower pitch and more resonance
    Regresses to higher pitch and straining especially at end of a phrase
Develops neuromuscular control to further refine and dissociate articulatory
    movements
    Chews with lips closed, less effortful rotary jaw movement, and more re-
        fined lateral tongue movement
    Drinks with more active and differentiated lip accommodation
    Moves articulators in more complex manner to blend sounds and form
        an increasing number of words (150–200)
    Regresses to exaggerated movement of articulators and overflow of move-
        ments in eyes and head when forming some words and phrases
Expands the structure and functional meaning of expressive language
    Impacts the meaning of a (holophrase) with intonations, facial expressions,
        and bodily language
    Progresses to combining two words in different semantic-syntactic rela-
        tionships reinforced by intonation and contrastable stress
    Orders a vertical sequence of words and two-word phrases to communicate
        a sentence-length meaning
    May progress to combining three words in a telegraphic sentence empha-
        sizing essential subject/verb/object segments
Thinks symbolically in an overliteral, self-centered way
    Centers content primarily on his needs and actions and immediate, con-
        crete events
    Speaks predominantly with a monologue quality, limited ability to address
        or adapt his utterance to the listener
Gradually decontextualizes and decentralizes language, more so toward end of
    stage
    Associates labels with an increasing number of two-dimensional represen-
        tations (pictures)
    Directs actions to another object upon request
    Searches for more absent inanimate and animate objects in expected loca-
        tions
    Labels an absent person or object associated with a visible cue—daddy
        when sees car
    Begins to use verbs that refer to an internal state
    Maintains a mental image to follow a two-part command

Description of Normal Cognitive Patterns

In the preceding stage the toddler assumed the role of a curious scientist who intentionally varied his action schemas to explore the novel features and potential of an object via tertiary circular reactions. He also came upon new means schemas through trial-and-error experimentation. The toddler had to act to think, groping his way to a solution through a series of approximations. As he practiced this new experimental approach, he became increasingly aware of causal sources outside himself, and the illusion of his own magical powerfulness began to wane.

A new cognitive process begins to evolve in this stage. The toddler develops the capacity to internally replicate schemas with symbolic images. He manipulates these inner images to think about actions without the support of external sensory-motor exploration. To use Piaget's terminology,[38] the toddler invents new means through mental combinations. Instead of resorting to visible, overt groping, the toddler internally experiments with a means to achieve the desired end result. He develops a mental plan prior to his overt action.

The budding attempts to experiment inwardly with words and visual images are fragile, and there is a transition period. The toddler may initially try to solve the problem with an old means schema, and he may also use another familiar schema, imitation, in the form of a motor symbol to support the fledgling internal process. For example, if an object is placed in a match box with the drawer closed except for a small slit, the toddler may try to obtain the object without enlarging the opening by placing his finger inside the slit or turning the box upside down. There is then a period of stillness, and the toddler opens and closes his mouth as he reflects on the problem. The mouth movement is a primitive signifier of the action that has to be performed to open the box and obtain the object. After using the imitation schema to help him think out the situation, the toddler places his finger in the slit and pulls the drawer open.[39]

The invention of new means through internal mental combinations represents the most advanced level of cognitive adaptations that the toddler achieves in this stage. This is not to imply that he no longer engages in sensory-motor exploration. The new process is still limited in scope, and the toddler may have to make some adjustments via external groping when he tries out his new mental plan. Also, if the problem situation is not closely tied to past experiences, the toddler falls back on trial-and-error experimentation just as an adult does when faced with a more novel situation. The toddler is a persistent and motivated problem solver, and he does not give up easily. If his new and old strategies are not effective, he requests help from his caregiver, who has become a reliable means to an end, when all else fails. There is a gradual increase in the toddler's proficiency as he practices using this more advanced level of thinking. He becomes less dependent on an imitative action (motor symbol) to help him think through the situation as inner symbols and images become more stable. He also executes his mental plan with less hesitancy and with less need for overt adjustments.

The toddler uses his new capacity to internally experiment with the interrelations between objects, reflected by less external groping. For example, he progresses to placing all the pegs in successive holes and placing elementary shapes in the correct holes and indentations without trial-and-error fitting and wasteful adjustments (hard pressing and turning). At the end of this stage the toddler may spatially arrange plates, cups, and spoons on a small table, place chairs up to the table, and place dolls on the chairs.[40] A representation of the spatial order and relationships of these objects evolves from the innumerable mealtime experiences.

There are also more periods of stillness when the toddler is engrossed in focused observation of objects and persons. He is less drawn to movement stimuli and more frequently tunes into relatively static social stimuli, that is, adult speech directed to him and also indirect conversations about him.[41] As discussed in the preceding section, he also enjoys looking at static pictures in a book.

The ongoing sensory-motor exploration, focused observations, and evolving representational skills expand the toddler's awareness of causal relationships. He begins to recognize the effect of an action of one object on another through spatial contact and the relationship of his own actions in a causal series. He can therefore use an intermediary tool as a means without the perceptual support of a demonstration or external groping. He also begins to infer a cause from observing its effect. If the toddler sees milk spilled on the floor, he looks for the upturned container. He likewise begins to foresee an effect from a cause. If the toddler is carrying an object or objects in both hands and comes to a door, he places one or both of the objects on the floor away from the path the door will follow, opens the door, and then picks up the object or objects. Although the notion of efficacy-phenomenalism continues to wane with new discoveries, the example cited earlier suggests that the toddler's fledgling internal experimentation may still be influenced by remnants of the notion. He possibly clings to the expectancy that the action of opening and closing his mouth will enlarge the opening of the match box. However, the toddler then figures out and executes the direct causal action.

The evolving representational intelligence reflects a more mature concept of the object. The toddler is beginning to accommodate to a symbol rather than to an event; to know about an object in his mind rather than through action. Toward the end of this stage the toddler fully realizes that an object has an existence of its own when not being observed, manipulated, or heard. The object has its own unique properties, occupies a space, and changes spatial positions relative to other objects. Likewise, the toddler realizes that he is an object among other objects. With this awareness, the toddler can flexibly follow the invisible displacement of objects, forming an elementary deduction of what took place out of sight.

The toddler embarks on the path to this end at the beginning of this stage, and he progresses through the same sequence that he followed in visible displacements. Thus, the same process occurs in motor and cognitive development when a new pattern evolves. A new function is expressed by an old form. When the caregiver introduces the toddler to the new game, she hides an object in her hand, releases the object under a cloth, and brings the closed hand back out. The toddler requests to look in the closed hand first. When the object is not there, he knows that it still exists and is someplace, and he looks under the cloth. The toddler begins to look directly under the cloth, and the caregiver progresses to alternate invisible displacements. The object is hidden in the caregiver's hand and placed under cloth B, and the toddler reverts back to an earlier search pattern and looks under cloth A where he last found the object. He then searches under cloth B. The toddler progresses to searching directly under the cloth where the closed hand disappeared. Now that he can reconstruct alternate invisible displacements, the toddler is ready to progress to sequential, invisible displacements. The object is hidden in the closed hand that is placed under cloth A. The closed hand is brought out and placed under cloth B to release the object, and the hand is closed under the cloth before it comes back out in view. The toddler repeats the old search pattern and looks under cloth A first and then cloth B. He progresses to searching directly under the cloth where the closed hand last disappeared in either direction by the end of this stage: H → A → B → C; A ← B ← C ← H.[42] Thus, the representation of a series of events can be played forward or backward. This physical plane of reversibility reflects increased cognitive flexibility and serves as a primitive precursor to later mental reversals involved with addition and subtraction.

The new ability to follow invisible displacements has functional significance in the here-and-now. The toddler can represent his own displacements in space. He points in the direction of his house, which is out of view, provided he is in familiar territory. The toddler has to have some concrete cues to conjure an image of the route he followed. He can also infer the invisible displacement of a ball and foresee the route it will take. The toddler takes a short-cut and meets the ball at its future location on the other side of the couch it rolled under.

It is evident that recall memory is replacing recognition memory, which relies on the actual presence of the person or object. This new form of memory enables the toddler to develop a very rudimentary awareness of the temporal duration of himself and other animate and inanimate objects. He recalls the recent displacement of persons and points in the direction of their disappearance. By the end of this stage, the toddler may point in the direction that a person disappeared two days earlier, reflecting an extended memory of the past. He is beginning to recognize in an elementary way that objects and events relate to each other in the sphere of time as well as space.

Imitation takes on a different form with the new capacity to evoke an image of an absent object and develop an internal mental plan. The toddler imitates actions he has observed a few hours earlier or the previous day. He also more readily imitates actions of persons when they are present now that he can replace external groping with an internal reorganization of schemas. The toddler may have to adjust his internal motor plan with some external groping to more precisely correspond his actions to that of the model. A higher-order representation of body parts allows the toddler to imitate invisible facial gestures more fluently.

The toddler expands his attempts to copy reality in other ways in this stage. He begins to imitate the actions of inanimate objects, for example, makes the sound of a motor when pushing his toy car, opens and closes his mouth to imitate the actions of a box. The toddler also begins to decentralize his actions by applying the imitation schema to a new context. He places the toy telephone and receiver up to the doll's ear and mouth.[43]

The new representational thinking allows the toddler to distort reality in the form of make-believe play. He begins to use one object to symbolize another object just as he uses a word as a symbol for an object. A stick becomes a microphone, and the toddler pretends to be a singer. A rock becomes a baby and a box a bed. Initially in this stage, the pretense is very elementary and only involves one schema. The toddler puts the doll in bed but does not cover it. Or he may apply schemas to an object in an unordered way, for example, combs the doll's hair and then puts the doll in bed. The toddler progresses to combining two sequential action schemas, which reflects a degree of internal preplanning. He places the doll in the bed and covers it.[44]

The toddler has come a long way in ordering the physical world. He singles out the parts of events that are predictable and repetitive, which leads to an inner sense of constancy or invariance. As discussed, the toddler orders words into the most regular grammatical sequence—agent/action/object—and he categorizes objects with similar physical properties by a name—chair. He continues to expand his perception of things that belong together in the common round of daily events—shoe and sock, flower and vase. The toddler also continues to group objects on the basis of their action potential or function, for example, things to stack, things to use in the bathtub.

The toddler combines objects in a form that Piaget referred to as a graphic collection. The form may remind him of something—aligned blocks become a train. The toddler mentally planned to align the blocks; the train just emerged much as objects emerge in doodling. He may also align two or more like objects together—two red blocks. The toddler then vacillates between focusing on the aligning action and putting like things together. For example, he ignores the remaining two red blocks and adds cars. Even though the toddler can now hold an image in his head, he still cannot stably hold a higher level grouping rule in his head over time. The criteria fluctuate at this point. The toddler is influenced both by the appearance of things and the immediacy of the situation, including the proximity of objects. He is likely to be more consistent if there is a strong perceptual draw, for example, blocks the same size and color and an assortment of totally unrelated objects. The toddler's fledgling categorization is also based on absolute terms. An object either belongs or it does not belong.[45] He cannot as yet order reality in a qualitative, relational way—big, bigger, biggest.

The toddler is a neophyte again embarking on years of developing adaptations that are increasingly less tied to overt actions. At this point in time, he can only internally replicate simple concrete action sequences that he just performed or is about to perform. Thus, the toddler is just beginning to make the transition from active testing of reality to thinking and talking about reality. Just as with motor patterns, he has to repeat the process and reconstruct the concepts of space, time, causality, and all of the other cognitive adaptations in a symbolic plane. However, a projection into the future should not detract from the progress that the infant and toddler have made during the sensory-motor period of cognitive development that culminates in this stage as shown in Table 2-24.

Description of Normal Affective Patterns

As the toddler elatedly focused on practicing his motor skills and testing physical realities in the preceding stage, the delicate and blissful balance of oneness and separateness began to tilt in the latter direction. The toddler's growing awareness of his separateness catalyzed a transition to what Mahler, Pine, and Bergman[46] term the rapprochement subphase. The toddler felt a need to confirm the bond with his caregiver more actively, and he wooed her by sharing his discoveries and

**TABLE 2-24 Evolvement of cognitive patterns
(Fifth Stage)**

Begins to internally replicate simple concrete action sequences
  Develops capacity to represent schemas in form of symbolic images
  Inwardly experiments with images and invents new means through mental combinations
  Initially supports fledgling internal process with familiar imitation schema (motor symbol) and some external groping
Represents actions with more stable mental images
  Develops internal mental plan with less reliance on an imitative action—motor symbol
  Executes mental plan with less hesitance and need for external adjustments
Internally experiments with interrelations between objects
  Replicates spatial arrangements in his head with the support of some external groping
  Progresses to spatially arranging objects without external adjustments—places elementary shapes in correct indentation
Conceptualizes object as separate, permanent entity that relates to other objects in sphere of space and time
  Begins to know about an object in his mind, inferring its itinerary and location
  Reconstructs alternate and then sequential invisible displacements
  Progresses to searching directly where object was last invisibly displaced in forward or reverse direction
  Keeps mental tab on his own displacement in familiar environment
  Begins to recall past events—direction of another person's earlier disappearance
Develops higher-order awareness of causal relationships
  Recognizes effect of action of one object on another through spatial contact
  Infers a cause from observing its effect
  Foresees an effect from a cause
  Continues to gradually give up notion of efficacy phenomenalism
Adapts self to reality in more complex and internalized ways
  Internally reorganizes schemas to more readily imitate actions of model
  More flexibly transfers imitative action to another context—places comb in doll's hand
  Imitates action of an object—sound of car motor
  Imitates actions of model not present in perceptual field—deferred imitation
Distorts reality in beginning symbolic play
  Uses one object to symbolize another object—stick becomes microphone
  Limits pretense to one schema initially—sings in stick microphone
  Progresses to mentally preplanning and combining two schemas—sings in stick microphone, bows
Orders reality in expanded categories and beyond confines of his own actions
  Groups more objects on basis of action potential or function—things used in sandpile
  Forms more relationships of objects and events that belong together—shoe and sock
  Orders words into the most regular grammatical sequence
  Categorizes objects possessing similar properties with a word label
  Begins to categorize objects on the basis of perceptual likeness—criteria fluctuates

new developmental skills in a more socially, interactive way. There was a toning down of the toddler's activity level and mood—a calm before the ensuing storm.

With the evolvement of new cognitive capacities in this stage, the toddler can no longer stave off the reality that he is a coherent, separate object with his own space filling properties. His elated mood even more so gives way to a realistic awareness of himself as a relatively small, helpless, separate person—the world is not his oyster after all. Thus, the toddler's illusions of omnipotence and grandeur begin to crumble, and he enters what Mahler, Pine, and Bergman term the rapprochement crisis. The longitudinal observations of the above investigators and Ainsworth and associates[47] suggest that the nature of the mother/child relationship is a very influential factor in determining the intensity of the toddler's anxiety during this unstable period.

There is a core pattern characterized by inconsistent and confused behavior that leaves the caregiver reeling at times. The toddler vacillates between attempting to undo separateness and maintain an illusion of oneness with a significant person at one extreme and asserting his autonomous selfhood and ability to manage on his own at the other extreme. The toddler becomes increasingly concerned about his caregiver's whereabouts expressed by shadowing or clinging behavior, which alternates with distancing to protect his autonomy. He may rather recklessly dart off, expecting to be swooped up, which he then resists. He also becomes increasingly demanding of his caregiver's attention in an ordering way, as if he is attempting to maintain an appendage tie.

The toddler becomes more vulnerable and less impervious to frustration, especially when there is added physiologic stress such as fatigue or hunger. There is a rapid swing of moods, and escalated tension has to be dissipated by stronger means at times. The toddler has a temper tantrum, which he may also see as a way of not surrendering his selfhood to the big adult. When the tantrum is over, the toddler feels a sense of inner release and is ready to forgive and forget. There may be a recurrence of sleep disturbances just as there may have been during the second stage when the toddler began moving off the lap.

Negativism increases as a way to define autonomy, and the toddler even says no when he means yes. He is imitating the power and authority of the parents to find his space and boundary, which is a precursor to taking on his parents' rules as his own. No-saying is therefore a precursor to the more accommodating yes, which evolves in full bloom during the next stage. The toddler primitively expresses his autonomy and self differentiation by asserting possessive rights—mine. This is a precursor to a higher level understanding of the difference between mine and yours in the preschool years. The toddler may begin to use pronouns in this stage, but this does not mean that he has the capacity to view himself conceptually as an I and recognize that he is a you to all other I's. He is just beginning to absorb the meaning of a separate identity. The pronouns are embedded in set phrases and echolalic speech, and me and you are confusingly reversed at times.

As discussed in an earlier section, the toddler is egocentric in that he cannot view things from another person's perspective. His constant talking about what he is doing reflects a lack of differentiation between social and private forms of language. The line is still blurred between thinking to oneself and sharing one's thoughts with another person. The toddler also has difficulty postponing gratification of his needs until his caregiver completes what she is doing. He only rudimentarily realizes that his caregiver has a life of her own with separate interests and plans that are not always congruent with his.

Although the toddler is egocentric, he senses the need for a social relationship with another human. He continues to woo his caregiver, seeking assurance that the attachment bond still exists, that he will not be abandoned now that he is separate. The toddler may more insistently express a need to share his discoveries and new skills. Mahler, Pine, and Bergman and Matas, Arend, and Sroufe[48] observed that the toddler who had developed a trusting relationship with his caregiver experienced less conflict during this unstable period and was more socially responsive and compliant. The toddler was especially cooperative when there was a clear adaptive advantage, such as a need for his caregiver's assistance with a problem.

Compliance is expressed in another way. The toddler is beginning to rudimentarily internalize the rules and limits established by his parents and regulate his behavior via his new language skills. He reaches toward the flower in the vase and then says no, either aloud or to himself.[49] However, the toddler is becoming more clever in dealing with some unpopular rules. This cleverness stems from his new representational intelligence, which allows him to foresee an effect from a cause. The toddler yells that he has an owee after being put to bed, which tricks the caregiver into getting him out of bed for the Band-Aid routine. He not only stalls a totally unfair bedtime, but he also plays with his truck one more time on the way back.

As the toddler plays the conflict of oneness and separateness in outer physical space, he is really attempting to establish an optimal emotional space between his inner image of self and caregiver. The toddler needs a representation of his caregiver to provide an increasing sense of emotional constancy, and he also needs to preserve space for his own image and the growth of his self concept during ensuing stages of development.[50] In the course of playing the drama in the physical space, the toddler determines the optimal distance he can comfortably

DEVELOPMENTALLY DISABLED INFANTS AND TODDLERS

stray away from his caregiver. He becomes more willing to leave for longer periods as he develops an increased ability to sustain a symbolic picture. He goes outdoors and over to a familiar person's house to associate with other adults or children. He derives pleasure from asserting his autonomy and socially interacting with other persons, and the change also provides respite from the struggles with his caregiver.

As he becomes more aware that another child has a separate existence, the toddler has a desire to mirror the other child in terms of imitating his actions and wanting what he has, which leads to some aggressive acts. Peer interaction is therefore still dependent on the security base and mediation of the adult. The interaction is also still limited in scope, centering on actions and objects rather than verbalization, because of the toddler's limited social language skills.[51] However, he is beginning to develop a primitive capacity for empathy, which can be expressed in a positive or negative way. The toddler becomes more excitable and aggressive when another child cries, or he may give him his soothing blanket.

Although the toddler is increasingly willing to leave his caregiver on his own, he may resist being left by her even more so during this stage when he is experiencing peak separation anxiety. If he has become attached to more than one person, he may protest being left by any one of them. The resistance possibly centers on the meaning of the departure. The toddler senses that his caregiver has a right to her separate space. There may also be a fear of abandonment not totally assuaged by the new representational thinking. The toddler is not completely secure that the relationship continues to exist despite periods of absence. He is still dependent on a certain degree of proximity, which he wants to actively determine. Instead of a low-key response as in the preceding stage, the toddler may attempt to avoid a mood of sadness by unfocused and scattered bursts of activity.

Mahler, Pine, and Bergman, and Ainsworth and associates observed that if the toddler was securely attached to his caregiver, he became increasingly more adept at coping with separation during this stage. The toddler developed the capacity to conjure a more stable and positive image of his caregiver in her absence. He was also able to cope with the milder distress by engaging in symbolic play. The toddler mothered his teddy bear to recapture his caregiver's comforting presence and re-enacted the appearance and disappearance sequence with ball play. He also greeted his caregiver on her return and sought proximity. The securely attached toddler was less apt to split his mother into a good and bad love object and react ambivalently toward her or ignore her.

There may be an increase in stranger anxiety during this unstable period, which can be expressed by turning away from the stranger or seeking proximity to the caregiver. Or the toddler may react with milder coy behavior characterized by simultaneous smiling and averting his gaze. The intensity of the reaction will no doubt be determined by the degree to which the toddler feels that he is in control of the encounter and the availability of his caregiver.

Now that the toddler is delineating his self boundary, he becomes very possessive of all the parts of his body. He even more persistently wants to do and not be done to. If the caregiver absentmindedly pulls the toddler's pants up, he pulls them down and back up again. He may insist on attempting to perform skills beyond his ability, such as tie his shoes. The toddler's desire to do for himself is matched by increased adaptiveness using an intermediary tool. He inserts the spoon in his mouth without turning it and with less spillage because of a beginning radial-palmar orientation, and he also holds the cup in one hand and adjusts the tipping angle. The toddler sets utensils back down on the surface versus handing them to his caregiver or throwing them, but he still becomes playful with his food after hunger has abated. By the end of this stage, the toddler may motor plan movements to undress himself and possibly even put on easy garments. He rudimentarily washes his own hands and may attempt to bathe himself.

Sensations of bladder, rectal, and genital pressure become more localized in this stage as the myelinization of newer pathways moves in a caudal direction. The toddler experiences more intense pleasure from genital manipulation, and he also experiences an urge to urinate or defecate and finds that he can begin to control these urges. However, boundary formation is not delineated to the point that the toddler can completely separate excretions (urine and feces) from body parts such as his penis, arm, and leg. If some part of the body can be emptied out and disappear, possibly an arm, leg, or other part will drop off and disappear also. Herein lies the danger of the toddler's new representational thinking without all the restraints of reality. His selfhood becomes just as dependent on claiming the excretions from his body, and the bowel movement may become the focal point. There is the potential of holding back because of the fear of losing a precious part of himself or of being dominated by the will of others. By the end of this stage the toddler may rudimentarily differentiate between body parts and body excretions.[52]

The toddler is actively establishing what belongs to self in the process of forming his own identity. He is also beginning to sense sex and gender differences in a very primitive way, and the toddler groups his father and mother in different classes. Lamb[53] found that the male toddler was becoming more attached to his father, mirroring his behavior and bodily movements, whereas the female toddler did not express a clear-cut attachment preference. Mahler, Pine, and Bergman observed that toddlers often discovered an anatomic difference midway in this stage. The investigators also observed that some female toddlers expressed more signs of stress in this stage, which may be related to the new discovery. The sense of not having, not possessing an important body part may enhance the characteristic deflated mood. The female toddler was more demanding of her mother's attention and reacted

TABLE 2-25 Evolvement of affective patterns (Fifth Stage)

Perceives himself as a separate person with his own space filling properties
    Experiences increased anxiety as he senses his smallness and helplessness
    Becomes more vulnerable and less impervious to frustration
    Dissipates escalated tension with more frequent temper tantrums
Expresses anxiety by more overt attachment behaviors at one end of the spectrum
    Becomes increasingly concerned about his caregiver's whereabouts, expressed by shadowing and/or clinging behavior
    Becomes increasingly demanding of the caregiver's attention and involvement in discoveries and new skills
    Resists being left by the caregiver more strongly, possibly reacting with unfocused and scattered bursts of activity
    May express heightened stranger anxiety, turning away or seeking proximity to the caregiver
Expresses anxiety by more overt assertions of his autonomy at other end of the spectrum
    Darts off rather recklessly expecting to be swooped up which is resisted
    Becomes more negativistic and assertive of possessive rights—mine
    Becomes more insistent in his desire to perform daily care routines
Becomes increasingly aware that another child is a separate entity
    Imitates the other child, wants what he has
    Empathizes with another child in a primitive way
    Continues to center the interaction on actions and objects versus verbalization
Senses bodily functions more discriminatorily with increased sensory maturation
    Begins to localize sensations of bladder, rectal, and genital pressure
    Senses an urge to urinate and defecate and begins to control the urge
    May begin to differentiate secretions from body parts at the end of stage
Primitively senses sex and gender differences
    Groups his mother and father in different classes
    Becomes more attached to his father and more imitative of his behavior if toddler is a male
    May discover anatomic differences
Uses representational thinking to mediate his behavior in new ways by end of stage
    Begins to rudimentarily internalize rules and limits and regulate behavior via inner language
    Voluntarily leaves caregiver for longer periods, deriving sustenance from an internal symbolic image
    Uses symbolic play as a means to cope with being left by the caregiver

more ambivalently toward her than the male toddler. This behavior was interpreted as holding her mother accountable for the missing part.

As shown in Table 2-25, everyone weathers the storm, and the toddler moves on in the process of becoming a separate, sociable being. The internal image of his caregiver is becoming more stable and will provide him with a beginning sense of emotional constancy that he can draw upon as he expands his relationships with other children and adults in the preschool years. The toddler is also developing pride in the ownership of his body, which frees him to use his body in pleasurable ways. He leaves this stage with the idea that although he is a small, separate person, he can make it on his own two feet within the context of a loving relationship with his parents. He is ready to move on to the next phase and consolidate his individuality.

GROWTH-FOSTERING ENVIRONMENT

The Master Chef can be thrown into a tailspin by the changeable palate of the diner. He may order his favorite dish and then reject it. Or the dish may be savored one day and pushed aside the next. At times it is impossible to please him no matter what is served. Translating the symbolism to the real environment, the toddler's inconsistent behavior rattles the nerves of even the most patient caregiver at times. She can experience a see-saw of emotions herself, ranging from a feeling of rejection, irritation, anger, invasion of her personal space, to warmth, joyfulness, and pride. However, if the caregiver values her own selfhood and autonomy and has experienced growth in the parenting role, she will be able to weather the storm.

She helps the toddler move through this more stressful period with empathic understanding and predictable emotional availability. The caregiver inhibits a tendency to reject the toddler when he rejects her nurturing gestures. She also inhibits a tendency to escalate her negativism in response to what seems like his never-ending no's. She realizes that this only makes the toddler feel more vulnerable, and he escalates negativism to protect his autonomy. Instead, the caregiver uses her adult flexibility and ingenuity to minimize situations that threaten the toddler's budding selfhood. The caregiver presents him with two equally acceptable options: "Do you want an apple or an orange?" She also uses an enticing lure that feeds into the toddler's new deferred imitation skills: "Mmm good lunch! Choo-choo to your chair." The caregiver gives the toddler a fair warning versus abruptly interrupting an activity: "Time to get out. Tell the duck bye-bye." She tries to maintain an unhurried atmosphere, which reduces tension and allows the toddler to actively participate in his daily routine and practice doing for himself.

The caregiver flexibly interrupts what she is doing for a short interval, within realistic limits, to respond to what can seem like a never-ending report of the toddler's activity. She senses when an expressive statement will suffice and when the toddler wants her to share the joy of his discovery more actively or lend a helping hand with a problem situation. The caregiver provides the minimal assistance that maintains the toddler's interest in the problem-solving process. She does not take over nor does she disparage the toddler's strategies, which will make him feel even more helpless and small. If the toddler views his caregiver as a helpful and accessible resource, there is a positive carryover in terms of his attitude toward other adults.[54] Her involvement also gives added meaning to the toddler's skills and discoveries.

The toddler becomes increasingly more verbal during interactive periods, and the caregiver becomes somewhat less verbal to sensitively give the toddler an opportunity to practice his expanding communicative skills. The caregiver still tailors the complexity of her verbalization to the toddler's developmental level, staying about six months ahead of him in the length of her utterance and grammatical form. The adaptation provides modeling for continued progress and also facilitates processing of what is presently being said. The toddler does not have to extract the meaning and grammatical rules from the long, complex sentences in adult conversation.[55]

The broader environment is also mediated to facilitate the beginning conceptualization of agent/action/object roles. The level of noise and confusion is controlled, and certain aspects of the environment are kept relatively constant, which helps the toddler form linguistic associations between persons, objects, and locations.[56,57] The associations are also facilitated by the caregiver's vocal intonation, which focuses the toddler's attention on certain aspects of an event and reaffirms her emotional involvement.

The daily interaction in the home environment fosters language development in other ways. The caregiver just naturally extends the toddler's utterance during care routines. For example, if the toddler says "Up!", she says "Ted up." The caregiver also helps the toddler put his thoughts into words—"Your tummy hurts?" She unconditionally accepts communicative attempts including syntactic and phonologic errors, realizing that the utterance is correct from the toddler's point of view. The caregiver takes advantage of situations that help the toddler practice decoding language. She continues to enlist his assistance in the role of fetcher, using a simple command. The caregiver progresses to a two-part command toward the end of this stage to give the toddler an opportunity to practice maintaining an inner replica of the verbal direction for a longer period, in keeping with his new way of thinking.

The caregiver also facilitates gradual decontextualization by requesting objects that are in different locations including another room.

Spontaneous play periods continue to provide a golden opportunity to associate language with pleasurable interaction. The caregiver playfully enters into the toddler's game of nonsense sounds. She also continues to blend repetition and novelty, just as she did in early infancy, by engaging the toddler in games that superimpose variation on a linguistic theme: "Where's your nose? Where's your toes?" A response is facilitated through gestures, repetition, and contrasting stress.

Thus, there is a flow of interaction in the natural context catalyzed by the toddler's intrinsic motivation and curiosity and the caregiver's sensitive involvement. This perpetuation of the affective bond is balanced by the caregiver's emotional willingness to also let go and gently nudge the toddler along the separation/individuation path. The caregiver places limits on her responsiveness to the toddler's demands for attention. She does not passively become an extension of her child, fulfilling his every wish, nor does she become a long-suffering victim of his inconsistent behavior. The caregiver protects the space that rightfully belongs to her and other family members, and the toddler sometimes gets what he wants and sometimes he does not. In this way the caregiver is helping the toddler acquire a beginning sense of proportion in terms of his selfhood and power. She is also helping the toddler modify his rigid, self-centered view of the world.

The caregiver is confronted with willfulness and persistence at times, because the toddler is not easily distracted from a want in this stage. She simply explains the limitation, attempts to redirect the toddler's attention to something else, and matter-of-factly removes him from the situation if necessary. The caregiver is aware of the toddler's new ability to resort to trickery, and she thwarts his efforts to prolong bedtime or alter other consistent rules. The caregiver remains calm when the toddler reacts with a temper tantrum, and she accepts his overtures for assurance that he is still loved after the tension has been discharged. The caregiver maintains a temporal rhythm in the daily schedule to prevent excessive fatigue, hunger, and other physiologic stresses that fuel the escalation of inner tension. She also mediates overstimulation from too much noise and chaotic activity.

The house and yard are safety proofed to the point possible again in this stage so the toddler has freedom to explore under the minimally intrusive but watchful eye of the caregiver. He comes upon varied situations that require problem solving: he cannot turn his wagon around in the narrow hall, dough is stuck on the cookie cutter, and so on. The toddler practices using his new way of thinking when past experiences suffice as the basis for internally developing a means to solve the problem. Otherwise, he falls back on external groping. As mentioned earlier, the caregiver serves as a consultant only if the toddler needs assistance. She also catalyzes an inference of the cause of an observed effect. For example, when the toddler sees jelly spilled on the floor, the caregiver poses the question, "What happened?"

With freedom to explore in the house and yard, the toddler has sufficient space to express his propensity for action and self mastery. He practices motor skills and experiments with the space-filling properties of himself and objects by pulling and pushing a wagon, cart, or box with a rope attached, and toting objects from point to point. The toddler senses movement and the gravitational force in varied ways by riding his Wonder Horse, riding piggy back with the caregiver in an upright and quadruped position, swinging, learning to go down the slide, and engaging in a ring-around-the-rosy game. The toddler may also enjoy riding on the merry-go-round platform at the park, spinning on the sit-n-spin, and riding the hoppity-hop more toward the end of this stage. His individual tolerance for vestibular input is still observed and respected.

The caregiver encourages continued practice in mapping different arrangements with objects: stacking, nesting, aligning, piling together, rotating, reversing, placing contents in a container. She provides the toddler with small boxes, old books, tile or lighter brick, spools, small plastic bottles, cosmetic jars, sticks, and different sized measuring cups, boxes, bowls, and pans with lids. The toddler also has access to odds-and-ends objects in a drawer. The size of the objects is monitored to prevent choking. Different types of containers and tools are provided for sand and water play—empty cans and plastic bottles, funnel, strainer, small pitcher, spatula, serving spoon, soup ladle, slotted spoon.

The toddler enjoys receiving a commercial toy on a special occasion, which adds variety to the above forms of exploration. The following is a limited sampling of the array of choices: blocks in different shapes, sizes, and colors; toy poker-chip caddy with the basic shapes; different colored circles that fit on a dowel (Add-a-Rack); wooden train in parts; barn with animals; one-piece puzzles progressing to two or even more pieces; busy bath; toy phonograph.

The toddler is also encouraged to observe his parents and siblings and become involved in activities as the basis for imitation and identification. For example, he watches his mother's cookie baking session and provides assistance by adding some of the ingredients and rolling and cutting a piece of dough. The toddler begins to recognize habitual associations between persons, objects, and locations, and he forms functional groupings. He also has an observational and experiential base for a deferred imitation at another time during the day or the next day. The caregiver catalyzes an image with a statement, "You made cookies." She also fosters the transference of an imitative action to another object by giving the toddler a doll, dish, and spoon, and other similar props.

These props, coupled with the caregiver's encouragement of free exploration, fosters make-believe play as a respite from reality testing. The caregiver catalyzes pretense at times with a suggestive statement, "Mommy is hungry," which leads to a cook who makes block soup. Later in this stage the caregiver says, "Mommy needs bread. Drive the car to the store." The toddler may straddle the chair and steer to the store. The caregiver spurs the evolvement of sequential actions with a cue: "Fasten the seat belt," or "Turn the key." The toddler may then imitate the action before he begins to steer and make a motor sound.

The caregiver may naturally engage the toddler in the old shell game involving invisible displacement. She closes her hand over an object and then places both closed hands together. The toddler looks in the hand where he saw the object disappear. The caregiver then places the hands behind her, transfers the object to the other hand, and brings the closed hands back into view. The toddler looks in the hand where he found the object the first time, and he then looks in the other hand. The caregiver varies the game by placing the object in her closed hand, releasing it in a pocket, and bringing the closed hand back out. When the toddler finds the object, the caregiver places her closed hand in another pocket. She progresses to placing her closed hand in one pocket, bringing the closed hand out, releasing the object in another pocket, and bringing the closed hand out. During dressing, the caregiver invisibly displaces an object under different articles of clothing, progressing through the sequence described in the section on cognitive patterns. The toddler develops the capacity to mentally search forward and backward. He also still enjoys hide-and-seek games and may keep his eyes closed while the caregiver or sibling hides.

The caregiver fosters representational thinking in other ways. She elicits the toddler's help searching for her glasses, keys, or other familiar items. She also looks at a book with the toddler and begins to read him simple stories, which feeds into his developmental tasks during this stage. The symbolism and fantasy provide distance; yet the toddler is simultaneously experiencing closeness sitting on his caregiver's lap or right next to her.

As mentioned earlier, the caregiver tries to maintain a schedule that allows the toddler to practice taking possession of his own body. She also observes signs of readiness to control urination and defecation and plays on the toddler's budding independence and desire to imitate. However, toilet training does not become an issue or battleground during this stressful period. The caregiver realizes that if she is patient and lets the toddler get the idea that his body is indeed his own, he will be more willing to part with the products at the right time in the right place. The caregiver mediates the toddler's observance of toilet flushing if he expresses fear or anxiety either in relation to his own products or those of another person.

Mahler, Pine, and Bergman emphasize the father's important role during this stage if the mother is the primary caregiver. He provides empathetic emotional support to his wife versus seeing her as the villain causing conflicts. He also provides a less ambivalent, alternative relationship for the toddler, which is characterized by the same empathy and emotional support that the mother provides. He becomes actively involved in the growth-fostering experiences that have been described in this section when he is home, adding a unique style to the activity and relationship.

The parents encourage the toddler's interest in other children and adults by taking him to the grocery store, to visit neighbors, friends, and relatives, and on other social outings. The father or mother allows the toddler to experiment with the optimal distance and time that he can comfortably be away from a significant person. He has the freedom to leave their side when he feels ready and return at intervals in the setting away from home. The parents also calmly and matter-of-factly leave the toddler at times to establish a right to their personal space. However, they make every effort to leave the toddler with a familiar person who will calmly respond to his possible restlessness or inconsistent behavior. The parents nudge rather than push the toddler into the space that rightfully belongs to him.

FRAMEWORK FOR ASSESSING ABERRANT DEVELOPMENTAL AND INTERACTIVE PATTERNS

In keeping with the assessment framework throughout the stages, it is important to focus on the effect that the toddler's disability has on his development during this more vulnerable period. How does his disability influence the separation/individuation process? How does his expression of the rapprochement crisis affect his relationship with the caregiver(s) and other family members? In what ways does the toddler's disability continue to impede or alter his interaction with the sensate world?

If the toddler has experienced a nurturing relationship with his parents and other family members in the previous stages of development, he has an inner source of emotional sustenance in the form of pleasurable feeling modes. Thus, he can draw upon both inner and outer sources of support during this more unstable period. If the parents have a positive image of selfhood and a support system, they also have both inner and outer resources to draw upon. They can continue to reach out and foster their child's development and coping strategies with empathic understanding and emotional availability. The toddler musters all his strengths to move forward in the process of becoming a separate being. He begins to develop a compass of his own to the extent possible.

Effect of a Disturbed Relationship

However, if the toddler has not sensed his caregiver's predictable emotional availability during the preceding stages, he may experience relatively marked anxiety when he begins to sense more fully his own separateness. The toddler has a strong survival need for proximity to another human regardless of the strength of the relationship, and he seeks assurance that he will not be abandoned. If the caregiver is predominantly unresponsive or is inconsistently responsive to the toddler's rapprochement behaviors, this escalates his anxiety. He may whine and cling to his caregiver or shadow her every move. The toddler may resort to very overt behaviors to elicit her attention if not her involvement: interruption of the caregiver's activity (throwing her book on the floor), spilling food on the floor and stomping on it, or a prolonged temper tantrum. He may alternate between excessive wooing and excessive negativism or excessive shadowing and more reckless darting away. The toddler may experience rather marked sleep disturbances at night, and he may have a low frustration level during the day. He is overreliant on the caregiver for assistance in a problem situation, yet he may swing 180 degrees and resist her assistance. The toddler's abrupt shift may be spurred by the caregiver's insensitivity to his cues and awkward timing or her inability to read his vague cues. He may be very noncompliant, because he sees no adaptive advantage to being cooperative.

The toddler may strongly resist being left by his caregiver because of the fear of abandonment. His inner representation of her is too fragile to be sustained during her absence. Or the toddler cannot maintain a positive image of his caregiver, and he is more apt to split the good and bad mother. The surrogate caregiver may become the bad mother who can do nothing right. Or the surrogate caregiver may become the good mother, and the toddler passively snuggles in her lap and willingly eats any food offered. The toddler may ignore his caregiver when she returns or angrily resist her overtures. Or he may ambivalently begin to seek proximity and then veer away.[58]

On the other hand, the toddler may not resist being left with even a strange person in a strange environment if he has not experienced a sense of closeness with his caregiver. He willingly interacts with the stranger, or he may direct his attention to objects, talking to himself with a sober facial expression. The toddler may withdraw into a world of his own and rock his body, stare at himself in a mirror, and engage in other self-centered behaviors, or he may crawl into a small enclosure to derive some sense of closeness and security. The toddler's inner representation of nurturing experiences or objects is still not coherent enough to substitute one object for another and act out his wishes with symbolic play, for example, mother a doll. He may exhibit some of the above withdrawal behaviors even when his caregiver is present, if he has given up seeking her emotional investment in his activities and assurance of her love.

The caregiver's own self identity may be blurred as an outgrowth of her caregiving environment as a child. Or the emotional impact of the diagnosis of a developmental disability may affect the caregiver's image of herself. She is struggling with the value of her own selfhood and personal space at the very time it is important that she protect and maintain her space and understand the child's attempts to define his space. The caregiver may overreact to the toddler's rejection of her nurturing approaches and reciprocate by rejecting his overtures. She may become threatened by his negativism, which triggers an escalation of her no's and don'ts and elicits a cycle. The caregiver may sense a need to assert power, which results in a predominantly negative, emotional tone and frequent restrictions. The toddler is denied the right to practice self assertion, which is a part of the process of establishing his own space in the world.

If there is a troubled relationship, the toddler's sensate world will continue to be more devoid of meaning. He lacks the curiosity, focused interest, desire to communicate, and typical drive to make sense of the world.[59] He does not have the catalyst of a responsive environment. However, an aberrant response pattern may have been instrumental in determining the nature of the environment. As discussed in preceding stages, it is no doubt impossible to sort out the interplay between the toddler's disability, his behavioral pattern, and his caregiver's behavioral pattern.

Effect of an Aberrant Response Threshold

The toddler with a very permeable stimulus barrier may be especially vulnerable during this more stressful period. He expresses his heightened instability with more rapid mood swings and frequent temper tantrums. The toddler may insist on being picked up, and he then senses a lack of pleasure from physical contact and angrily struggles to get back down. The escalated anxiety may also be expressed by unprovoked aggression toward the caregiver, other family members, and other children or autoaggressive behavior, for example, head banging, self biting, or scratching. The toddler becomes more destructive of toys because of his low frustration level and increased strength. He cannot interact with objects and other environmental stimuli with the level of explorative skill and orderliness typical of this stage. The toddler's movement pattern may become even more overactive and disorganized in an attempt to discharge tension from emotions that he has difficulty understanding and modulating. He wiggles all over in response to stimuli, which can be frustrating to the whole family at mealtime. His constantly moving feet kicks another member, and he spills food and breaks objects. The toddler may have to be removed to his room, or he may leave the table in tears.

The toddler's erratic behavior may especially tax the coping capacity of the primary caregiver. She may alternate between tuning in to his needs and tuning him out from sheer exhaustion. Or she monitors his behavior in a restrictive way. The tension can lead to disintegration of the caregiver's behavior when the toddler needs the mediation of her calmness and wholeness. If the caregiver's tension frequently escalates to degrading comments and physical punishment, this can make the toddler feel more insecure and powerless, which will reactivate the cycle of mounting tension and need for discharge. The toddler's behavior may lead to intense stress within the family unit and even to abuse.

If the toddler has a more nonpermeable stimulus barrier, his behavioral pattern may take on a new dimension during this stage. The caregiver may sense an abrupt change if the toddler becomes more assertive, especially if he has been very easy going and rather passive in nature. She may have difficulty shifting gears and allowing the toddler to express willfulness and negativism and practice doing for himself. The caregiver is used to engineering stimulus events, and she is too helpful. The toddler may resist his caregiver's intrusiveness in a more passive-aggressive manner than the reactive toddler. He withdraws from an activity and lies on the floor, refusing to get up. When the caregiver stands him up, he lies down again. He is more apt to be termed stubborn.

Or it may be that the toddler's expressions of anxiety are relatively attenuated and more easily overlooked. He cannot muster a high enough level of physiologic arousal to escalate his assertive or rapprochement behaviors, or he lacks the energy to persist. His signals are too vague to evoke a change in the caregiver's interactive approach that would foster his fragile attempts to engage in the drama of oneness and separateness. If the caregiver has become more burned out from attempts to increase the stimulus level of the environment, the toddler may have a lot of empty time again in this stage when no animate or inanimate event arouses him, and he continues to turn inward to his own body. If an object catches his interest, the toddler may predominantly engage in repetitive and gross exploration. He still has a limited ability to pursue novelty and explore objects in a more differentiated way, especially without the emotional investment and mediation of the caregiver.

Effect of an Overintrusive Environment

There is again the extreme of the overnurturing caregiver who delays the rapprochement crisis. She fulfills the toddler's every need and perpetuates the illusion that she is an extension of him. Or the caregiver may invest too much energy in the toddler's development in a doting and intrusive way, and she becomes very anxious when he begins to develop more independent skills. The transition may conjure fears of the child's vulnerability as a separate person if the caregiver lacks faith in the child's ability to develop a compass of his own to any degree. The caregiver may express her anxiety by becoming the shadower. She feels the need to control the toddler's behavior, solving problems before he even has a chance to recognize the frustration. The caregiver focuses on certain criteria for the toddler's experiences and performance versus sharing his explorative activities and discoveries. She also maintains possession of the toddler's body, controlling his daily care routines. The toddler may pay the price for his caregiver's love by surrendering his will. The caregiver remains omnipotent; the toddler accommodates his actions to her smiling approval.

Effect of Sensory Impairments

As in other stages, it is important to assess the effect of a known sensory loss, and it is also important to recognize behaviors that may reflect a dysfunction of the sensory system. Some of the descriptive information in this section of the preceding stage is still relevant. The focus of the following discussion will be on additional expressions of an impairment that may affect development in this stage.

VISUAL IMPAIRMENT. If the toddler has a total loss of vision or a severe visual impairment, he may not begin to walk until the end of this stage or on into the third year.[60] Even if he begins walking in the first part of this stage, he may not attain other mobility skills (running, kicking, jumping), because he lacks the most efficient sense for spatial orientation. Practice with a lower mobility pattern, creeping, facilitates increased stability in the shoulder girdle and arm and also intertwines with other maturational processes to foster higher order discrimination and integration of tactile, proprioceptive, and auditory input. The toddler explores objects with less fumbling movements. However, he still has to test reality in a more proximal and piecemeal way; external groping is a necessity. Thus, the toddler continues to live in a narrower sensate world, which limits exploration of the spatial, temporal, and causal relationships between animate and inanimate objects, including himself as an object.

The construction of the object world, representational thinking, and self differentiation may continue to evolve more slowly compared with the norm even with early intervention. The toddler can only feel himself. He cannot see a replicate, whole body image in the mirror, and he cannot see the mirrored actions of other humans. He cannot tune into the more subtle visual stimuli that allow the toddler with an intact visual sense to imitate precisely another person and identify with him. Since the toddler does not have a visual image as the basis for inserting objects in elementary play schemas, his imitative behavior does not take on new dimensions. He very probably will not begin to direct his actions to another object, nor does he substitute one object for another in make believe play.

The toddler with a severe visual impairment may expressively use language in a self-centered way to label a need or want within the same timetable as the sighted toddler, but his vocabulary of words is more limited. It takes him longer to learn about unique properties with the other senses as the basis for categorizing objects via a label. Evolvement to the two-word stage will probably be somewhat delayed,[61] because the toddler lacks the most efficient visual-auditory link to perceive agent/action and action/object sequences, such as "Car go." He has to derive the relationship by associating a temporal sequence of sounds with past proximal experiences riding in a car. Since the toddler has no awareness of two-dimensional representations of three-dimensional objects, this affects an aspect of language development. Obviously, he cannot point to or label a picture, and he may not enjoy listening to simple stories at the end of this stage.

If the toddler has a dysfunction of the visual system rather than a severe visual loss, his exploratory behavior continues to be less elaborate and adaptive. He may have an impairment in one or more of the following components: acuity, convergence, figure-ground discrimination, figural unity, or coordination of eye and head movements. Although a definitive diagnosis of causal sources cannot always be established, the functional effects are observable. The toddler continues to have difficulty exploring the unique visual characteristics of objects. He also has difficulty mapping objects in different arrangements to study and internalize their spatial relationships and to come upon graphic forms and perceptual likenesses. The toddler may lack sufficient control of eye movements to visually focus on actions and events in his environment for long periods. He alternates between focusing and darting his eyes, or a short period of still, focused attention alternates with restless darting around the room. The toddler may have difficulty maintaining a stable image on the retina when walking and running and during other movements, which affects his ability to perceive the relationship of his body to objects in space. He frequently bumps into things.

AUDITORY IMPAIRMENT. If the toddler has a permanent hearing loss or if he continues to have recurrent bouts of otitis media, he also exists in a sensate world that is narrower in scope. The toddler cannot hear the intonation patterns that give a combination of words a certain meaning, nor does he hear the regularities in the grammatical structure. He lacks the basis for organizing events that he sees in a linguistic agent/action/object sequence; time is to audition what space is to vision. He watches the car drive away, but he cannot auditorally and temporally represent the visible displacement by a word order—"Car go." Even if the toddler has an intermittent loss, he still lacks the adequacy and constancy of auditory input to associate with visual, proprioceptive, and tactile input to form an expanding vocabulary of words.[62] Attempted speech may be distorted and flat and thus very difficult to understand. The toddler cannot effectively coordinate intonational variations, facial expressions, and words to get his message across.

As the toddler explores the world with other senses, internal images become more coherent, and he will probably begin thinking in a more representational way if the central nervous system is intact. He can conjure images of objects, actions, and needs, but his expressive language ability lags far behind. He cannot communicate his thoughts in an effective way, which causes frustration and perpetuates passivity. The toddler senses that he has limited ability to control his environment and interact with his caregiver in a socially positive way.

The caregiver has expended a lot of energy in attempts to communicate with her child over the months, relying heavily on the context, gestures, and more intrusive physical manipulation at times to get her message across. The caregiver may have become so used to dominating the interaction that she has difficulty changing her pattern and tuning in to the toddler's infrequent attempts to assume the role of initiator. She misses opportunities to nudge him out of a passive role. The one-sided nature of the interaction may gradually drain the caregiver's cup, and she interacts with her child less as he gets older, in contrast to the typical trend. The diminished emotional investment enhances the toddler's dependency, and he has a need to remain in rather close physical proximity to his caregiver, although he seldom attempts to interact with her.[63]

If there is a related vestibular dysfunction, the toddler has the added stress of being unsure of where his body is in space. This further decreases his ability to adaptively cope with the environment. The toddler's behavior may be characterized by restless movement, distractibility (because cognitive energy has to be directed to postural adaptations), decreased ability to modulate emotional states (because of a lack of inner centeredness or homeostasis), frequent temper tantrums, and inflexibility that may be termed stubborness.[64] Coupled with the inner stress is the limited ability to communicate with himself either internally or via a monologue because of the language delay. He therefore lacks another means of controlling his own behavior. There is the potential of shaping a relationship with his caregiver, which is characterized by negativism and restrictiveness.

The toddler may not have a hearing loss, but he cannot centrally process auditory input in an organized way. He may not be able to tune out irrelevant background noise (tick of a clock) and focus on speech sounds. The toddler may have difficulty following the pitch pattern and temporal sequence of words, which interferes with abstracting grammatical regularities, conceptualizing agent/action/object roles, and reconstructing the order of essential words in echolalic speech. If self-hearing is delayed because of a faulty feedback mechanism, the toddler cannot simultaneously compare the sound he is making with oral movements at that point in time, which interferes with his ability to modify sounds and more closely approximate words.

The toddler may have adapted over the months by becoming less and less interested in auditory stimuli, characterized by infrequent attentive listening. However, he cannot close his ear the same as he can close an eye, although the toddler may attempt to do so by placing his hands over his ears at times, especially when there is a lot of noise and confusion in the room. The stress from his attempts to turn annoying auditory input off or his struggle to make sense of auditory input may be manifested by overactivity, distractibility, inconsistency, irritability, noncompliance, a low level of social responsiveness, and a budding negative sense of self.[65] Thus, the attachment and individuation process may be at risk just as it is in the case of the toddler who has a hearing loss.

A dysfunction of the auditory sense may be expressed in a different way. The toddler may enjoy certain strange noises, or he may listen to noise or make noises seemingly to entertain himself rather than to make sense of the input in a cognitive way. Or he may enjoy making loud noises.

VESTIBULAR IMPAIRMENT. A vestibular impairment may be intertwined with a visual or auditory impairment as discussed above, or a dysfunctional vestibular sense may place a burden on another system. If the toddler cannot accurately sense gravitational shifts and where his body is in space from vestibular receptors, he has to rely more heavily on supplemental visual information which has even more importance in this stage. When the visual sense has to take on part of the function of another sense, this compromises the toddler's capacity to receive and process visual stimuli and focus his attention. DeQuiros[66] hypothesized that if conscious attention must be directed to maintaining balance in a position and when moving, there is a rechanneling of cognitive energy and a delay in the evolvement of representational thinking.

The toddler also compensates for weaker equilibrium reactions by tensing his body and widening his base of support, which interferes with the evolvement of a more adaptive walking pattern, with beginning proximal rotation and a narrower, rudimentary heel-toe gait. He continues to seek a dependable center of gravity, and he may avoid or reluctantly become involved in certain activities, such as going up and down a hill on a walk or going down the slide. The toddler may become car sick very easily, and he may not be able to ride in a boat, which creates problems on family outings.

On the other hand, the receptors may only respond to more intense vestibular input. The toddler may spin and whirl more than is typical at this age or jump a lot. He may especially enjoy the spinning and abrupt starts, stops, and directional changes involved in an amusement park ride; he resists getting off when the other member of the family feels very overloaded.

TACTILE AND PROPRIOCEPTIVE IMPAIRMENT. If the toddler has a dysfunction of the tactile or proprioceptive system, he will continue to have difficulty timing and differentiating movements, which affects his ability to imitate an expanding number of words and word combinations and test reality in more complex ways. A relatively limited and unstable repertoire of sensory-motor explorative schemas will no doubt affect the toddler's capacity to represent actions with symbolic images and develop a mental plan.

An impairment of these two systems also places a burden on vision. The toddler has to look at what his extremity is doing when he imitates an action, and his approximation may remain more gross. He has to check where his foot is when climbing or he will miss his mark. The toddler also has to visually monitor placement of body parts when undressing, and he has more difficulty learning self-help skills.

If certain sensations continue to be unpleasant, the toddler may perceive his environment as threatening, which elicits evasiveness, overreactiveness, overactivity via flightlike behavior, and/or aggressiveness, such as pushing or hitting. A protective demeanor limits the toddler's experiences at the very time they should be expanding. He may avoid exploring sand, dough, and other textures or going barefoot. The toddler may stay in the periphery to avoid contact with other children, and he may be fearful of pets. He may limit the variety in his menu because of sensitivity to certain textures. However, it may be that the toddler is rejecting certain odors or tastes rather than or as well as the texture because of sensitivity to gustatory or olfactory input. He may smell food before eating it.[67]

Summary

The toddler with a sensory impairment does not perceive the vivid and enlivened world that the toddler with unblunted senses perceives. Nor can he respond to the sensate world in as integrated a manner. There is something amiss in one or more of the following functions: his ability to attend to stimuli, receive stimuli, integrate stimuli, or act upon his environment in an adaptive way. There may be an imbalance with one sense performing its function and the function of another sense, and it is impossible to do two jobs and maintain an optimal level of performance. Or there may be a processing problem. The toddler cannot tune in to one instrument in the orchestra, placing it in the foreground. Or the toddler can only attend to one instrument rather than the whole orchestra. Or he can only attend to music with a slower tempo. The toddler's inner image of the sensate world is no doubt less coherent and stable, which delays the evolvement of some or all aspects of representational thinking. Or the new way of thinking may be fragile and has to be supported with a motor symbol or some external groping for a longer period of time.

The toddler may feel even more helpless than is typical of this stage. Or he may be a troubled child, because he cannot understand and control what his nervous system is doing to him. He may easily become disoriented because of a diminished or distorted sense of his own displacements in space relative to other objects and his home. Thus, his journey along the separation/individuation path is also in jeopardy.

Effect of Motor Impairments

As was discussed in the preceding stage, the toddler with abnormal muscle tone may use compensatory patterns to assume the upright position and walk, and there may be an observable improvement in the quality of his gait as the result of practice. However, abnormal tone very probably will delay or negate evolvement of a heel-toe pattern. The toddler cannot blend stability and mobility and dissociate movements to flex one joint and extend an adjacent joint and then reverse the pattern. The toddler also lacks sufficient midline stability to provide the background for beginning pelvic and thoracic rotation.

EFFECT OF HYPERTONIA ON MORE ADAPTIVE MOTOR PATTERNS. If the toddler has hypertonia, the compensatory walking patterns described in the preceding stage may not improve or may become more exaggerated because of the stress of maintaining his balance against the force of gravity. The toddler may also develop contractures. However, there is a possibility that the gait will become less compensatory over a longer time span as the result of maturational changes and facilitative therapy approaches. Even so, taking one example of a child who has more involvement in the lower extremities, excess tone limits the extent of improvement. The knee does not fully extend and the ankle does not dorsiflex at the end of the swing phase, and the toe comes in contact with the surface instead of the heel. The knee then

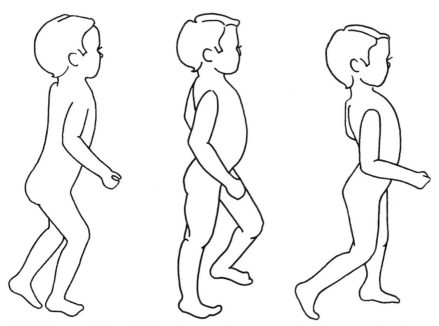

FIGURE 2-61. If the child has hypertonia and more involvement in the lower extremities, excess tone inhibits the evolvement of a beginning heal-toe gait and pelvic and thoracic rotation.

hyperextends during the stance phase in response to full weight bearing because of a strong positive support reaction. Late in the stance phase there is lack of complete hip, knee, and ankle extension and external rotation to push the foot off and provide propulsion to the step. The hip, knee, and ankle flex almost simultaneously for the swing phase instead of sequentially: knee, hip, and then ankle. This results in a diminished amplitude of flexion and a shorter stride. The child flexes the lateral surface of the trunk to help bring the swing leg around because of the lack of beginning pelvic rotation, which is also a contributing factor in shortening the stride. There is still a lurching movement to help bring the body forward, which increases the lordotic curve. The arms assume a protective medium guard or low guard position and move together versus beginning reciprocation. The walking pattern is illustrated by Figure 2-61.

When the child attempts to run, the stress increases the compensatory pattern. The base of support widens, and the trunk tilts more forward. There is lack of extension of the push-off leg and minimal flexion of the swing leg to propel the body upward and forward, and both feet may not leave the surface in a brief nonsupport phase. The stress may elicit regression from whole foot contact to only toe contact with the surface. The arm on the same side as the swing leg exaggeratedly extends backward to offset the forward momentum. The other flexed arm fixates in a protective position versus the typical alternate movement in closer toward the midline of the body. The shoulder also becomes more tense and shrugged in response to the stress (Fig. 2-62A).

The child cannot shift weight to one leg and maintain his balance to effectively kick a ball. He more or less walks into the ball, pushing it forward with whatever part of his plantarflexed foot comes in contact with it. The stress elicits an increased positive support reaction in the extended leg, increased hip flexion in the kicking leg, and a more exaggerated anterior tilt of the pelvis. The child cannot extend his leg to complete the arc of the kicking motion. There is increased tension in the shoulders and associated flexor tone in the arm opposite the kicking leg, reflected by adduction and internal rotation (Fig. 2-62B).

The child works against himself when he attempts to jump. The crouching movement increases flexor tone characterized by adduction, internal rotation, and flexion of the hips and knees (Fig. 2-62C). The child cannot completely move out of the flexion to extend his legs in a thrusting action, and his feet do not clear the surface or just barely clear the surface (Fig. 2-62D). One or both arms fixate in a medium guard position with exaggerated shrugging of the shoulders.

If the toddler has less involvement in the upper extremities, he will probably be able to throw and even catch a ball in a relatively

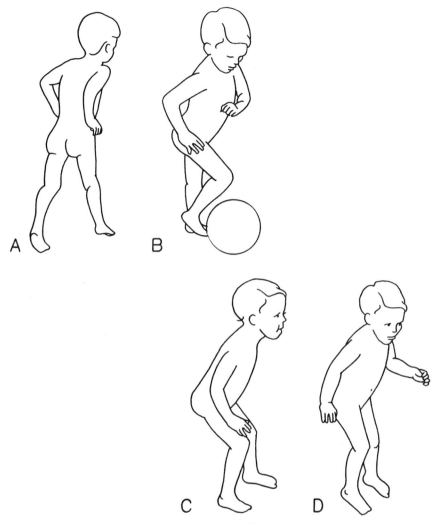

FIGURE 2-62. (A) Running, (B) kicking, and (C and D) jumping movements intensify compensations if the child has hypertonia.

functional way. However, if he has a flexor pattern that more equally involves the upper and lower extremities as illustrated in Figure 2-49C and D, Stage IV, the toddler will have difficulty engaging in ball play. As he brings his flexed arm back in readiness to throw the ball, his head flexes forward; and the other arm flexes in an associated reaction (Fig. 2-63A). The toddler cannot completely extend his elbow during the throwing action because of excessive use of flexor muscles, and the movement arc is limited. The fingers exaggeratedly extend in an avoid-

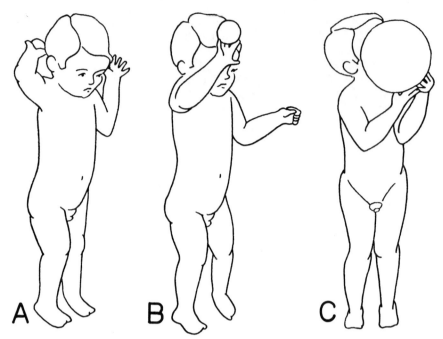

FIGURE 2-63. There is excessive use of flexor muscles during ball play if the child has hypertonia with a predominant flexor pattern.

ance reaction during the release (Fig. 2-63B). When the toddler attempts to catch a ball, there may be an avoidance reaction expressed by a slight backward leaning of the trunk or head retraction; and the toddler turns his head away or closes his eyes even before the ball arrives. He may sense that he will not be able to trap the ball against his chest, or he may have difficulty perceiving the moving ball. The arms quickly pull into flexion which pushes the ball up against his face or off to the floor (Fig. 2-63C).

EFFECT OF HYPOTONIA ON MORE ADAPTIVE MOTOR PATTERNS. If the toddler has hypotonia, the walking gait very probably will improve with practice. However, the qualitative changes are not comparable with those of the nondisabled toddler within the same time span. There is still some fixation in the midline to compensate for lack of normal proximal stability, which delays the evolvement of beginning pelvic and thoracic rotation. Lack of background stability in the leg, ankle, and foot delays the evolvement of a rudimentary heel-toe gait. Just as with the toddler who has hypertonia, there is incomplete extension of the hip, knee, and ankle at the end of the stance phase to push the foot off and provide propulsion to the step. The hip flexes excessively during the swing phase, compared with the norm for this stage, and the leg is still somewhat externally rotated with out-toeing. The less direct posterior-anterior movement shortens the stride. The body inclines forward with a somewhat lurching movement toward the end of the swing phase, which increases the lordotic curve. Most of the foot comes in contact with the surface instead of just the heel because of incomplete extension of the knee and dorsiflexion of the ankle. The leg then extends or hyperextends after the foot contacts the surface. The upper extremities are held at the side or in a low guard position, and the shoulders are rounded because of weak scapular muscles. The arms may extend backward in a compensatory movement when the pelvis tilts more forward. The walking pattern is illustrated in Figure 2-64.

When the toddler attempts to run, the stress elicits a wider base of support and increased out-toeing. Leg movements are minimally propulsive because of the lack of complete extension of the push off leg and minimal flexion of the swing leg, and both feet may not leave the surface in even a brief, nonsupport phase. Thus, the primitive run is more like a hurried walking gait with stiff leg movments and an increased waddling effect in the hips. The shoulders shrug and the upper extremities move to a medium guard position because of increased instability, which limits the alternate movement of the arms (Fig. 2-65A).

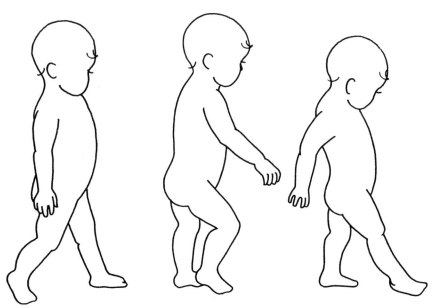

FIGURE 2-64. If the child has hypotonia, lack of adequate background stability delays the evolvement of a beginning heel-toe gait and thoracic and pelvic rotation.

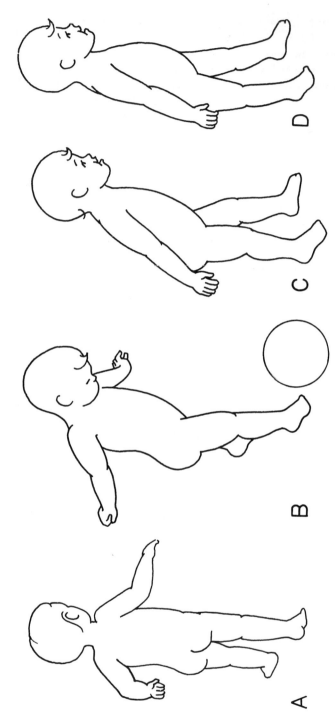

FIGURE 2-65. The toddler with hypotonia (*A*) runs with a stiff waddling gait and predominantly uses extensor muscles when attempting to (*B*) kick and (*C* and *D*) jump.

The toddler uses extensor muscles to compensate for weaker flexor muscles in an attempt to kick the ball. He moves the ball with a pushing action of the extended leg and slightly plantarflexed foot, which barely clears the surface; the arc and force of the primitive kick is therefore very limited. There is a counterproductive backward winging of the extended arms because of the imbalanced use of extensor muscles and weak equilibrium reactions (Fig. 2-65B).

The toddler also primarily uses extensor muscles when attempting to jump. He crouches by flexing only the hips, locking the more unstable and hyperflexible knees in extension (Fig. 2-65C). The toddler then extends the hips and hyperextends the knees in an attempted jump, but the feet do not leave the surface, because proximal hip flexion is the only source of leverage (Fig. 2-65D).

Weaker muscles in the shoulder girdle limit the thrust of the throwing action during ball play. The toddler cannot bring his flexed arm back far enough to position the ball in line with or behind his shoulder (Fig. 2-66A). This limits the excursion of the posterior-anterior arm movement, and the ball is more or less dropped downward as the elbow extends and the body moves forward (Fig. 2-66B). Weaker shoulder and upper extremity muscles also interfere with maintaining the arms in an extended, readiness position to catch a ball. The arms begin to drift farther apart and possibly downward, and the ball slips between them (Fig. 2-66C). A response latency is a limiting factor, even

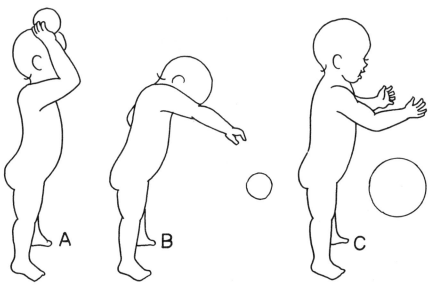

FIGURE 2-66. Ball play is hampered by weak muscles and poor timing if the toddler has hypotonia.

if the arms remain in position. The toddler cannot time the elbow flexion to successfully trap the ball.

EFFECT OF FLUCTUATING TONE ON MORE ADAPTIVE MOTOR PATTERNS. The child with athetosis may develop increased postural stability and balance as he practices walking over a number of years. This is evident in one example of a child who has a fluctuating tonal pattern with a predominance of hypotonia. There is an improvement in the walking gait in this stage (Fig. 2-67) compared with the preceding stage (see Fig. 2-50C and D). However, the child still lacks the background components to simulate the adult gait. Although there is a decrease in the high-stepping effect, the leg still externally rotates as it comes forward, rather than moving in a more posterior-anterior plane. This is due to the fact that the child still has to rely on lateral trunk flexion to help bring the leg forward; proximal fixation prevents the evolvement of pelvic rotation. Most of the foot contacts the surface rather than the heel because of incomplete extension of the knee. The support leg still hyperextends, and the foot does not begin to push off

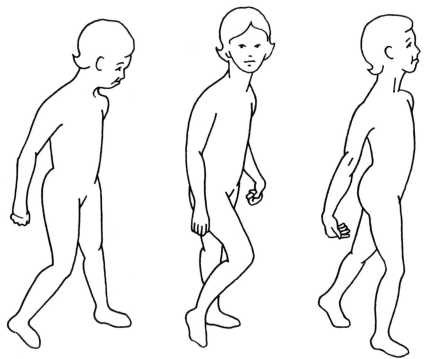

FIGURE 2-67. The child with fluctuating tone cannot grade and dissociate movements to walk with a beginning heel-toe pattern and pelvic rotation.

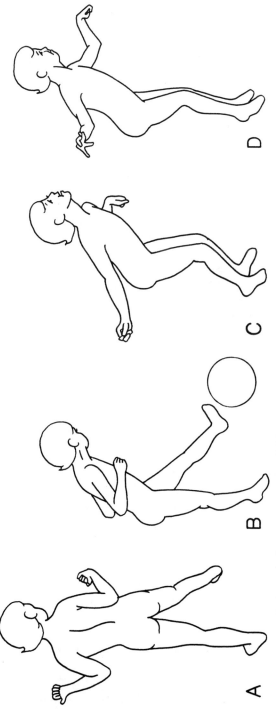

FIGURE 2-68. The stress of (A) running, (B) kicking, and (C and D) jumping elicits compensatory fixation and aberrant movements of the upper extremities.

at the end of the stance phase. The trunk leans somewhat forward during the swing phase, which tilts the pelvis anteriorly. The head extends and the arms also extend backward in a chainlike reaction at the end of the swing phase to offset the forward shift, which exaggerates the lordotic curve.

There is considerable regression when the child attempts to run. The base of support widens considerably, and the child shifts his weight to one side, moves the opposite leg, and then shifts his weight to the other side to regain his balance. Thus, the leg movements are stiff and abrupt, and the arms assume an aberrant protective position to compensate for the lack of proximal stability. (Fig. 2-68A).

Because the child has difficulty grading and dissociating movements, he keeps his leg extended to kick the ball, and there is also increased extension in the support leg, which places the weight more on the toes. If the child attempted to flex one leg in a preparatory movement, this very probably would elicit flexion of the support leg. The postural instability increases bodily tension, which hyperextends the neck and juts the chin forward, and the flexed arms also fixate in an adducted position. There is an exaggerated forward deviation of the trunk during the kicking movement (Fig. 2-68B).

The child flexes at the hips more so than the knees when he minimally crouches in readiness to jump, and the knees come closer together to provide distal stability. The head compensates by extending backward in an exaggerated way with the chin pointed upward. The one arm also extends backward (Fig. 2-68C). There is incomplete extension of the hips and knees during the take off, and the feet do not clear the surface or barely clear the surface. The arms move up in an aberrant high guard position because of immature equilibrium reactions (Fig. 2-68D).

The child with fluctuating tone has difficulty engaging in ball play because of more involvement in the upper extremities. Lack of proximal stability in the shoulder girdle limits the backward movement arc of the flexed arm during the readiness phase (Fig. 2-69A). The arm then moves from flexion to the other extreme of extension, and the ball is more or less dropped with an exaggerated hyperextension of the fingers, which reflects poor integration of the avoidance response (Fig. 2-69B). An unsuccessful attempt to catch a ball can elicit regression to abrupt, disorganized movements and asynchronous timing (Fig. 2-69C).

Summary of Effect of Compensatory Movement Patterns

When the above described patterns are compared with the patterns of a child who does not have a disability (Fig. 2-70), it is evident that there

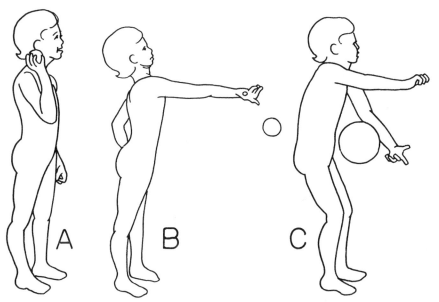

FIGURE 2-69. Ball play is hampered by the poor grading and control of movements in the upper extremities.

is a qualitative difference. The child with a motor impairment has to concentrate more intently on maintaining his balance and the upright position when walking, running, and performing other movements. The higher energy cost is evident in the muscular fixation, effortful and wasteful movements, and the strained facial expression. When physiologic demands exceed the adaptive capacity of the body, the child runs out of oxidative fuel, and there is more use of aneorobic pathways. Thus, he tires very quickly and has a limited ability to focus on environmental events as he walks because of the rechanneling of cognitive energy. The child may also have difficulty keeping up with the activity level of other children, and he has to pull back in the role of an observer, or he is left behind. He may become frustrated with his attempts to imitate the movement patterns of another child. I have observed that some children avoid motor play even in this stage, as if they already sense failure in a primitive way rather than an increasing sense of mastery of their body. This perception affects the child's budding sense of self.

There is also a difference in the way the child with a disability perceives his body. Parts of the body and interconnections between them are not as vividly sensed, or they are sensed in a different way. The child may not have as stable an inner referent of himself as an object that occupies a segment of space and moves from one position to

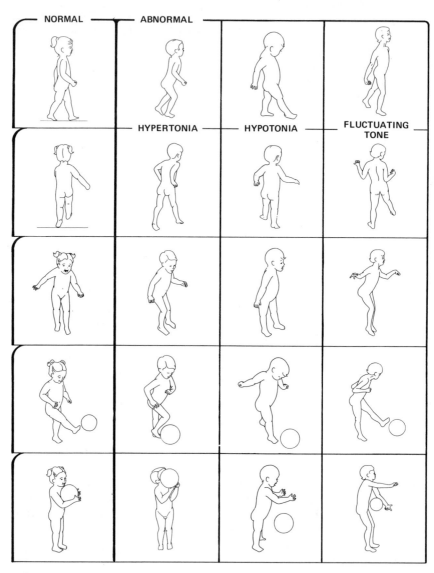

NORMAL ——— ABNORMAL ———

HYPERTONIA ——— HYPOTONIA ——— FLUCTUATING TONE

FIGURE 2-70. Compensatory motor patterns are compared with normal patterns.

DEVELOPMENTALLY DISABLED INFANTS AND TODDLERS

another relative to other objects. More limited and less focused mobility experiences may also interfere with the full awareness that an object is an independent entity that continues to exist in time and space over various visible and invisible displacements.

EFFECT OF MOTOR IMPAIRMENTS ON EXPLORATIVE SCHEMAS. If the walking gait is still characterized by midline instability and weaker equilibrium reactions, the upper extremities are not completely freed from a postural role, and the child may remain locked in at a lower skill level for a rather long period of time. When a child with hypertonia attempts a new skill (manipulate a crayon), there may be marked regression to a tight ulnar-palmar grasp. There is also an overflow of increased tone in the other upper extremity and other parts of the body. If there is prolonged, excessive use of flexor muscles, the grasp may remain primitive.

If the child cannot dissociate movements of the forearm and wrist from the shoulder and upper arm (supinate and pronate), and he lacks stability on the ulnar side of the hand as the background for regulating mobility on the radial side, his repertoire of schemas remains narrower in scope. He cannot experiment with the relationship between objects and means-end relationships in more complex and varied ways. The child has difficulty adding a new horizontal spatial dimension to his arrangements (aligning) if his hand remains in the palmar orientation. He therefore misses opportunities to come upon graphic forms and the notion of sameness when two like objects end up adjacent to each other. If the child cannot dissociate the movements and functions of the two hands and use one hand as a stabilizer and one hand as a mobilizer, he cannot adaptively stir the cake dough, grind the food, and help his caregiver with other similar activities. The toddler may also have difficulty coordinating the movements of the two sides of the body to clap to music and catch the ball.

Incomplete integration of reflexes interferes with exploration in a number of ways. If righting reactions are still strong, the toddler may feel a need to hold on to the chair with one hand when sitting because of the possibility that, if he turns his head or shoulder, the rest of the body will follow, and he will fall off the chair. Thus, one hand has to remain in a support role. If the STNR has not been fully integrated, flexion of the head will elicit flexion of the arms and extension of the legs, which interferes with sitting at a table with other family members to engage in an activity and to eat with a spoon. If the toddler has a persistent ATNR on the right, he will use his left hand, because it is easier to use the arm that is flexed to manipulate objects.

More limited reality testing and trial-and-error experimentation may delay the evolvement of a new approach—invention of a means through mental combinations. I have observed that if the child with hypertonia is encouraged to conserve energy and point where he wants the block, circle, or other object placed, he very often will persist in his attempts to place the object himself. It may be that he still has too fragile an inner referent of actions to internally experiment with the relationship between objects and develop a mental plan. The child may sense that he still needs to actively experiment to organize more stable inner images; he is not cognitively ready to be the Director. There is also the possibility that he is asserting his desire to do things himself.

EFECT OF MOTOR IMPAIRMENTS ON ORAL AND RESPIRATORY PATTERNS. As discussed previously, the toddler with a motor impairment does not walk with the ease and flexibility that characterizes the normal pattern at the end of this stage. There is more fixation of the shoulders, trunk, and hips, and the head is either flexed or extended. The tension limits the movement of the ribs and the front portion of the mouth, and the effort shortens the interval of sustained activity, which would strengthen ventilatory muscles. Also, if the toddler cannot blend stability and flexibility to begin dissociating the thorax from the pelvis when he walks, he very probably will have difficulty coordinating the respiratory muscles in a teamwork fashion as was discussed in the preceding stage. Nor can he control the movements of the smaller and faster acting thoracic muscles in more discrete ways.

Thus, there is a lack of background components for more refined intermeshing of breathing and phonation. If the respiration rate remains over 30, this very noticeably interferes with the toddler's ability to expand the expiratory phase.[68] An immature respiration pattern and neuromuscular control also limit the toddler's ability to momentarily increase the subglottal pressure to stress a syllable or word and enhance the meaning of his utterance. If the movement of the articulators is restricted or distorted by the position of the head, their role in regulating the air stream is compromised, which affects the formation or quality of certain sounds. An increased workload is also placed on the immature respiratory system.

Postural tension coupled with weak neck muscles may interfere with the formation of the supralaryngeal vocal tract and the descension and mobility of the larynx. The voice may remain higher pitched and less resonant, and vowels may continue to have a more nasal quality, which can be related to other factors. Defects of the oral-facial structure and hypotonia of the muscles responsible for the velopharyngeal closure is associated with Down syndrome, and children with this disability often have a hypernasal voice. Hypertrophied tonsils can reduce oral sound pressure levels.[69]

Just as the toddler has difficulty coordinating the movements of respiratory muscles to regulate the air pressure, he likewise has difficulty executing more complex, synergistic, articulatory movements to form an increasing number of words. There may be very exaggerated associated movements in the head and neck and a lot of concurrent body movement. The toddler tires quickly from the effort of talking. Chewing also requires more effort if the rotary jaw movement is not refined, and the toddler quickly experiences fatigue and lack of results when he attempts to eat a more textured food. He discards the carrot after a few bites.

The energy factor affects language development in another way. As discussed earlier, the toddler is not as attuned to stimuli when he is walking if conscious attention has to be directed to postural adaptations. He does not see as many novel objects and events more apt to elicit vocalization, if only an exclamation. The toddler, therefore, misses golden opportunities to attract his caregiver's attention and elicit a label for a new discovery. If the toddler fatigues more quickly, this discourages taking him on errands and other outings, and his range of experiences is more narrow. The results of a study of children with Down syndrome[70] suggest that the child's vocabulary is more influenced by his environmental experiences, whereas the structure of his utterance (ability to combine words) is related to his cognitive level.

Intertwined sensory and motor impairments limit the toddler's repertoire of explorative schemas, which no doubt affects the evolvement of representational thinking. If the toddler cannot follow invisible displacements of objects, internally experiment with means-end relationships, and substitute one object for another in beginning symbolic play, he may have a more limited ability to use words as a tool for social interaction.[71,72] He remains in the habitual labeling stage and is more dependent on perceptual and motor supports. As an example, the disabled toddler is more apt to label the present object, whereas the nondisabled toddler begins to refer to a past experience that was in some way related to the stimulus. He says "Daddy" when he sees a car versus just saying "car."

FRAMEWORK FOR HABILITATIVE APPROACHES

It is evident from the discussion thus far that this may be a stressful period for both the developmentally disabled child and family members. The stress will be compounded if there are other environmental factors that consume energy, such as financial strain, change in place of employment of one or both parents, or change in residence. The parents may request more intensive professional intervention, especially if the family has a weak support network. The intervener may sense that one or both parents has a need for someone to nourish their selfhood and help them work through internal struggles regarding their individuality and right to personal space. The parents may also need help from an outsider to provide the right level of emotional support, which gently nudges the child along the separation/individuation path.

It is even more important that the child have exploratory freedom in this stage not only to process stimulation at his own pace but also to practice being the mediator and introducer of events. New experiences will only facilitate the transition to a more advanced state of knowing if existing internal referents can impart meaning to the novelty. If the caregiver accepts this tenet, she will be more apt to tune in to the child's interests. She realizes that if she attempts to artificially force or mimic development, the child will be trained to submissively give the appropriate behavioral response in a specific instance with little transfer effect. Or the child may attempt to exercise his will by rejecting control and the learning experience. An elementary suggestion such as encouraging the caregiver to face her child as much as possible during interaction may increase her sensitivity to his cues and needs.

If the environment provides interesting objects and events mediated by the emotional availability and adaptiveness of the caregiver, and if the child has the freedom to pace his involvement, I have observed growth in terms of increased curiosity, goal-directed behavior, and autonomous function. The child engages in a particular activity for a more sustained period of time, because interest is the motivating factor. He also develops the ability to provide his own buffer by withdrawing to the periphery or to his room for a period of time until he can pull himself together. He then returns and explores the sensate world in a more ordered and cohesive manner. However, if the child is very reactive or very unresponsive to his environment, the external mediation burden increases considerably to maintain the right match between the stimulation level and the child's response threshold. There are realistic limits in terms of the caregiver's energy and ongoing adaptability even with the availability of suggestions such as those provided in Chapter 3.

Also, it is not realistic to always be emotionally available. It can be even more of a challenge to allow the toddler with a disability to practice rapprochement behaviors and willfulness without allowing him to perpetuate the illusion of omnipotence. The toddler's self-centered wishes can best be toned down by the reasonableness of the caregiver, which is an impossibility at times, because no one is infallible or always in control of his emotions. If the child has frequent temper tantrums on outings, especially when he is physically larger than his mental age, this can humiliate the caregiver. She is then more vulnerable, and her behavior may disintegrate. When the caregiver falls apart, this enhances the child's sense of smallness and insecurity. The intervener can help the caregiver evaluate circumstances that escalate tension within herself and the child. The intervener can also discuss a tendency to resort to food as an appeaser and means of control during this stage and the implications. Frequent snacking disrupts physiologic rhythms, thereby fueling stress reactions, and there is the problem of weight gain with some developmentally disabled children.

The philosophical framework discussed in the above paragraphs provides the basis for habilitative approaches that will be described in this stage. Just as is the case with the nondisabled toddler, the focus is on fostering a more functional pattern, a more functional communicative repertoire, more elaborate explorative schemas, a transition to representational thinking, and movement along the separation/individuation path.

Approaches to Foster a More Adaptive Walking Pattern and Explorative Schemas

Approaches will be outlined in this section to facilitate the following habilitative outcomes if the toddler has hypotonia or immature motor development.

- Develops increased strength in antigravity flexor and extensor muscles.
- Adjusts to a gravitational shift with a more mature equilibrium response in the lower positions.
- Develops increased flexibility in the trunk and pelvis.
- Develops increased stability and flexibility in the knee, ankle, and foot.
- Refines the movements of the lower extremities to walk with a beginning heel-toe gait.
- Develops increased strength and endurance in ventilatory muscles.
- Becomes more assertive in possessing his own body.
- Uses walking as a functional means to an end.
- Invents means through mental combinations with progressively less external adjustments.
- More fully recognizes the causal effect of one object on another and one part of an object on another.
- Arranges objects in more complex forms.
- Expands groupings of objects, actions, and events that functionally belong together.
- Begins to categorize objects on the basis of sameness.
- Deferably imitates actions.
- Associates an expanded number of objects with labels.
- Synchronizes movements in a more rhythmic way.

Specialized therapy will no doubt be required again in this stage to foster a more adaptive walking gait if the toddler has hypertonia or fluctuating tone. If the toddler has hypotonia or immature motor patterns, a complement of activities may foster more functional mobility. However, the caregiver adaptively modifies her approach in keeping with the toddler's developmental level. She uses modeling and environmental cues as a catalyst more so than physical contact to support the toddler's enhanced desire to possess his body. If he is still rather passive, this new approach very possibly will foster more active mediation of physical contact. The caregiver may have to fall back on some approaches in the preceding stage that involve proximal contact if the toddler has a severe visual impairment. He cannot see modeling or a visual lure, and a sound cue may not be an effective substitute at times.

There may be a need to engage the toddler in activities in lower positions to improve the quality of background components, especially if the disability was not identified early. Midline stability and a more erect upright posture are dependent on the balanced strength of flexor and extensor muscles, and rotation can only be superimposed on axial stability. More well-developed extensor muscles also serve as a background for the evolvement of the heel-toe pattern. The hip and knee must extend to push the foot off the surface with more of a thrust at the beginning of the swing phase and to place the heel in contact with the surface at the end of the swing phase.

The toddler may enjoy the following activities to strengthen antigravity extensor muscles, especially if he is allowed to assume the pivot prone position in a more independent way. He lies on his stomach over a low hassock or padded bench or box with his hands and knees in contact with the floor. The toddler is then encouraged to practice deferred imitation and fly like a bird or plane (Fig. 2-71A). The caregiver or sibling may have to provide perceptual cues by modeling the action. If the toddler has difficulty raising his arms and legs simultaneously, he can assume the position in segments. The toddler pulls the cord of a Mattel talking toy, which elicits a pivot prone position of the upper extremities and awareness of the causal effect of one part of an object on the other part (Fig. 2-71B). He is then encouraged to raise his legs to hit a ball with a bell inside or another sound-producing object suspended by the caregiver (Fig. 2-71C). A body action becomes the causal agent via direct spatial contact with the object. The toddler is also encouraged to pull a weighted wagon, box, or other object and pull another person forward in a "Row-Row the Boat" game.

The toddler is simultaneously engaged in activities to facilitate balanced strength in antigravity flexor muscles. He may enjoy imitating a modified hide-and-seek game. The caregiver or sibling acts as a model hiding her face by curling up with the arms crossed in the

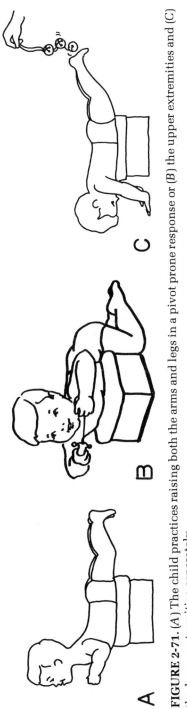

FIGURE 2-71. (A) The child practices raising both the arms and legs in a pivot prone response or (B) the upper extremities and (C) the lower extremities separately.

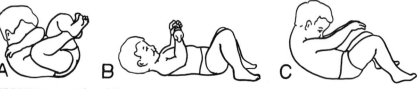

FIGURE 2-72. The child engages in activities to increase the strength in anti-gravity flexor muscles.

midline and the legs flexed up on the trunk. The toddler likewise hides his face (Fig. 2-72A). If the flexor muscles are too weak, he will no doubt have difficulty imitating the position. There is also the possibility that the inner representation of his body is not coherent enough to bring all the parts together. However, his attempt to hide will strengthen the muscles. The toddler is also encouraged to lie on his back and use an intermediary tool as a means to create an interesting effect, for example, push the toy apparatus which blows up balloons (Fig. 2-72B). If this is too difficult, the toddler can push a toy accordion or push prickly blocks together. These movements provide resistance to flexor muscle activity, and the toddler is also motivated to oppose the force of gravity and keep his head flexed to watch what he is doing. He is encouraged to experiment with an intermediary tool in another way. The toddler lies on his back and hits a suspended ball with a cardboard roll, which also elicits neck flexion. He gradually begins to develop a mental plan reflected by less external trial-and-error experimentation.

The toddler may enjoy other activities that strengthen the flexor muscles. The caregiver encourages him to become involved in an exercise session that includes a modification of the sit-up. She models sitting with the head and knees flexed and the extended arms forward in a *relaxed* position. The caregiver reclines back a short way and then sits back up keeping her head and knees flexed and the upper back curled. The toddler imitates the sit-back and gradually reclines farther as the flexor muscles strengthen (Fig. 2-72C). He is also encouraged to push a weighted wagon, box, or other object. He may come to the end of a narrower hall and start to pull the object backward. If he then goes around to the other side and pushes it, this reflects a beginning capacity to internally experiment with a means to achieve the desired result.

Stronger proximal muscles provide a more stable base for beginning pelvic and thoracic dissociation as the toddler walks, which has a counterbalancing effect. Another equally important substrate is flexible rotational movements in the lower positions. If this is lacking, the toddler is encouraged to continue engaging in motor play, which in-

DEVELOPMENTALLY DISABLED INFANTS AND TODDLERS

volves rolling over a hump (sofa pillow, his caregiver's body) or up an incline (old mattress at an angle, small hill outdoors). He may respond to the suggestion that he roll like the ball that the caregiver propels up the incline. The toddler may also enjoy rolling in a Wonder Bread barrel lined with a carpet sample. Refinement of the reciprocal and rotational combat crawl movements is fostered by encouraging the toddler to crawl on his stomach through box or bench tunnels to find a surprise at the other end, and the toddler may also imitate a lizard that he saw on an outing. The caregiver or sibling may need to provide some modeling to help him conjure an image of the movement. The toddler may be willing to sit on a small beach ball and twist to music, which involves pelvic and thoracic rotation (Fig. 2-73A), or he can twist to music when kneeling if the ball surface is too unstable. The oblique muscles are also activated by encouraging the toddler to pull the string on the Mattel talking toy, pull pop beads apart, and pull the rope in a tug-of-war game in a diagonal plane.

Since a beginning lateral pelvic shift accompanies rotation in the normal walking gait by the end of this stage, the toddler is involved in activities that increase the flexibility of lateral pelvic movements. He is enticed to lift one buttocks cheek when sitting on the ball or on a pillow by suggesting that a mouse is going to nip his bottom or another similar ruse (Fig. 2-73B). The movement also strengthens the lateral trunk muscles, which increases midline stability.

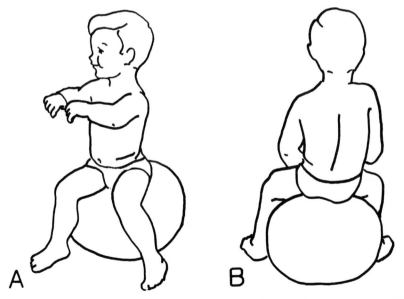

FIGURE 2-73. The child (A) dissociates pelvic and thoracic movements and (B) shifts the pelvis laterally on the ball.

More mature antigravity adjustments in the lower positions is an important background component for a more adaptive walking pattern. If the toddler still has immature equilibrium reactions in the sitting position, he is encouraged to sit on a piece of foam for an interval to look at a book with the caregiver or watch Sesame Street (Fig. 2-74A). When he has adjusted to the foam surface, he may sit on a T-stool, which should be high enough so the knees and hips are flexed at a right angle and the feet are on the floor (Fig. 2-74B). The above positions will also facilitate a more erect posture if the toddler has a tendency to slump. He may enjoy bouncing to his caregiver's song or other music when sitting on an inflatable clown, which also facilitates a more erect posture and adjustments to a gravitational shift. However, bouncing on an inflatable clown may elicit internal rotation at the shoulders and hips if the toddler with an immature motor pattern has a tendency to tense the body. The activity will therefore not elicit a more flexible equilibrium response and should be discontinued. This response may also signify abnormal tone associated with undiagnosed pathology.

The ability to dissociate the knee and ankle movements in a rudimentary heel-toe gait is dependent on background stability and flexibility in the hip, leg, ankle, and foot. Squatting therefore continues to be an important activity. The caregiver requests that the toddler

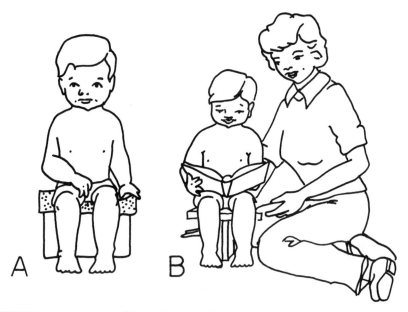

FIGURE 2-74. An unstable surface facilitates a more erect sitting posture and equilibrium responses.

help pick up objects indoors, and she also gives him a bucket to pick up rocks, leaves, sticks, and other objects outdoors. When the toddler sits down to rest, he may align the objects he has collected, place them in piles, or group them in other ways, possibly with some like objects together. The toddler may also enjoy walking, bouncing, and falling on an old mattress or large pillows. The added resistance of the uneven surface and the bouncing provide proprioceptive input through joint compression that elicits increased neuronal activity and muscle tone. The bouncing also provides vestibular input. Again, the activity should be discontinued if the hips and legs internally rotate. A dorsiflexion and plantarflexion movement of the ankle is elicited by having the toddler sit on a small ball with his feet on the surface and rock back and forth (Fig. 2-75).

More adaptive movements of the leg and foot are dependent on the caudal emergence of newer, more direct tactile and proprioceptive pathways and the modification of protective responses. When it is felt that the toddler has a more discriminative sense of where the leg and foot are in space and is capable of more adaptive motor planning, the caregiver encourages him to climb up more steps, climb on new pieces of playground equipment, and walk in areas where there is more surface variability. The toddler also sees new objects to explore and associate with a label as he moves in a new terrain. A sibling encourages the toddler to somewhat imitate stilt walking by walking in tissue boxes on different surfaces. The adaptation requires motor planning and helps the toddler control random, scattered movement if he is overactive.

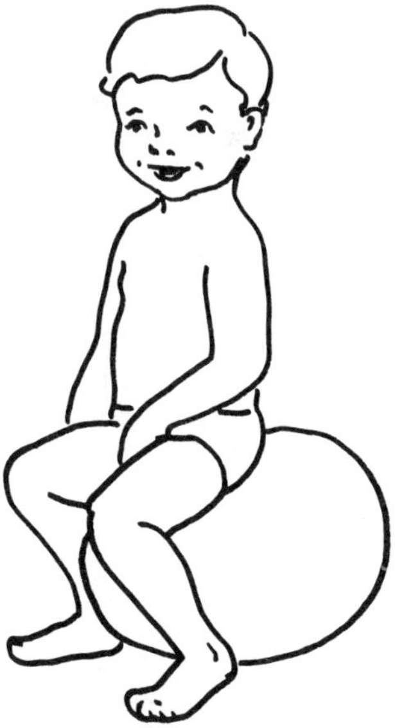

FIGURE 2-75. A forward and backward rocking movement on the ball facilitates increased flexibility in the ankles.

As the toddler's walking gait becomes less compensatory, he may meet the minimum criterion of a running gait with both feet leaving the surface for a brief nonsupport phase. The caregiver can help the toddler who is blind gain courage to run by holding both of his hands while moving backward. The toddler then senses that someone else is charting the space ahead. The caregiver gradually decreases her support by holding only one hand and then letting go of both of the toddler's hands as she moves backward. She also holds the toddler's hands to help him get the feel of jumping. Irrespective of the disability, the toddler may feel more comfortable kicking a ball down on his knees initially. A large light ball that compresses somewhat on contact may be easier for the child to kick in both the kneeling and upright position.

As movements become less wasteful and effortful, the toddler will no doubt remain involved in activities for a longer period of time, which increases the strength and endurance of ventilatory muscles. Physical fitness is a very popular movement, but there has to be a more cautious approach when the child has a developmental disability. Regular medical follow-up is important to identify cardiovascular abnormalities, respiratory infections, and other health problems that decrease the child's ability to physiologically adapt to increased energy demands. Another impediment is an emotional set that has evolved from unpleasurable experiences. The toddler ends an activity when he experiences even mild discomfort, because this sensation conjures an image of past events. Because many children enjoy the water, swimming very often is the activity that most effectively encourages the sustained involvement necessary for an aerobic form of exercise. There is also less likelihood of muscular and structural strain due to gravitational resistance. Practice with breath control is an added payoff as the toddler shortens the inspiration and lengthens the expiration. However, this activity may be contraindicated if tubes have been inserted to treat recurrent otitis media or there are other health problems.

Summary

If the toddler's walking pattern becomes less compensatory and he develops increased endurance, more conscious attention can be focused on stimuli and events in the environment. The toddler has more energy to follow his caregiver and other family members around the house and observe what they are doing and identify with them. Now that his hands are freed from a fixated, protective role, he can carry out a mental plan to obtain a no-no by lugging a chair over to the cupboard if there are corresponding advances in cognitive development. He can also stand by the caregiver's chair and demonstrate a new explorative discovery or enlist her assistance with a problem. The toddler becomes a more helpful assistant during daily routines, and he expands his groupings of things that belong together. He also uses walking as a means to engage in higher-order search behavior, inferring where his caregiver or a misplaced toy might be—their invisible displacement. He can direct more attention to his own displacements, and the toddler remembers where he came from in a familiar environment. Thus, he is more oriented in time and space. The toddler is taken on errands and other outings more frequently, which expands his sensate world and socialization with adults and other children.

Adaptation of Equipment to Provide a Source of Mobility and Expand Experiences

Again in this stage the child's level of motor functioning may lag behind other areas of development, and he is dependent on an assistive device to move about and explore the world. The team collaborates with the parents to determine the most appropriate mode of assistance. Important parameters to consider were discussed in this section of the preceding stage. It is even more important that the child is able to independently get on and off a device himself, if at all possible, to foster autonomous function. There is a dilemma if he needs something on the device to improve the position (abductor wedge on a belly board) which prevents him from assuming a more independent role. All aspects of development must be considered. Again, a device is not developmentally functional if the effort of mobility consumes so much energy that the toddler cannot focus on environmental stimuli, which is the primary reason for moving about.

Equipment should also be designed to support the child's expressed desire to do for himself. There are many suggestions in the book written by Finnie[73] of ways to position the child and use adaptive equipment that foster increased involvement in undressing, self feeding, and other care needs. Socialization is an important aspect of the separation/individuation process, and some adaptations should encourage imitation and identification with other children. A seat can possibly be devised for the swing and wagon, and a tricycle or other wheeled toy should also be modified if at all possible.

Approaches to Foster More Complex Explorative Schemas

More adaptive manipulative schemas is an important by-product of the above activities that facilitate a more functional walking gait, because the upper extremities are freed from a protective role. The caregiver can also involve the toddler in activities that foster increased strength in the shoulder girdle, arm, and ulnar side of the hand. With a background of stability, the toddler can begin regulating movements of the radial fingers to explore objects in more complex ways, such as aligning objects and operating the toy cash register. The toddler with hypertonia or fluctuating tone should only be involved in the activities under the direction of a therapist.

If the toddler has hypotonia or immature motor development unrelated to abnormal tone, he may enjoy some or all of the following activities. He is encouraged to assume the forearm support position and pull pop beads or prickly blocks apart or squirt water from a flexible, plastic spray bottle. The caregiver or a sibling may have to assume the same position and become involved in the activity to foster imitation. At other times during the day, the toddler can help his caregiver mist the plants with an atomizer. He can also rinse soap off his body with water from a spray bottle during the bath and play with a large sponge, which will elicit a squeezing action. The toddler may enjoy pushing objects into clay, and he may place some like objects together. The caregiver capitalizes on the toddler's interest in toting by giving him a suitcase to carry around and a bucket filled with objects that provide more weight and resistance.

If the toddler has difficulty coordinating the movements of the two arms to trap a ball, clap to music, and engage in other bilateral activities, practice may be helpful. He is encouraged to imitate rolling cookie dough, and this activity may facilitate deferred imitation and substitution of one object for another. The toddler rolls out play dough at a later time. He is encouraged to hold the handle of a weighted sander with both hands and help sand the board under supervision. The toddler may also enjoy all or some of the following activities involving bilateral coordination: holding the handle bars with the hands and pushing with both feet on a tricycle, holding the handles with the hands and bouncing up and down on a hoppity hop, pushing away from the wall with both hands when prone on a scooter board if one is available. Reciprocal movements of the upper extremities are facilitated by turning the sit-n-spin and pushing around in a circle when prone on a Lazy Susan platform or scooter board. Some children with a disability have difficulty operating the sit-n-spin and become discouraged.

The above activities involve proprioceptive, tactile, vestibular, visual, and auditory input. It is not just a matter of developing background stability to regulate mobility or to get the two hands moving together. More advanced explorative schemas also involve higher-order discrimination and integration of sensory input. The toddler has to have accurate information and a functional feedback mechanism as the basis for adjusting hand and finger movements to accommodate to the properties of the object and perform the intended action. If the toddler is exposed to a sensate world that he can relate to in a pleasurable way for the most part, this no doubt facilitates more organized processing of sensory stimuli versus reinforcement of avoidance behaviors. With support from the intervener, the caregiver more sensitively reads the toddler's cues, and she does not force him to engage in an activity that provides unpleasurable sensations. She also attempts to protect him from well-meaning but intolerable touch, such as tickling, hair tossling. If noxious stimulation cannot be avoided, the caregiver prepares the toddler for the coming event as much as possible. She becomes more understanding of overreactions and responds calmly rather than with punishment or humiliating remarks, such as "Don't be such a baby!" Sensitive mediation gives the toddler a sense of control over his body and exploration versus a feeling that he is a helpless victim of his environment.

The toddler is also supported in his adaptive substitution of one sense for another. In one study[74] approaches that were designed to remediate a weakness actually improved the function of a more intact sense. These findings suggest that the emphasis should be on strengths. However, Ayres[75] found that sensory input from one modality may increase receptivity to input and the processing capabilities of another sensory modality, that is, if the child has a learning disability. Ayres hypothesized that one component of the sensory system provides a substrate for the higher-order functioning of another component. There is much to be learned about the sensory system and the effects of input.

Adaptation of Objects and Experiences to Foster Explorative Schemas

The toddler may engage in some explorative activities only if objects are adapted or the experience is engineered in a certain way, which places an added burden on the caregiver. However, the increased responsiveness and involvement of the child is perceived by some caregivers as a fueling reciprocation. Ways to adapt objects and foster displacement schemas were outlined in this section of the preceding stage. These suggestions can also be used in this stage to encourage continued practice mapping objects in different arrangements and groupings. The caregiver provides additional assistance to facilitate arranging the objects in a new horizontal orientation—aligning. She gives the child objects that are easy to manipulate and access to a well-defined track, for example, long narrow box, edge of the table, window sill.

The caregiver catalyzes an expansion of functional categories by giving the child a selected assortment. She provides objects that lend themselves to stacking (plastic cubes) and three or four objects that do not lend themselves to stacking (small doll, car, spoon). On another day the child is given objects that lend themselves to aligning (large spools) with a long, narrow box and objects that lend themselves to nesting (three bowls of different sizes). It is interesting to see if he aligns the spools and nests the bowls or interacts with them in a different way, which should be accepted. The child may align magnets on the refrigerator, placing two or more alike ones together or group them in other ways. On some days, the child is given a pile of objects that relate to one another in the natural environment: shoe and sock, baby bottle and doll, keys and purse. He may interact with the objects in a way that reflects his recognition of paired relationships, for example, places the keys in the purse.

If the child has limited opportunity to run into problem situations because of mobility restrictions or difficulty focusing his attention, practice with means schemas may be facilitated by creating situations. When the child is relaxed in his bath, the caregiver places objects that float (ping pong ball, boat) and objects that do not float (golf ball, clean rock) in the water. One or more of the objects are placed out of reach. She places a fish net, large spoon, and spatula either in a can or in her hand. The child may experiment with the different tools as a means to retrieve the objects. At another time during the day the caregiver gives the child different-sized pans with lids and objects that fit in some of the pans and not in others. He is given objects that are easy to handle if hand movements are very clumsy, for example, bean bags, larger spools, easily graspable bottles. It is interesting to see how much trial-and-error experimentation the child engages in to fit objects in the pans and fit the right lids on the pans. The caregiver also remembers to especially encourage the motor involved child to observe her problem-solving approaches: bang a jar on the table to loosen the tight lid, stuff objects in a box to make them fit. An electronic device was described in the preceding stage to allow the child to operate switches as a means to elicit different effects. Very possibly the practice will lead to the development of means through mental combinations without the support of trial-and-error experimentation. The caregiver inhibits any tendency to interrupt the thinking process by providing suggestions.

The caregiver facilitates inferring a cause from an effect by standing behind the child and directing the beam of a flashlight in front of him, rolling a ball within view, and exposing him to other similar experiences. He may look for the source. She also places tape over one of the rings that fit on the plunger dowel described in the preceding stage. The child may attempt to cram the ring on the dowel, or he may notice the tape and put the ring aside indicating that he is aware of a hindrance to an end, or he may even more adaptively try to remove the tape. The toddler who is blind may not attempt to place the ring on the dowel when he feels the tape. The caregiver catalyzes an inference of a cause from an auditory effect by saying, "What do you hear?" when Daddy's truck stops in the driveway. The toddler who is blind may begin initiating interaction by saying "Hi" when he hears footsteps and the door shut.

Repetition may help the child make the transition to higher-order search behavior involving invisible displacements. The caregiver places an object in her hand in view of the child, closes her hand, and leaves the object under an easily grasped towel. If the child looks in the hand but not under the cover, the caregiver does not show him the object under the cover. She repeats the invisible displacement with several other objects. If the child continues to look in the hand each time, the caregiver removes the cover and becomes excited about finding all the objects. The child may begin to see the connection with this added help. When the object is invisibly displaced again, he glances at the hand and then focuses on the towel, which he removes. The eye movements alone are an indication that the child with a motor impairment is following the invisible displacement. He can actively engage in search behavior when objects are invisibly displaced if a mechanism has been set up whereby he can activate an easy switch to lift the screens.

Displacements have always been invisible for the child who is blind. Hiding activities are engineered to elicit more adaptive tactual search behavior which reflects his awareness of the permanence of objects. The caregiver makes a sound with a toy, hides it under a box, and stacks another box on top. If the toddler sustains his tactual search after not finding the object under the first box, this is an indication that he knows the object is permanent and is someplace. The caregiver progresses to stacking two boxes on top of the box that the object is hidden under. The caregiver also places two objects that are shaped differently and that sound differently under a cover. She then places a sound-making object that the toddler has been interacting with under the cover. If the toddler looks surprised when he picks up one of the other two objects and continues to search for the object he was interacting with, this is again an indication that he can maintain an image of a certain object and knows it is someplace.

If the caregiver brings props to the child, this may stimulate decentralization and the substitution of one object for another. He is given a fatter dowel and a doll with hair. The caregiver also makes her hair readily available and further catalyzes applying an action to a new context with a suggestion if necessary, "Comb Mommy's hair." A comb is provided if the child needs the actual object, but the dowel is placed in view, which may facilitate using the comb and then the dowel. The child may also attempt to place the comb in the doll's hand, making the doll the passive agent of an action.

Ball play encourages social interaction with the caregiver and also helps the child deal with separation anxiety when she leaves by acting out the disappearance and reappearance sequence. The child with fluctuating tone can handle a heavy ball more easily, whereas the child with hypertonia can more easily handle a smaller, light ball. A bean bag may be easier to throw and catch, irrespective of the nature of the child's disability. If the child cannot track a ball moving in the air, it is rolled along the surface. The path of the ball then becomes two dimensional in terms of speed and direction. The trajectory is also more easy to follow if the ball is a bright color that contrasts with the surface or has a bell inside, if the child has a severe visual impairment. With practice playing with a ball, the child may not have to actually see the trajectory. When the ball disappears behind the caregiver's back, he foresees that it will appear on the other side of her, and he looks toward the future position.

Labeling pictures in a book and listening to a very elementary story allows the toddler to experience closeness and distance simultaneously. He possibly can visually make sense of only one large object on a page with a plain background. The caregiver can color single objects in a coloring book, if she cannot find a book featuring one familiar, lifelike object on a page. A series of objects can also be arranged on subsequent pages for a simple story. A toddler with a severe visual impairment may respond to a simple story that centers on a familiar object and includes the child's name. The caregiver can also add touch and movement input. A child with severe mental retardation very possibly will not progress to the point that he can use pictures to represent persons and objects in his environment or think representationally in other ways.[76]

In the course of adapting objects and events in a more circumscribed way, the caregiver must not lose sight of the importance of broader environmental parameters. In a study of children with Down syndrome,[77] a lower developmental performance was associated with poor organization of the physical and temporal environment, a lesser number of appropriate objects to interact with, and less maternal involvement. Experiences must be organized around a social and spatial/temporal base.

Approaches to Foster Language Development

It also seems reasonable to maintain a broader view in terms of the intertwined effect that all the above activities have on language development. If the toddler can move about and explore objects in more adaptive ways, he is doing more to talk about, and speech is primarily tied to actions again in this stage. The toddler practices being the agent of actions, and he more clearly perceives that other persons are separate and can serve as an agent of actions. He also experiences more and more effects that actions have on objects in a means-end relationship. The toddler may find that single words are no longer adequate to express thoughts and an elementary conceptualization of roles that evolve from experiences. There is an increasing emphasis on the motivational, personal, and social aspects of speech rather than just syntax and semantics.[78]

The caregiver is no doubt the most powerful motivator of language. If she sensitively responds to the toddler's attempts to communicate within reasonable limits, she provides him with the optimal means to elicit her emotional investment in his activities and needs. However, a less contingent approach may have its origin in the early infancy period based on Field's findings.[79] If the mother was less attentive and sensitive to her infant's cues, she was more directive and less contingent when the infant became a toddler. She also posed more questions possibly to elicit feedback that would verify the child's comprehension. The child was less verbal, had a smaller working vocabulary, and vocalized in a shorter utterance. Researchers are beginning to look at the role of parental speech in language development. Does the language acquisition problem stem at least in part from a deviant model who does not yoke to the child's developmental level?

It is a challenge to stay in tune with the developmentally disabled child's cognitive level and his processing rhythm. The caregiver may find it difficult to allow time for the toddler to express his thoughts, inhibiting a tendency to provide words or fill in words too quickly, which can deny him the opportunity of combining words himself. Yet, it is also important that the caregiver know when to intervene and help the toddler put his actions, feelings, desires, and observations into words. The caregiver may also have difficulty remaining in the periphery and allowing the toddler to talk to himself and play with words and phrases rather than succumbing to an urge to dominate the nature of the content. In a quest to catalyze talking of any kind, the caregiver may be tempted to engage the toddler in labeling games of objects and pictures that have little or no meaning in his concrete world rather than grounding verbal experiences in reality. As discussed earlier, the developmentally disabled child may be even more reliant on the immediate perceptual field and concrete actions to determine the meaning of words.

The caregiver may also be tempted to encourage the toddler to form isolated sounds and place his tongue in a specific location. Yet, even the toddler without a disability cannot separate a syllable into a consonant and vowel in this stage. A word involves a blend and flow of sounds, and a particular sound is not made with the articulator in one exact position. The placement varies depending on the sound preceding and following.[80] The caregiver can engage the toddler in games involving syllables, for example, "This is the way we say bee bee," and other nonsense sounds (boe boe).

Rhythmic activities may help the toddler organize and synchronize his speech, facial expressions, head movements, and body position changes just as the nondisabled toddler does. The activities may also enhance his awareness of pitch and stress patterns and other salient features in the structure of his language. He is encouraged to bounce or sway his body or shake an instrument in rhythm with the caregiver's song. The toddler is also involved in games involving a sequence of movements: Ring-Around-the-Rosey, London Bridges, This is the Way We Wash Our Clothes. Some of the activities described earlier encourage rhythmic movement.

The length of the toddler's utterance may be regulated by a much more mundane but equally important factor such as the lung volume. The ventilatory muscles will become stronger and more fatigue-resistant as the child engages in more sustained activity such as swimming, and the vital capacity will likewise increase. The caregiver can also engage the toddler in activities to help him learn to use the ventilatory muscles more adaptively. He may imitate a deeper inspiration and slower expiration in yoga breathing, especially if he hums during the expiration. The caregiver can also encourage the toddler to imitate her simulation of yawning movements. She sits and flexes and abducts her arms, placing her hands behind her head. The caregiver inhales as she pulls the hands back, elevates the rib cage, and arches the back. The caregiver then exhales as she flexes the head and thoracic area, adducts and extends the arms, and leans forward to place the elbows between the abducted knees. A fanning of the air in front of the toddler's nostrils may also elicit a deeper inspiratory movement.

If there is no speech, this does not infer that there is no internal language, especially if the child's nonverbal signals indicate otherwise. The caregiver and interveners continue to explore the child's language-learning capacity—signing, T-K speech, or other modes. In one study[81] the developmentally disabled children were able to sign in a phrase much earlier than they could expressively combine two words. These findings suggest that sign language is easier to learn and use in a functional way.

The child with a severe motor impairment may learn to use an elementary communication board with pictures of familiar persons and objects. This may be the most effective option because the child does not feel pressured to attempt to speak and experience failure over and over when he cannot get his message across. Instead, he senses the power of communication. The caregiver is also sensitive to the child's gestures, because a communication board cannot accompany him everywhere. Also, the board has to remain limited in scope in keeping with the child's budding level of representational thinking. His eyes may brighten or he may smile when he wants more carrots, to go to grandmother's, or engage in his environment in other ways. Averting his gaze or a sober expression signals lack of interest and disengagement. The child may learn to shake his head in a "no" gesture, although a head shake for "yes" will probably not evolve in this stage. A particular child enjoyed a game with his parents that gave him a sense of power and fostered increased interest in communication. Whichever parent he looked at as he smiled would blow the "doopity doo"—a sound instrument rigged up by connecting plastic plumbing pipes together.

Approaches to Foster Self Awareness and Autonomous Function

The toddler becomes more aware of the wholeness and centeredness of his body as he engages in activities that increase midline stability and activities that involve bodily contact with the floor (rolling up an incline). He also becomes more aware of individual parts as movements become more flexible. The perineal muscles are strengthened when he squats, belly crawls through a tunnel, and tenses and releases muscles during genital play. There is a possibility that sensory input from these experiences influences the maturation of the newer posterior column, medial lemniscal pathways that transmit more localized information to the higher levels. The toddler more discriminantly perceives sensations in the lower part of his body, including the urge to urinate and defecate and sensations during the actual elimination.

Self-representation is also tied to the emergence of other parameters of development according to the results of a study by Mans, Cicchetti, and Sroufe.[82] The child with Down syndrome recognized himself as a separate person within the normal child's timetable, if the mental age was used as the criterion. Thus, the separation/individuation process represents a complex interplay between an affective attachment, maturational changes, and environmental experiences. There no doubt has to be a coalescence of the toddler's awareness of separateness, a desire to possess his body as his own, and an ability to plan movements before he begins to assert his autonomy in more definite ways during daily care routines. If the child is pressured to do for himself before he is developmentally ready, he will perform the skills in a programmed way with heavy reliance on extrinsic motivational forces.

An approach that completes toilet training in a day or week also has implications in terms of readiness. If the toddler is only vaguely aware of bodily sensations because of delayed maturation of the newer pathways, he is unlikely to realize that the bowel movement or urine belongs to him, and he will not be able to associate an urge with the actual act. Elimination functions may also be very irregular. It becomes a matter of programmed training or hit-and-miss elimination when the child is placed on the potty. If the disabled toddler is becoming aware of his separateness and senses a need to possess his body, there is a possibility that the potty will become a battleground. Submission to the will of the caregiver can be at the expense of healthy self-assertion and a sense of pride in the ownership of his body. No one really wins if toilet training is embedded in a negative and tense context.

Need for Alternate Care Resources

The developmentally disabled child may remain in this stage for a rather long period or never progress beyond this stage. If the child remains egocentric in that he cannot see another person's viewpoint and if he continues to engage in the conflictive drama of oneness and separateness over a prolonged period, this can place chronic adaptive demands on family members. There may be an even more urgent need to share the role of caregiving with another resource. Or the parents may feel that the toddler is ready to relate to other adults and children in a group session in an early intervention program. However, Blehar[83] found that children who were first enrolled in a day care program at two or three years of age cried more during separation, resisted the caregiver on reunion, and were more wary of strangers than children cared for at home. The investigator proposed that it may be more difficult for a child to adjust to long absences from his caregiver at this age. He may interpret this as abandonment at a time when he needs increased assurance of his caregiver's love.

Although the above study involved children who do not have a disability, the results suggest that a transition period should be encouraged when a new caregiving resource is used. As an example, if the toddler is enrolled in an early intervention program or a special education class and the caregiver is not employed, she is encouraged to stay in the corner of the room, an adjacent bathroom, or an office area. The child is then free to leave and return to her at his own pace. When the child is comfortable remaining with other adults and children for a longer period of time, he no doubt will be ready for his caregiver to leave him. He has been allowed to gradually determine the optimal distance in the new environment. If he has pleasant experiences, this can help him cope with hospital admissions and other more stressful separation episodes.

It is more of a challenge to meet the environmental needs of each child in a program setting. If the child has lived in a home with a low level of stimulation or if he is reactive to stimuli, the new environment may be too noisy and confusing for him whereas the level is just right for another child. There is also a challenge in terms of the child's need for a relationship with a significant adult. The toddler in this stage still does not have the repertoire of verbal skills to elicit and maintain more elaborate social interchanges with peers as discussed earlier. There is a trend to more emphasis on the emotional aspects of the child's development in whatever setting he is in. Adults are beginning to look at both the soma and soul of the child.

REFERENCES: INTRODUCTION

1. STOCKMEYER, SA: An interpretation of the approach of Rood to the treatment of neuromuscular dysfunction. Am J Phys Med 46:900, 1967.
2. LORIA, C: Relationship of proximal and distal function in motor development. Phys Ther 60:167, 1980.

REFERENCES: FIRST STAGE

1. COMPARETTI, AM: Postural Reflexes in Normal and Abnormal Motor Development: Implications for Intervention. Presentation at Thirty-Third Annual Meeting, American Academy for Cerebral Palsy and Developmental Medicine, San Francisco, September, 1979.
2. GILFOYLE, EM AND GRADY, AP: Cognitive-perceptual-motor behavior. In: WILLARD, HS AND SPACKMAN, CS (EDS): Occupational Therapy. JB Lippincott, Philadelphia, 1971, p 401.
3. FIORENTINO, MR: Reflex Testing Methods for Evaluating CNS Development. Charles C Thomas, Springfield, Ill, 1978.
4. HAYNES, U. A Developmental Approach to Casefinding: Among Infants and Young Children. Health, Education, and Welfare, (HSA) 79-5210, Bethesda, Maryland, 1979.
5. WYKE, B: The neurological basis of movement—A developmental review. In: HOLT, K (ED): Movement and Child Development. JB Lippincott, Philadelphia, 1975, p 19.
6. BRAZELTON, TB: Neonatal Behavioral Assessment Scale. JB Lippincott, Philadelphia, 1973, p 13.
7. GILFOYLE AND GRADY, op. cit.
8. STOCKMEYER, SA: A sensorimotor approach to treatment. In: PEARSON, PH AND WILLIAMS, CE (EDS): Physical Therapy Services in the Developmental Disabilities. Charles C Thomas, Springfield, Ill, 1972, p 186.
9. STOCKMEYER, SA: An interpretation of the approach of Rood to the treatment of neuromuscular dysfunction. Am J Phys Med 46:900, 1967.
10. WEEKS, ZR: Effects of the vestibular system on human development: Part 1. Overview of functions and effects of stimulation. Am J Occup Ther 33:376, 1979.

11. Goodkin, F: *The development of mature patterns of hand-eye coordination in the human infant.* Early Human Devel 4:373, 1980.

12. Bower, TGR: *A Primer of Infant Development.* WH Freeman, San Francisco, 1977, p 26.

13. Burton, LW, Castle, P, and Held, R: *Observations on the development of visually-directed reaching.* Child Devel 35:349, 1954.

14. Ammon, JE and Etzel, ME: *Sensorimotor organization in reach and prehension: A developmental model.* Phys Ther 57:7, 1977.

15. Burton, Castle, and Held, op. cit.

16. Stockmeyer, op. cit.

17. Lieberman, P, Crelin, ES, and Klatt, DH: *Phonetic ability and related anatomy of the newborn and adult human, neanderthal man, and the chimpanzee.* Am Anthropol 74:287, 1972.

18. Lieberman, P: *On the Origins of Language.* Macmillan, New York, 1975, p 113.

19. Buhr, RD: *The emergence of vowels in an infant.* J Speech Hear Res 23:73, 1980.

20. Thach, BT: *Morphologic zones of the human fetal lip margin.* In: Bosma, JF (ED): *Fourth Symposium on Oral Sensation and Perception.* US Department of Health, Education, and Welfare, Bethesda, Maryland, 1973, p 96.

21. Brown, JV: *Non-nutritive sucking in great ape and human newborns: Some phylogenetic and ontogenetic characteristics.* In: Bosma, JF (ED): *Fourth Symposium on Oral Sensation and Perception.* US Department of Health, Education, and Welfare, Bethesda, Maryland, 1973, p 118.

22. Sameroff, A: *Reflexive and operant aspects of sucking behavior in early infancy.* In: Bosma, JF (ED): *Fourth Symposium on Oral Sensation and Perception.* US Department of Health, Education, and Welfare, Bethesda, Maryland, 1973, p 135.

23. Campbell, D: *Sucking as an index of mother-child interaction.* In Bosma, JF (ED): *Fourth Symposium on Oral Sensation and Perception.* US Department of Health, Education, and Welfare. Bethesda, Maryland, 1973, p 152.

24. Newth, CJL: *Recognition and management of respiratory failure.* Pediatr Clin North Am 26:617, 1979.

25. Muller, NL and Bryan, AC: *Chest wall mechanics and respiratory muscles in infants.* Pediatr Clin North Am 26:503, 1979.

26. Krieger, I: *Studies on mechanics of respiration in infancy.* Dis Child 105:439, 1963.

27. Muller and Bryan, op. cit.

28. Curzi-Dascalova, L and Plassart, E: *Respiratory and motor events in sleeping infants: Their correlation with thoracico-abdominal respiratory relationships.* Early Human Devel 2:39, 1978.

29. Newth, op. cit.

30. BRYAN, AC: *Diaphragmatic fatigue in newborns.* Am Rev Res Dis 119:143, 1979.

31. ERIKS, J: *Infant "talk".* In: *Learning Resource Manual.* Nursing Child Assessment Satellite Training Project, University of Washington, 1979, p 170.

32. STERN, D: *The First Relationships: Infant and Mother.* Harvard University Press, Cambridge, Mass., 1977, p 47.

33. EISENBERG, RB: *Auditory Competence in Early Life: The Roots of Communicative Behavior.* University Park Press, Baltimore, 1976, pp 10, 139.

34. DECASPER, AJ AND FIFER, WP: *Of human bonding: Newborns prefer their mothers' voices.* Science 208:1174, 1980.

35. CONDON, WS AND SANDER, LN: *Neonate movement is synchronized with adult speech: Interactional participation and langauge acquisition.* Science 183:99, 1974.

36. ARMITAGE, SE, BALDWIN, BA, AND VINCE, MA: *The fetal sound environment of sheep.* Science 208:1173, 1980.

37. WILDER, CN: *Respiratory Patterns in Infants: Birth to Eight Months.* University Microfilms, Ann Arbor, 1973.

38. CURZI-DASCALOVA AND PLASSART, op. cit.

39. CURZI-DASCALOVA, L: *Thoracico-abdominal respiratory correlations in infants: Constancy and variability in different sleep stages.* Early Human Devel 2:25, 1978.

40. SHARP, JT, et al: *Relative contributions of rib cage and abdomen to breathing in normal subjects.* J Appl Physiol 39:608, 1975.

41. KEENS, TG AND JANUZZO, DC: *Development of fatigue-resistant muscle fibers in human ventilatory muscles.* Am Rev Resp Dis 119:139, 1979.

42. MULLER AND BRYAN, op. cit.

43. BOYDEN, EA: *Notes on the development of the lung in infancy and early childhood.* Am J Anat 121:749, 1967.

44. GEORGE, SL: *A longitudinal and cross-sectional analysis of the growth of the postnatal cranial base angle.* Am J Phys Anthropol 49:171, 1978.

45. KENT, RD: *Anatomical and neuromuscular maturation of the speech mechanism: Evidence from accoustical studies.* J Speech Hear Res 19:421, 1976.

46. BUHR, op. cit.

47. SMITH, BL AND OLLER, DK: *A comparative study of pre-meaningful vocalizations produced by normally developing and Down's syndrome infants.* J Speech Hear Dis 46:46, 1981.

48. BUHR, op. cit.

49. SMITH AND OLLER, op. cit.

50. MENYUK, P: *The role of distinctive features in children's acquisition of phonology.* J Speech Hear Res 11:138, 1968.

51. KENT, op. cit.

52. SHEPPARD, WC AND LANE, HL: *Development of the prosodic features of infant vocalizing.* J Speech Hear Res 11:94, 1968.

53. STERN, op. cit.

54. MILLER, JF ET AL: *Language comprehension in sensorimotor stages V and VI.* Speech Hear Res 23:284, 1980.

55. BANKS, MS: *The development of visual accommodation during early infancy.* Child Devel 51:646, 1980.

56. GOREN, CC, SARTY, M, AND WU, PYK: *Visual following and pattern discrimination of face-like stimuli by newborn infants.* Pediatrics 56:544, 1975.

57. KLAUS, M: *Basic biopsychosocial process of bonding.* Presentation at conference: *Unexpected Risks for the High Risk Infant, the Newborn, the Parents, and the Staff.* Los Angeles, California, October, 1977.

58. FLAVELL, JG: *The Developmental Psychology of Jean Piaget.* Van Nostrand, Princeton, New Jersey, 1963, p 138.

59. BOWER, TGR: *Heterogeneous summation in human infants.* Animal Behav 14:395, 1966.

60. WEIZMANN, F, COHEN, LB, AND PRATT, RJ: *Novelty, familiarity, and the development of infant attention.* Devel Psychol 4:149, 1971.

61. FRIEDMAN, S: *Newborn visual attention to repeated exposure of redundant vs. "novel" targets.* Perception and Psychophysics 12:291, 1972.

62. SELF, PA: *Control of infant visual attending by auditory and interspersed stimulation.* Monographs Society Research Child Development 39:16, 1974.

63. UZGIRIS, IC AND HUNT, JM: *Attentional preference and experience: II. An exploratory longitudinal study of the effect of visual familiarity and responsiveness.* J Genet Psychol 117:109, 1970.

64. BURTON, CASTLE, AND HELD, op. cit.

65. FLAVELL, op. cit., p 124.

66. BURTON, CASTLE, AND HELD, op. cit.

67. BOWLBY, J: *Attachment and Loss (vol. 1): Attachments.* Basic Books, New York, 1969, p 273.

68. ARONSON, E AND ROSENBLOOM, S: *Space perception in early infancy: Perception within a common auditory-visual space.* Science 172:1161, 1971.

69. MARTIN, RM: *Effects of familiar and complex stimuli on infant attention.* Devel Psychol 11:178, 1975.

70. WETHERFORD, JJ AND COHEN, LB: *Developmental changes in infant visual preferences for novelty and familiarity.* Chld Devel 44:416, 1973.

71. SIGMAN, M AND PARMELEE, AH: *Visual preferences of four-month-old premature and full-term infants.* Child Devel 45:959, 1974.

72. MAHLER, MS, PINE, F, AND BERGMAN, A: *The Psychological Birth of the Human Infant.* Basic Books, New York, 1975, p 41.

73. STERN, op. cit., p 25.

74. BRAZELTON, TB: *Early parent-infant reciprocity.* In: BRAZELTON, TB AND VAUGHN, V (EDS): *The Family: Can It Be Saved.* Yearbook Medical Publishers, Chicago, 1976, p 133.

75. Spitz, RA: *The First Year of Life.* International University Press, New York, 1965, p 139.

76. Brazelton, op. cit., 1976, p 137.

77. Ibid., 1976, p 138.

78. Ricks, M, Krafchuk, E, and Tronick, E: *A descriptive study of infant-mother face to face interaction at 3, 6, and 9 months of age.* Presentation at Biennial Meeting, Society for Research in Child Development, San Francisco, March, 1979.

79. Wolf, PH: *Observations on the early development of smiling.* In: Foss, BM (ed): *Determinants of Infant Behavior, Vol 2.* John Wiley & Sons, New York, 1963, p 113.

80. Bowlby, op. cit., p 266.

81. Lamb, ME: *Separation and reunion behaviors as criteria of attachment in mothers and fathers.* Early Human Devel 3:329, 1979.

82. Chibucos, TR and Kail, PR: *Longitudinal examination of father-infant interaction and infant-father attachment.* Merrill-Palmer Quarterly 27:81, 1981.

83. Stern, op. cit., p 16.

84. Lewis, M and Goldberg, S: *Perceptual-cognitive development in infancy: A generalized expectancy model as a function of the mother-infant interaction.* Merrill-Palmer Quarterly 15:81, 1969.

85. Pederson, FA, Rubenstein, JL, and Yarrow, LJ: *Infant development in father absent families.* J Genet Psychol 135:3, 1979.

86. Clark, DL, Kreutzberg, JR, and Chee, FKW: *Vestibular stimulation influence on motor development in infants.* Science 196:1228, 1977.

87. Korner, AF, and Thoman, EB: *Visual alertness in neonates as evoked by maternal care.* J Exper Child Psychol 10:67, 1970.

88. Lewis and Goldberg, op. cit.

89. Stern, op. cit., p 91.

90. Yarrow, LJ and Goodwin, MS: *Some conceptual issues in the study of mother-infant interaction.* Am J OrthoPsychiatr 35:473, 1965.

91. Sameroff, AJ: *Caretaking or reproductive casualty? Determinates in developmental deviancy.* In: Kearsley, RB and Siegal, IE (eds): *Infants at Risk: Assessment of Cognitive Functioning.* Halstead Press, New York, 1979, p 79.

92. Donovan, WL, Leavitt, LA, and Balling, JD: *Maternal physiological response to infant signals.* Psychophysiol 15:68, 1978.

93. Barnard, KE and Eyres, SJ: *Child health assessment: part 2: The first year of life.* DHEW Publications, No. HRA 79-25, 1979.

94. Thoman, EB, Becker, PT, and Freese, MP: *Individual patterns of mother-infant interaction.* In: Sackett, GP (ed): *Observing Behavior: Vol. I: Theory and Applications in Mental Retardation.* University Park Press, Baltimore, 1978, p 95.

95. Fraiberg, S: *Insights From the Blind.* Basic Books, New York, 1977, p 275.

96. Chee, FKW, Kreutzberg, JR, and Clark, DL: *Semicircular canal stimulation in cerebral palsied children.* Phys Ther 58:1071, 1978.

97. KANTNER, RM, ET AL: *Effects of vestibular stimulation on nystagmus response and motor performance in the developmentally delayed infant.* Phys Ther 56:414, 1976.

98. GOODKIN, op. cit.

99. ILLINGWORTH, RS: *Delayed visual maturation.* Arch Dis Child 36:407, 1961.

100. MIRANDA, SB AND FANTZ, RL: *Recognition memory in Down's syndrome and normal infants.* Child Devel 45:651, 1974.

101. LASKY, RE AND KLEIN, RE: *Fixation of the standard and novelty preference in six-month-old well- and malnourished infants.* Merrill-Palmer Quarterly 26:171, 1980.

102. THOMAN, EB AND BECKER, PT: *Issues in assessment and prediction for the infant born at risk.* In: FIELD, T (ED): *Infants Born at Risk.* SP Medical and Scientific Books, New York, 1979, p 461.

103. MULLER AND BRYAN, op. cit.

104. BRYAN, op cit.

105. VOYSEY, M: *A Constant Burden: The Reconstitution of Family Life.* Routledge & Kegan-Paul, Boston, 1975, p 39.

106. SAMEROFF, op. cit., 1979.

107. WHITE, BL AND HELD, R: *Plasticity of sensorimotor development in the human infant.* In: ROSENBLITH, JF AND ALLINSMITH, W (EDS): *The Causes of Behavior II: Readings in Child Development and Educational Psychology.* Allyn & Bacon, Boston, 1966, p 60.

108. WHITE AND HELD, op. cit.

109. BELL, SM AND AINSWORTH, MDS: *Infant crying and maternal responsiveness.* Child Devel 43:1171, 1972.

110. MULLER AND BRYAN, op. cit.

111. FARBER, SD AND HUSS, AJ: *Sensorimotor Evaluation and Treatment Procedures for Allied Health Personnel.* The Indiana University Foundation, Indianapolis, 1974, p 90.

112. HUSS, AJ: *Touch with care or a caring touch?* Am·J Occup Ther 31:11, 1977.

113. SMITH, KU AND HENRY, JP: *Cybernetic foundations for rehabilitation.* Am J Phys Med 46:379, 1967.

114. WACHS, TD: *Proximal experience and early cognitive-intellectual development: The physical environment.* Merrill-Palmer Quarterly 25:3, 1979.

115. GOULD, V: *Cognitive development.* In: FREEMAN, J, ET AL. (EDS): *ADAPT: A Developmental Curriculum.* Health and Welfare Agency. State of California, 1975, p 161.

116. THOMAN AND BECKER, op. cit.

117. MULLER AND BRYAN, op. cit.

118. HUTCHINSON, AA, ROSS, KR, AND RUSSELL, G: *The effects of posture in ventilation and lung mechanics in preterm and light-for-date infants.* Pediatrics 64:429, 1979.

119. FLEMING, PJ, ET AL.: *The effects of abdominal loading on rib cage distortion in premature infants.* Peditrics 64:425, 1979.

REFERENCES: SECOND STAGE

1. STOCKMEYER, SA: *A sensorimotor approach to treatment.* In: PEARSON, PH AND WILLIAMS, CE (EDS): *Physical Therapy Services in the Developmental Disabilities.* Charles C Thomas, Springfield; Ill, 1972, p 186.

2. STOCKMEYER, SA: *An interpretation of the approach of Rood to the treatment of neuromuscular dysfunction.* Am J Phys Med 46:900, 1967.

3. GILFOYLE, EM AND GRADY, AP: *Cognitive-perceptual-motor behavior.* In: WILLARD, HS AND SPACKMAN, CS (EDS): *Occupational Therapy.* J. B. Lippincott, Philadelphia, 1971, p. 401.

4. STOCKMEYER, op. cit., 1972.

5. BOSMA, JF: *Anatomic and physiologic development of the speech apparatus.* In: TOWER, DB: *The Nervous System Vol. 3: Human Communication and Its Disorders.* Raven Press, New York, 1975, p 469.

6. HEIN, A AND HELD, R: *A neural model for labile sensorimotor coordinations.* In: BERNARD, EE AND KARE, MR (EDS): *Biological Prototypes and Synthetic Systems. Vol. 1.* Plenum Press, New York, 1962, p 71.

7. HALVERSON, HM: *Variations in pulse and respiration during different phases of infant behavior.* J Genet Psychol 59:259, 1941.

8. MULLER, NL AND BRYAN, AC: *Chest wall mechanics and respiratory muscles in infants.* Pediatr Clin North Am 26:503, 1979.

9. BOYDEN, EA: *Notes on the development of the lung infancy and early childhood.* Am J Anat 121:749, 1967.

10. HAPPENBROUWERS, T, ET AL: *Polygraphic studies of normal infants during the first sixth months of life. II. Respiratory rate and variability as a function of state.* Pediatr Res 12:120, 1978.

11. CURZI-DASCALOVA, L: *Thoracico-abdominal respiratory correlations in infants: Constancy and variability in different sleep states.* Early Human Devel 2:25, 1978.

12. MULLER AND BRYAN, op. cit.

13. WILDER, CN: *Respiratory patterns in infants: Birth to eight months.* University Microfilms, Ann Arbor, 1973.

14. GEORGE, SL: *A longitudinal and cross-sectional analysis of the growth of the postnatal cranial base angle.* Am J Phys Anthropol 49:171, 1978.

15. RUTHERFORD, D: *Auditory motor learning and the acquisition of speech.* Am J Phys Med 46:245, 1967.

16. BOSMA, J: *Assessment and prognosis of oral pharyngeal dysfunction in cerebral palsy.* Presentation Thirtieth Annual Meeting, American Academy for Cerebral Palsy, Los Angeles, 1976.

17. BUHR, RD: *The emergence of vowels in an infant.* J Speech Hear Res 23:73, 1980.

18. LIEBERMAN, P: *On the Origins of Language.* Macmillan, New York, 1975, p 114.

19. LIEBERMAN, P: *Speech Physiology and Acoustic Phonetics.* Macmillan, New York, 1977, p 184.

20. SMITH, BL AND OLLER, DK: *A comparative study of pre-meaningful vocalization produced by normally developing and Down's syndrome infants.* Speech Hear Dis 46:46, 1981.

21. WILDER, op. cit.

22. WILSON, WR: *Auditory fusion in infants—A means of assessing one aspect of central auditory function.* SENTEC, Sixth Annual Meeting, Santa Barbara, California, 1978.

23. MERKLEY, FA: *Consideration of the developmental sequence of speech, language and feeding and the infant with delay in these areas.* In: FREEMAN, J, ET AL: *ADAPT: A Developmental Curriculum.* Health and Welfare Agency, State of California, 1975, p 103.

24. FLAVELL, JH: *The Developmental Psychology of Jean Piaget.* Van Nostrand, Princeton, New Jersey, 1963, p 101.

25. PIAGET, J AND INHELDER, B: *Memory and Intelligence.* Basic Books, New York, 1973, p 3.

26. JACKSON, E, CAMPOS, JJ, AND FISCHER, KW: *The question of decalage between object permanence and person performance.* Devel Psychol 14:1, 1978.

27. FRAIBERG, S: *Libidinal object constancy and mental representation.* The Psychoanalytic Study of the Child, XXIV, International Universities Press, New York, 1969, p 31.

28. BOWER, TGR: *A Primer of Infant Development.* WH Freeman, San Francisco, 1977, p 115.

29. UZGIRIS, IC AND HUNT, JM: *Assessment in Infancy: Ordinal Scales of Psychological Development.* University of Illinois Press, Urbana, 1975, p 115.

30. MAHLER, MS, PINE, F, AND BERGMAN, A: *The Psychological Birth of the Human Infant.* Basic Books, New York, 1975, p 53.

31. BOWER, op. cit., p 114.

32. RUTTER, M: *Maternal deprivation, 1972–1978: New findings, new concepts, new approaches.* Child Devel 50:283, 1979.

33. LAMB, ME: *Separation and reunion behaviors as criteria of attachment in mothers and fathers.* Early Human Devel 3:329, 1979.

34. CHILBUCOS TR AND KAIL, PR: *Longitudinal examination of father-infant interaction and infant-father attachment.* Merrill-Palmer Quarterly 27:81, 1981.

35. KAPLAN, LJ: *Oneness and Separateness: From Infant to Individual.* Simon & Schuster, New York, 1978, p 140.

36. MAHLER, PINE, AND BERGMAN, op cit., p 221.

37. UNMANSKY, R: *The hand sock: An artificial handicap to prehension in infancy, and its relation to clinical disuse phenomena.* Pediatrics 52:546, 1973.

38. STERN, D: *The First Relationships: Infant and Mother.* Harvard University Press, Cambridge, Mass., 1977, p 21.

39. YARROW, LJ, ET AL: *Dimensions of early stimulation and their differential effects on human development.* Merrill-Palmer Quarterly 18:205, 1972.

40. KAPLAN, op. cit., p 153.

41. CICCHETTI, D AND SROUFE, LA: *The relationship between affective and cognitive development in Down's syndrome infants.* Child Devel 47:920, 1976.

42. MIRANDA, SB AND FANTZ, RL: *Recognition memory in Down's syndrome and normal infants.* Child Devel 45:651, 1974.

43. CICCHETTI AND SROUFE, op. cit.

44. STERN, op. cit., p 105.

45. MAHLER, PINE, AND BERGMAN, op. cit., p 111.

46. FRAIBERG, S: *Insights From the Blind.* Basic Books, New York, 1977, p 277.

47. RUTHERFORD, op. cit.

48. WILDER, op. cit.

49. FAULKNER, JA: *The diaphragm as a muscle.* Am Rev Resp Dis 119:89, 1979.

50. BRYAN, AC: *Diaphragmatic fatigue in newborns.* Am Rev Resp Dis 119:143, 1979.

51. DERENNE, JP, MACKLEM, PT, AND ROUSSOS, C: *The respiratory muscles: Mechanics, control, and pathophysiology, part III.* Am J Resp Dis 118:581, 1978.

52. KEENS, TG, ET AL.: *Cellular adaptations of the ventilatory muscles to a chronic increased respiratory load.* J Appl Physiol 44:905, 1978.

53. CRICKMAY, MC: *Speech Therapy and the Bobath Approach to Cerebral Palsy.* Charles C Thomas, Springfield, Ill, 1966, p 122.

54. FREEMAN, J: *Motor development.* In: FREEMAN, J, ET AL.: *ADAPT: A Developmental Curriculum.* Health and Welfare Agency, State of California, 1975, p 25.

55. HEIN AND HELD, op. cit.

56. FINNIE, NR: *Handling the Young Cerebral Palsied Child at Home.* EP Dutton, New York, 1975, p 217.

57. KEENS, TG AND IANUZZO, DC: *Development of fatigue-resistant muscle fibers in human ventilatory muscles.* Am Rev Resp Dis 119:139, 1979.

58. KEENS, TG: *Exercise training programs for pediatric patients with chronic lung disease.* Pediatr Clin North Am 26:517, 1979.

59. MERKLEY, op. cit.

60. STOCKMEYER, op. cit., 1967.

61. LOHREY, B AND BAUMANN, JU: *Normal and abnormal mobility from 2 to 15 years.* Presentation at Thirty-Third Annual Meeting, American Academy for Cerebral Palsy and Developmental Medicine, September, 1979.

62. HEIN AND HELD, op. cit.

63. HEIN, A AND HELD, R: *Dissociation of the visual placing response into elicited and guided components.* Science 158:390, 1967.

64. LEBOYER, F: *Loving Hands.* Alfred A. Knopf, New York, 1978.

65. FRAIBERG, op. cit, 1977, pp 162, 201.

66. ANDERSON, CW: *Attachment in daily separations: Reconceptualizing day care and maternal employment issues.* Child Devel 51:242, 1980.

67. RUTTER, op. cit., 1979.

68. VANDELL, DL, WILSON, KS, AND BUCHANAN, NR: *Peer interaction in the first year of life: An examination of its structure, content, and sensitivity to toys.* Child Devel 51:481, 1980.

REFERENCES: THIRD STAGE

1. STOCKMEYER, SA: *An interpretation of the approach of Rood to the treatment of neuromuscular dysfunction.* Am J Phys Med 46:900, 1967.
2. WILDER, CN: *Respiratory Patterns in Infants: Birth to Eight Months.* University Microfilms, Ann Arbor, 1973.
3. HALVERSON, HM: *Variations in pulse and respiration during different phases of infant behavior.* J Genet Psychol 59:259, 1941.
4. DERENNE, JP, MACKLEM, PT, AND ROUSSOS, CH: *The respiratory muscles: Mechanics, control, and pathophysiology, Part II.* Am Rev Res Dis 118:373, 1978.
5. DERENNE, JP, MACKLEM, PT, AND ROUSSOS, CH: *The respiratory muscles: Mechanics, control, and pathophysiology, Part III.* Am J Resp Dis 118:581, 1978.
6. MULLER, NL AND BRYAN, AC: *Chest wall mechanics and respiratory muscles in infants.* Pediatr Clin North Am 26:503, 1979.
7. DERENNE, MACKLEM, AND ROUSSOS, op. cit., 1978, p 373.
8. SHARP, JT, ET AL: *Relative contributions of rib cage and abdomen to breathing in normal subjects.* J Appl Physiol 39:608, 1975.
9. HIXON, TJ, MEAD, J, AND GOLDMAN, MD: *Dynamics of the chest wall during speech production: Function of the thorax, rib cage, diaphragm, and abdomen.* J Speech Hear Res 19:297, 1976.
10. PROCTOR, DF: *Breathing mechanics during phonation and singing.* In: WYKE, B: *Ventilatory and Phonatory Control Systems.* Oxford University Press, New York, 1974, p 39.
11. HALVERSON, op. cit.
12. BUHR, RD: *The emergence of vowels in an infant.* J Speech Hear Res 23:73, 1980.
13. BOSMA, JF: *Anatomic and physiologic development of the speech apparatus.* In: TOWER, DB: *The Nervous System, Vol. 3: Human Communication and Its Disorders.* Raven Press, New York, 1975, p 469.
14. BUHR, op. cit.
15. RANKIN, J AND DEMPSEY, JA: *Respiratory muscles and the mechanisms of breathing.* Am J Phys Med 46:198, 1967.
16. NELSON, K: *Who talks, what do they say, and why—A functional interpretation of individual differences in the transition to language.* Presentation, Biennial Meeting, Society for Research on Child Development, San Francisco, March, 1979.
17. LARGO, RH AND HOWARD, JA: *Developmental progression in play behavior of children between nine and thirty months. II. Spontaneous play and language development.* Devel Med Child Neurol 21:492, 1979.

18. BLOOM, L, LIGHTBOWN, P, AND HOOD, L: *Structure and variation in child language.* Monographs of the Society for Research in Child Development 40(2), 1975.

19. MILLER, JF, ET AL: *Language comprehension in sensorimotor stages V and VI.* J Speech Hear Res 23:284, 1980.

20. CICCHETTI, D AND SROUFE, LA: *The relationship between affective and cognitive development in Down's syndrome infants.* Child Devel 47:920, 1976.

21. KENT, RD: *Anatomical and neuromuscular maturation of the speech mechanism: Evidence from acoustic studies.* J Speech Hear Res 19:421, 1976.

22. FLAVELL, JH: *The Developmental Psychology of Jean Piget.* Van Nostrand, Princeton, New Jersey, 1963, p 109.

23. YARROW, LJ, ET AL: *Dimensions of early stimulation and their differential effects on human development.* Merrill-Palmer Quarterly 18:205, 1972.

24. LeCOMPTE, GK AND GRATCH, G: *Violation of a rule as a method of diagnosing infants' levels of object concept.* Child Devel 43:385, 1972.

25. LARGO, RH AND HOWARD, JA: *Developmental progression in play behavior of children between nine and thirty months. I: Spontaneous play and imitation.* Devel Med Child Neurol 21:299, 1979.

26. MAHLER, MS, PINE, F, AND BERGMAN, A: *The Psychological Birth of the Human Infant.* Basic Books, New York, 1975, p 111.

27. STERN, D: *The First Relationship: Infant and Mother.* Harvard University Press, Cambridge, Mass., 1977, p 105.

28. MILLER, ET AL, op. cit.

29. SCHAFFER, HR AND EMERSON, PE: *The development of social attachments in infancy.* Monographs Society Research Child Development, Vol. 29, No. 3, Serial No. 94, 1964, p 70.

30. AINSWORTH, MDS, ET AL: *Patterns of Attachment: A Psychological Study of the Strange Situation.* Halstead Press, New York, 1978, p 271.

31. Ibid, p 261.

32. Ibid, p 312.

33. MAHLER, PINE, AND BERGMAN, op. cit., p 56.

34. GREEN, JA, GUSTAFSON, GE, AND WEST, MJ: *Effects of infant development on mother-infant interactions.* Child Devel 51:199, 1980.

35. AINSWORTH, ET AL, op. cit., p 184.

36. BUCHWALD, JS: *Central features of nervous system organization.* J Phys Med 46:88, 1967.

37. GOLDBERG, S AND LEWIS, M: *Play behavior in the year old infant: Early sex differences.* Child Devel 40:21, 1969.

38. KAPLAN, LJ: *Oneness and Separateness: From Infant to Individual.* Simon & Schuster, New York, 1978, p 144.

39. YARROW, ET AL, op. cit., 1972.

40. STEVENSON, MB AND LAMB, ME: *Effects of infant sociability and the caretaking environment on infant cognitive performance.* Child Devel 54:340, 1979.

41. BARNARD, KE AND EYRES, SJ: *Child health assessment Part 2: The first year of life.* DHEW Publication, No. HRA 79-25, 1979.

42. SERAFICA, FC AND CICCHETTI, D: *Down's syndrome children in a strange situation: Attachment and exploration behaviors.* Merrill-Palmer Quarterly 22:137, 1976.

43. CICCHETTI AND SROUFE, op. cit.

44. Ibid.

45. SERAFICA AND CICCHETTI, op. cit.

46. BERRY, P, GUNN, P, AND ANDREWS, R: *Behavior of Down's syndrome infants in a strange situation.* Am J Mental Deficiency 85:213, 1980.

47. DOWNS, MP: *The interaction of critical periods with critical conductive losses.* Presentation at Sixth Annual Meeting, SENTEC, Santa Barbara, California, December, 1978.

48. LOHREY, B AND BAUMANN, JU: *Normal and abnormal mobility from 2 to 15 years.* Presentation at Thirty-Third Annual Meeting, American Academy for Cerebral Palsy and Developmental Medicine, San Francisco, 1979.

49. KAWAMURA, Y AND MORIMOTO, T: *Neurophysiological mechanisms related to reflex control of tongue movements.* In: BOSMA, JF (ED): *Fourth Symposium on Oral Sensation and Perception.* US Department of Health, Education, and Welfare, Bethesda, Maryland, 1973, p 206.

50. SMITH, BL AND OLLER, DK: *A comparative study of premeaningful vocalizations produced by normally developing and Down's syndrome infants.* J Speech Hear Dis 46:46, 1981.

51. STEVENSON AND LAMB, op. cit.

52. LENCIONE, RM, HOWARD, J, AND TROWBRIDGE, K: *A study of two sets of identical twins, male and female, in infancy: A comparison of developmental growth in all areas with special emphasis on language.* Presentation at Thirtieth Annual Meeting, American Academy of Cerebral Palsy, Los Angeles, California, September, 1976.

53. KAUFFMAN, IB AND RIDENOUR, M: *Influence of an infant walker on onset and quality of walking pattern of locomotion: An electromyographic investigation.* Perceptual and Motor Skills 45(Part 2):1323, 1977.

54. McCALL, RB: *Exploratory manipulation and play in the human infant.* Monographs of the Society for Research in Child Development 155(2), 1974.

55. AINSWORTH, ET AL, op cit., p 164.

56. CICCHETTI AND SROUFE, op. cit.

57. HOCK, E: *Working and nonworking mothers and their infants: A comparative study of maternal caregiving characteristics and infant social behavior.* Merrill-Palmer Quarterly 26:79, 1980.

58. PIPER, MC AND RAMSAY, ML: *Effects of early home environment on the mental development of Down's syndrome infants.* Am J Mental Deficiency 85:39, 1980.

REFERENCES: FOURTH STAGE

1. OTIS, AB: *Some ventilation-phonation-relationships.* In WYKE, B: *Ventilatory and Phonatory Control Systems.* Oxford University Press, New York, 1974, p 334.

2. HIXON, TJ, MEAD, J, AND GOLDMAN, MD: *Dynamics of the chest wall during speech production: Function of the thorax, rib cage, diaphragm and abdomen.* J Speech Hear Res 19:297, 1976.

3. KENT, RD: *Anatomical and neuromuscular maturation of the speech mechanisms: Evidence from acoustic studies.* J Speech Hear Res 19:421, 1976.

4. BUHR, RD: *The emergence of vowels in an infant.* J Speech Hear Res 23:73, 1980.

5. BENEDICT, H: *Early lexical development: Comprehension and production.* J Child Language 6:183, 1979.

6. McCUNE-NICOLICH, L: *The cognitive bases of relational words in the single word period.* J Child Language 8:15, 1981.

7. MILLER, JF, ET AL: *Language comprehension in sensorimotor stages V & VI.* J Speech Hear Res 23:284, 1980.

8. BLOOM, L, LIGHTBOWN, P, AND HOOD, L: *Structure and variation in child language.* Monographs of the Society for Research in Child Development 40(2), 1975.

9. NELSON, K: *Structure and strategy in learning to talk.* Monographs of the Society for Research in Child Development 38(1-2), No. 149, 1973.

10. McCUNE-NICOLICH, op. cit.

11. GREENFIELD, PM: *The role of perceptual uncertainty in the transition to language.* Presentation, Biennial Meeting, Society for Research in Child Development, San Francisco, 1979.

12. SNYDER, LS: *Communicative and cognitive abilities and disabilities of the sensorimotor period.* Merrill-Palmer Quarterly 24:161, 1978.

13. GREENWALD, CA AND LEONARD, LB: *Communicative and sensorimotor development of Down's syndrome children.* Am J Mental Deficiency 84:296, 1979.

14. HOWE, CJ: *Interpretive analysis and role semantics a ten-year misalliance?* J Child Language 8:439, 1981.

15. TWENEY, RD AND PETRETIC, PA: *On the comprehension of comprehension studies: A reply to Gleitman, Shipley, and Smith's (1978) criticism of Petretic and Tweney.* J Child Language 8;193, 1981.

16. GLEITMAN, LR, SHIPLEY, EF, AND SMITH, C: *Old and new ways not to study comprehension: Comments on Petretic and Tweney's (1977) experimental review of Shipley, Smith, and Gleitman (1969).* J Child Language 5:501, 1978.

17. CHAPMEN, RS AND MILLER, JF: *Word order in early two and three word utterances: Does production precede comprehension?* J Speech Hear Res 18:255, 1975.

18. WETSTONE, HS AND FRIEDLANDER, BZ: *The effect of word order on young children's responses to simple questions and commands.* Child Devel 44:734, 1973.

19. GOLINKOFF, RM: *The case for semantic relations: Evidence from the verbal and nonverbal domains.* J Child Language 8:413, 1981.

20. SLOBIN, DI: *They learn the same way all around the world.* Psychology Today 6:71, 1972.

21. STROHNER, H AND NELSON, KE: *The young child's development of sentence comprehension: Influence of event probability, nonverbal context, syntactic form, and strategies.* Child Devel 45:567, 1974.

22. BENEDICT, op. cit.

23. GLEITMAN, SHIPLEY, AND SMITH, op. cit.

24. MILLER, ET AL, op. cit.

25. SYNDER, op. cit.

26. HUTTENLOCHER, J: *The origins of language comprehension.* In: SOLSO, RL (ED): *Theories in Cognitive Psychology: The Loyola Symposium.* Halstead Press, New York, 1974, p 331.

27. SACHS, J AND TRUSWELL, L: *Comprehension of two-word instructions by children in the one-word stage.* J Child Language 5:17, 1978.

28. LARGO, RH AND HOWARD, JA: *Developmental progression in play behavior of children between nine and thirty months: II: Spontaneous play and language development.* Devel Med Child Neurol 21:492, 1979.

29. SCHACHTER, FF, ET AL: *Everyday preschool interpersonal speech usage: Methodological, developmental, and sociolinguistic studies.* Monographs of the Society for Research in Child Development 39(3), 1974.

30. HOLMBERG, MC: *The development of social interchange patterns from 12 to 42 months.* Child Devel 51:448, 1980.

31. WHITE, BL, ET AL: *Competence and experience.* In: UZGIRIS, IC AND WEIZMAN, F (EDS): *The Structuring of Experience.* Plenum Press, New York, 1977, p 115.

32. CORRIGAN, R: *Language development as related to stage 6 object permanence development.* J Child Language 5:173, 1978.

33. UZGIRIS, IC AND HUNT, JM: *Assessment in Infancy: Ordinal Scales of Psychological Development.* University of Illinois Press, Urbana, 1975, p 208.

34. LARGO AND HOWARD, op. cit.

35. FENSON, L AND RAMSAY, DS: *Decentration and integration of the child's play in the second year.* Child Devel 51:171, 1980.

36. MAHLER, MS, PINE, F AND BERGMAN, A: *The Psychological Birth of the Human Infant.* Basic Books, New York, 1975, p 69.

37. AINSWORTH, MDS, ET AL: *Patterns of Attachment: A Psychological Study of the Strange Situation.* Halstead Press, New York, 1978, p 278.

38. KAPLAN, LJ: *Oneness and Separateness: From Infant to Individual.* Simon & Schuster, New York, 1978, p 182.

39. YOUNG, G AND LEWIS, M: *Effects of familiarity and maternal attention on infant peer relations.* Merrill-Palmer Quarterly 25:105, 1979.

40. BRUNNER, JS: *The ontogenesis of speech acts.* J Child Language 2:1, 1975.

41. WACHS, TD: *Proximal experience and early cognitive-intellectual development: The physical environment.* Merrill-Palmer Quarterly 25:3, 1979.

42. MATAS, L, AREND, RA, AND SROUFE, LA: *Continuity of adaptation in the second year: The relationship between quality of attachment and later competence.* Child Devel 49:547, 1978.

43. SERAFICA, FC AND CICCHETTI, D: *Down's syndrome children in a strange situation: Attachment and exploration behaviors.* Merrill-Palmer Quarterly 22:137, 1976.

44. BERRY, P, GUNN, P, AND ANDREWS, R: *Behavior of Down's syndrome infants in a strange situation.* Am J Mental Deficiency 85:213, 1980.

45. SERAFICA AND CICCHETTI, op. cit.

46. MAHLER, PINE, AND BERGMAN, op cit., p 79.

47. DOWNS, MP: *The Interaction of Critical Periods with Critical Conductive Losses.* Presentation at Sixth Annual Meeting, SENTEC, Santa Barbara, California, December, 1978.

48. EILERS, RE AND OLLER, DK: *A comparative study of speech perception in young severely retarded and normally developing infants.* J Speech Hear Res 23:419, 1980.

49. TALLAL, P: *Rapid auditory processing in normal and disordered language development.* J Speech Hear Res 19:561, 1976.

50. GREENWALD AND LEONARD, op. cit.

51. SNYDER, op. cit.

52. DEMPSEY, JA AND RANKIN, J: *Physiological adaptations of gas transport systems to muscular work in health and disease.* Am J Phys Med 46:582, 1967.

53. OTIS, op. cit.

54. HIXON, MEAD, AND GOLDMAN, op. cit.

55. MULLER, NL AND BRYAN, AC: *Chest wall mechanics and respiratory muscles in infants.* Pediatr Clin North Am 26:503, 1979.

56. WAISBREN, SE: *Parents' reaction after the birth of a developmentally disabled child.* Am J Mental Deficiency 84:345, 1980.

57. VAN KLEECK, A AND CARPENTER, RL: *The effects of children's language comprehension level on adults' child-directed speech.* J Speech Hear Res 23:546, 1980.

58. SNYDER, op. cit.

59. DOWNS, op. cit.

60. RANKIN, J AND DEMPSEY, JA: *Respiratory muscles and the mechanisms of breathing.* Am J Phys Med 46:198, 1967.

61. GOLDMAN, M: *Mechanics of specific patterns of respiratory muscle dysfunction.* Am Rev Resp Dis 119:135, 1979.

62. FINNIE, NR: *Handling the Young Cerebral Palsied Child at Home.* EP Dutton, New York, 1975, p 257.

63. HOLMBERG, op cit.

64. YOUNG AND LEWIS, op. cit.

65. PIPER, MC AND RAMSAY, MK: *Effects of early home environment on the mental development of Down's syndrome infants.* Am J Mental Deficiency 85:39, 1980.

66. WACHS, op. cit.

67. WACHS, op. cit.

68. ZELLE, RS: *Early intervention: A panacea or an experiment?* Maternal Child Nurs 1(6):343, 1976.

REFERENCES: FIFTH STAGE

1. MURRAY, MP: *Gait as a total pattern of movement.* Am J Phys Med 46:290, 1967.

2. SCRUTTON, DR: *Footprint sequences of normal children under five years old.* Devel Med Child Neurol 11:44, 1969.

3. WICKSTROM, RL: *Fundamental Motor Patterns.* Lea & Febiger, Philadelphia, 1977, p 25.

4. MURRAY, op. cit.

5. OKAMOTO, T: *Electromyographic study of the learning process of walking in 1- and 2-year-old infants.* In: CERQUIGLINI, A, VENERANDO, A, AND WARTENWEILER, J: *Biomechanics III.* University Park Press, Baltimore, 1973, p 328.

6. WICKSTROM, op. cit., p 37.

7. HIXON, TJ, MEAD, J, AND GOLDMAN, MD: *Dynamics of the chest wall during speech production: Function of the thorax, rib cage, diaphragm and abdomen.* J Speech Hear Res 19:297, 1976.

8. HALVERSON, HM: *Variations in pulse and respiration during different phases of infant behavior.* J Genet Psychol 59:259, 1941.

9. WILDER, CN: *Respiratory Patterns in Infants: Birth to Eight Months.* University Microfilms, Ann Arbor, 1973.

10. HALVERSON, op. cit.

11. WILDER, op. cit.

12. BUHR, RD: *The emergence of vowels in an infant.* J Speech Hear Res 23:73, 1980.

13. KENT, RD: *Anatomical and neuromuscular maturation of the speech mechanism: Evidence from accoustic studies.* J Speech Hear Res 19:421, 1976.

14. BOSMA, JF: *Anatomic and physiologic development of the speech apparatus.* In: TOWER, DB: *The Nervous System, Vol. 3: Human Communications and Its Disorders.* Raven Press, New York, 1975, p 469.

15. BOSMA, J: *Assessment and prognosis of oral pharyngeal dysfunction in cerebral palsy.* Presentation Thirtieth Annual Meeting, American Academy for Cerebral Palsy, Los Angeles, 1976.

16. RUTHERFORD, D: *Auditory motor learning and the acquisition of speech.* Am J Phys Med 46:245, 1967.

17. MENYUK, P: *The role of distinctive features in children's acquisition of phonology.* J Speech Hear Res 11:138, 1968.

18. LEONARD, LB: *Language impairment in children.* Merrill-Palmer Quarterly 25:205, 1979.

19. SNYDER, LS: *Communicative and cognitive abilities and disabilities in the sensorimotor period.* Merrill-Palmer Quarterly 24:161, 1978.

20. BATES, E, ET AL: *From gesture to the first word: On cognitive and social prerequisites.* In: LEWIS, M, AND ROSENBLUM LA (EDS): *Interaction, Conversation, and the Development of Language.* John Wiley & Sons, New York, 1977, p 247.

21. MOSKOWITZ, BA: *The acquisition of language.* Scientific American 239:82, 1978.

22. RODGON, MM, JANKOWSKI, W, AND ALENSKAS, L: *A multifunctional approach to single-word usage.* J Child Language 4:23, 1977.

23. BLOOM, L, LIGHTBOWN, P, AND HOOD, L: *Structure and variation in language.* Monographs of the Society for Research in Child Development 40(2), 1975.

24. RODGON, MM: *Situation and meaning in one- and two-word utterances. Observations on Howe's "The meaning of two-word utterances in the speech of young children."* J Child Language 4:111, 1977.

25. SNOW, CE: *The uses of imitation.* J Child Language 8:205, 1981.

26. MOSKOWITZ, op. cit.

27. MILLER, JF, ET AL: *Language comprehension in sensorimotor stages V and VI.* J Speech Hear Res 23:284, 1980.

28. PARISI, D AND GIANNELLI, W: *Language and social environment at 2 years.* Merrill-Palmer Quarterly 25:61, 1979.

29. SCHACHTER, FF, ET AL: *Everyday preschool interpersonal speech usage: Methodological, developmental, and sociolinguistic studies.* Monographs of the Society for Research and Child Development 39(3), 1974.

30. SNYDER, op. cit.

31. HOWE, CJ: *Interpretative analysis and role semantics a ten-year misalliance?* J Child Language 8:439, 1981.

32. TWENEY, RD AND PETRETIC, PA: *On the comprehension of comprehension studies: A reply to Gleitman, Shipley, and Smith's (1978) criticism of Petretic and Tweney.* J Child Language 8:193, 1981.

33. GOLINKOFF, RM: *The case for semantic relations: Evidence from the verbal and nonverbal domains.* J Child Language 8:413, 1981.

34. MILLER, ET AL, op. cit.

35. GOLINKOFF, op. cit.

36. LARGO, RH AND HOWARD, JA: *Developmental progression in play behavior of children between nine and thirty months: II: Spontaneous play and language development.* Devel Med Child Neurol 21:492, 1979.

37. UZGIRIS, IC AND HUNT, JMV: *Assessment in Infancy: Ordinal Scales of Psychological Development.* University of Illinois Press, Urbana, 1975, p 121.
38. FLAVELL, JH: *The Developmental Psychology of Jean Piaget.* Van Nostrand, Princeton, New Jersey, 1963, p 118.
39. PIAGET, J: *The Origins of Intelligence in Children.* International University Press, New York, 1952, pp 337–338.
40. LARGO AND HOWARD, op. cit.
41. WHITE, BL, ET AL: *Competence and experience.* In: UZGIRIS, IC AND WEIZMANN, F (EDS): *The Structuring of Experience.* Plenum Press, New York, 1977, p 115.
42. CORRIGAN, R: *Language development as related to stage 6 object permanence development.* J Child Language 5:173, 1978.
43. FENSON, L AND RAMSAY, DS: *Decentration and integration of the child's play in the second year.* Child Devel 51:171, 1980.
44. Ibid.
45. GOULD, V: *Cognitive development.* In: FREEMAN, J, ET AL: *ADAPT: A Developmental Curriculum.* Health and Welfare Agency. State of California, 1975, p 161.
46. MAHLER, MS, PINE, F, AND BERGMAN, A: *The Psychological Birth of the Human Infant.* Basic Books, New York, 1975, p 76.
47. AINSWORTH, MDS, ET AL: *Patterns of Attachment: A Psychological Study of the Strange Situation.* Halstead Press, New York, 1978, p 177.
48. MATAS, L, AREND, RA, AND SROUFE, LA: *Continuity of adaptation in the second year: The relationship between quality of attachment and later competence.* Child Devel 49:547, 1978.
49. RUBIN, KH AND DYCK, L: *Preschoolers private speech in the natural setting.* Presentation Biennial Meeting, Society for Research in Child Development, San Francisco, March 1979.
50. KAPLAN, LJ: *Oneness and Separateness: From Infant to Individual.* Simon & Schuster, New York, 1978, p 191.
51. HOLMBERG, MC: *The development of social interchange patterns from 12 to 42 months.* Child Devel 57:448, 1980.
52. KAPLAN, op. cit., p 226.
53. LAMB, ME: *The development of mother-infant and father-infant attachments in the second year of life.* Devel Psychol 13:637, 1977.
54. SCHACHTER, ET AL, op. cit.
55. MOSKOWITZ, op. cit.
56. BLOOM, op. cit.
57. SACHS, J AND TRUSWELL, L: *Comprehension of two-word instructions by children in the one-word stage.* J Child Language 5:17, 1978.
58. MAHLER, PINE, AND BERGMAN, op. cit. p 99.
59. AINSWORTH, ET AL, op. cit., p 171.
60. FRAIBERG, S: *Insights From the Blind.* Basic Books, New York, 1977, p 19.
61. FRAIBERG, op. cit., p 246.

62. Downs, MP: *The Interaction of Critical Periods with Critical Conductive Losses.* Presentation at Sixth Annual Meeting, SENTEC, Santa Barbara, California, December, 1978.

63. Greenberg, MT and Marvin, RS: *Attachment patterns in profoundly deaf preschool children.* Merrill-Palmer Quarterly 24:265, 1979.

64. Jirgal, D: *Vestibular-Auditory Considerations.* Presentation Sensorimotor Integration Symposium, University of California, San Diego, July 1974.

65. Jirgal, op. cit.

66. de Quiros, J: *Diagnosis of vestibular disorders in the learning disabled.* J Learn Disabil 9:50, 1976.

67. Kinnealey, M: *Aversive and nonaversive responses to sensory stimulation in mentally retarded children.* Am J Occup Ther 27:464, 1973.

68. Crickmay, MC: *Speech Therapy and the Bobath Approach to Cerebral Palsy.* Charles C Thomas, Springfield, Ill, 1966, p 87.

69. Kline, LS and Hutchinson, JM: *Acoustic and perceptual evaluation of hypernasality of mentally retarded persons.* Am J Mental Deficiency 85:153, 1980.

70. Parisi and Giannelli, op. cit.

71. Leonard, op. cit.

72. Synder, op. cit.

73. Finnie, NR: *Handling the Young Cerebral Palsied Child at Home.* EP Dutton, New York, 1975.

74. Rampp, DL and Plummer, BA: *A Child in Jeopardy: Medical and Educational Profiles of Children with Auditory Processing Learning Disabilities.* Presentation Sixth Annual Meeting, SENTEC, Santa Barbara, California, December, 1978.

75. Ayres AJ: *Sensory Integration and Learning Disorders.* Western Psychological Services, Los Angeles, 1972, p 115.

76. Dixon, LS and Spradlin, JE: *Picture Representation Skills of Nonverbal Severely Retarded Adolescents.* Presentation, Biennial Meeting Society for Research in Child Development, San Francisco, 1979.

77. Piper, MC and Ramsay, MK: *Effect of early home environment on the mental development of down's syndrome infants.* Am J Mental Deficiency 85:39, 1980.

78. Schachter, et al, op. cit.

79. Field, TM: *Interactive patterns of pre-term and term infants.* In: Field, TM (ed): *Infants Born at Risk.* SP Medical and Scientific Books, New York, 1979, p 333.

80. Moskowitz, op. cit.

81. Kahn, JV: *A comparison of sign and verbal language training with nonverbal retarded children.* J Speech Hear Res 24:113, 1981.

82. Mans, L, Cicchetti, D, and Sroufe, LA: *Mirror reactions of Down's syndrome infants and toddlers: Cognitive underpinnings of self-recognition.* Child Devel 49:1247, 1978.

83. Blehar, MC: *Anxious attachment and defensive reactions associated with day care.* Child Devel 45:683, 1974.

Chapter 3

ENVIRONMENTAL AND HABILITATIVE APPROACHES TO MEDIATE THE ATTENTION LEVEL AND RESPONSE THRESHOLD

Raeone S. Zelle

CONCEPTUAL FRAMEWORK

The emphasis on stimulation in a generic sense is giving way to a more individualistic focus. There is a growing realization that ingredients in the environmental diet have to be blended in a certain way to nourish the development of a particular infant or toddler. The assumption that stimulation is synonymous with excitation is also giving way. It may be that the infant or toddler needs an environmental diet that has a calming effect. The more cautious trend has been catalyzed in part by recent advances in the technology of measurement. Although research findings create more questions than answers, it is evident that the response to a given stimulus is dependent on a number of factors: the modality of the stimulus, the spatial and temporal organization and intensity of the stimulus, the background of activities in the environment, and the state of especially the very young infant.

LEVEL OF RESPONSIVENESS AS A FUNCTION OF THE BEHAVIORAL STATE

A more dynamic and interrelated concept of the stimulus environment is also the outgrowth of some older research in the natural setting. Wolff[1] observed infants for long continuous periods, and he recognized the interplay between stimuli emanating from within the infant and external stimuli. This interplay determines the level of arousal and influences the nature of the infant's interaction with the animate and inanimate environment. In keeping with the model presented in the first part of Chapter 2, he also observed that the behavioral patterns of even the very young infant are grouped in more or less consistent constellations. The functional significance of a discrete behavior is inferred from the reciprocal relationship with other behaviors; it is a part of the whole. Wolff[2] classified the six configurations that he observed as states, and the descriptive labels reflect an arousal continuum.

STATE I: REGULAR SLEEP. The threshold to sensory input is high. Although intense internal or external stimuli can arouse the infant, he is undisturbed by the usual environmental activity. The muscle tone is low, and there is minimal diffuse motor activity. The eyelids are closed, and there are no spontaneous eye movements. The respirations are stable and rhythmic, and the skin is pale pink. The biologic clock naturally elicits the transition from this state.

Wolff observed a frequent occurrence of spontaneous behaviors during regular sleep, such as rhythmic mouthing (sucking), startles, erections, and sobbing inspirations. He hypothesized that there is a build up of neural energy that is discharged by these movements. Older research[3] supports Wolff's inference that these early rhythmic patterns influence the temporal ordering of later, more complex motor actions, for example, locomotion and speech. More recently, Delcomyn[4] presented a strong argument for a natural regulator that operates independent of sensory feedback. He postulated that the neuronal oscillator generates the proper sequence and rhythm of movement in repetitive behaviors, such as walking and breathing. Sensory input may interact with the neural oscillator to modulate the intrinsic patterns and shape the motor act.

STATE II: IRREGULAR SLEEP. The sensory threshold is less high, and the infant is more susceptible to internal and external stimuli. There is some increase in muscle tone, and periods of relative inactivity alternate with periods of phasic activity, such as movement of the extremities, more general stirring bodily movements, facial expressions. The rhythmic mouthing in State I changes to more gross movements of the tongue and jaw. The eyes are closed, and there are irregularly occurring rapid eye movements under the lids. The skin is predominantly a pale pink color but may become flushed during a spurt of movement. The respiration rate increases and becomes irregular.

There are alternating cycles of regular and irregular sleep, but the irregular sleep state predominates in the very young infant. Researchers question whether irregular sleep is a true sleep state and why the infant remains in this state for longer periods of time than in the other states. It may be that the lower level of activity conserves caloric energy in the growing infant or the state provides internal stimulation to the developing nervous system. Or it may be that the state reflects neocortical immaturity. There is lack of sufficient tonic inhibition originating from higher centers to maintain longer intervals of stability in the regular sleep and alert inactivity states.[5]

STATE III: DROWSINESS. There is a further decrease in the sensory threshold, and the infant is responsive to stimulation but often with a latency. The eyes open and close and have a dull appearance, and there are spurts of activity when the infant is waking up but rarely when he is falling asleep. The respiration rate is variable but usually regular. Stimulation frequently elicits a more alert state especially when the infant is awakening.

STATE IV: ALERT INACTIVITY. The eyes are open and the infant is awake with a bright, alert look. There is relative internal stability and minimal movement, including facial expressions. The infant is most attentive during this state in terms of his ability to selectively focus on external stimuli. Although he may turn toward a sound when he is in the drowsy and the other awake states (V and VI), his orienting response is of higher quality during this state. The pursuit of a visual stimulus occurs almost exclusively in this state. Wolff postulates that a vertical and horizontal pursuit movement of the head and eyes involves a reciprocal interaction between the infant and his external environment and is more adaptive than stereotyped responses such as swiping toward a noxious stimulus. Respirations are generally constant in amplitude and frequency, albeit more variable and rapid than in regular sleep.

STATE V: WAKING ACTIVITY. When internal or external stimuli become sufficiently intense, the inner stability begins to disintegrate. There is an increase in the arousal level characterized by frequent intervals of diffuse, phasic motor activity that varies in intensity and duration. The face may be relaxed or become tense in a cry-face expression, and the infant may fuss. The eyes are open but do not brighten because the higher level of variable, internal stimuli decreases the infant's ability to focus on external stimuli. The skin becomes flushed when the infant is active, and respirations are grossly irregular.

STATE VI: CRYING. The increased activity in the above state escalates to crying and vigorous, diffuse motor activity. The face is tense and flushed, and the eyes may be partially open or tightly closed. Since the infant is now experiencing very variable somatosensory input from his body movements and crying, he is capable of focusing only on the most overriding external stimuli. If the provoking stimulus persists, there may be a further escalation to uncoordinated thrashing and spasmodic, intense crying, which inundates the infant with intermittent proprioceptive, tactual, and auditory input. He cannot habituate because of the variation in the intensity and location of sensations. Thus, the excitable activity feeds itself, and only fatigue or the caregiver's intervention interrupts the cycle. There is a similarity between the infant's escalated response and the temper tantrum of a young child and the excess emotional excitability of an adult.

It is evident from the above descriptions that there is a hierarchical organization of states on a quantitative arousal continuum between sleep and wakefulness. The infant is most sensitive to discrete, external animate and inanimate stimuli midway along the continuum; he is much less responsive at both ends. However, the infant's responsiveness is also influenced by his interaction with the external environment, especially in the alert inactivity state. Certain stimuli appeal to him more than others or certain attributes of a stimulus have salience as discussed more fully in Stage I, Chapter 2. The amount of time the infant spends in a state and the transition from one state to another is also influenced by the mediation of external stimuli. Wolff observed a wide range of individual differences in the time that an infant remained in State IV. Some infants were able to remain alert and inactive for a 40-minute interval, which suggests a complex interplay between the infant's innate adaptiveness and the adaptiveness of his caregiver.

Wolff emphasized the importance of recognizing the affective significance of a configuration of behaviors in a particular state. The pattern influences the nature of the interaction with another human and thus acquires a social meaning. The infant who cries most of the time when he is awake will have a different social experience than the infant who can remain in an alert, inactive state for a 40-minute interval. Likewise, the emotional tone of his immediate environment will be different.

MATURATIONAL CHANGES IN STATE BEHAVIOR. At approximately four weeks of age, the infant is able to attend to environmental events while he is active; and the waking activity state (V) is renamed the alert activity state. Other maturational changes also occur during early infancy, which are very observable at approximately three months of age. There is increased consolidation of behavioral and physiologic parameters, which further delineates the states. The more predictable, integrated patterning is also reflected by the infant's increased ability to modulate behaviors within a state and modulate the transition from one state to another. This is manifested by the progressively longer periods of quiescence both in the regular sleep state and the alert inactive state reported by Parmelee and Stern.[6] Kleitman, a discussant of the published study, proposes that the ability to stay awake is what really reflects the maturation of the brain. The infant may sleep through the night at four to six weeks of age, but it is not until five to six years that he can sustain long, continuous wakeful periods. Wolff observed that increased periods of wakefulness and attention corroborate with the development of sensory pathways and organizational structures to process input. There is a rather marked increase in the interval of the awake alert state when the infant acquires more adaptive ways of eliciting and recapturing interesting spectacles.

The maturation of the central nervous system is a complex heterogenous process that is not fully understood. The changes may be an outgrowth of the formation and branching of dendrites, which increases the synaptic connections between neurons,[7] the clustering of dendrites in bundles which may provide a substrate for more extensive processing of information,[8] and the accelerated postnatal development of excitatory interneurons in the cortex, which decreases the response latency to stimuli. Purpura and Shofer[9] found that the inhibitory synaptic pathways are well developed in contrast to excitatory pathways in the cortex of the newborn kitten.

Related to the above underlying forces, the forebrain is becoming more developed and interconnected with the brain stem. Sterman[10] hypothesized that an inhibitory influence emanates from extrapyramidal structures and is relayed through the descending fibers of the reticular formation of the brain stem to modulate neuronal excitability. Behaviorally this evolving influence from the higher centers if reflected by the infant's increasing capacity to suppress voluntary phasic movements and engage in longer periods of sustained attention. The gradual waning of diffuse movement is also related to the myelinization of nerve fibers, which limits the spread of input. There is an oscillating balance between inhibitory and excitatory mechanisms that begins to come into play when the infant is approximately four to six weeks of age according to Metcalf's findings.[11]

Regulation of Inhibitory and Excitatory Influences

One of the oldest parts of the central nervous system, the reticular formation is felt to serve an integral regulatory function. The formation is a loose network of cells of all sizes and shapes that are located in the central core of the spinal cord, brain stem, midbrain, and thalamus. The afferent or sensory component is called the reticular activating system, which indirectly connects with the cerebral cortex. Ascending polysynaptic fibers terminate in thalamic nuclei, which sends fibers to other thalamic nuclei that directly project to widespread cortical areas. Fibers from the reticular formation also terminate in the hypothalamus. Collateral branches of fibers transmitting impulses from all the sensory systems project into this central area with the exception of the more discriminative tactile and proprioceptive input transmitted by the newer dorsal column pathways.[12] Fibers that originate in many areas of the cortex also terminate in the reticular formation and influence its performance, and there is a functional connection with the cerebellum. Because of the manifold sources of input, the old system is felt to be an important integrative center.[13]

In a general sense, the ascending impulses from this system have a facilitory and inactivating influence on neurons in the cortex. The system therefore plays an important role in the alternating patterns of sleep and wakefulness. During wakefulness, stimuli from this system facilitate a certain level of neuronal activity in the cortex to maintain the aroused state. Magoun[14] proposed that the system also subserves discriminative and differential activity at the higher cortical level. Because of the convergence of input upon common neuronal elements, the information that feeds into the reticular formation is nonspecific. The information is coded in this older integrative center in terms of its alerting potential. There is a general message sent to the cortex to become more attentive, because important, more specific information is being transmitted through more direct pathways. The increased excitation elicits an orienting response that increases the efficiency of the neuronal circuits and sets the stage for adaptive, discriminative perception of the input. This old system also interacts with more specialized neuronal systems to determine which input will be preeminent at the conscious level at a given point in time.[15] Other irrelevant forms of sensory input are not permitted to intrude during this interval of focused attention. If a stimulus continues repetitively, the level of attention decreases, and the input drops from the conscious level. Thus, habituation occurs. If there is a sudden change in the input (variation in the pitch or position of a sound) or a sudden cessation, the cortex is re-alerted.

The regulatory function of the reticular activating system is always under the influence of cortical processes. There is a built-in homeostatic mechanism to prevent overactivity and over-responsiveness of cortical neurons via an inverse inhibitory influence from the brain. This feedback has a braking effect on reticulocortical excitation.[16] The inverse corticoreticular influence is also responsible for the emotional and psychic effects on the level of arousal and attention.[17]

The efferent or motor component of the reticular formation consists of descending fibers that terminate on motor nuclei of cranial nerves and alpha and gamma motor neurons in the spinal cord. Impulses from large nuclei in the brain stem, the corpus striatum, cerebellum, and motor areas in the frontal lobe of the cortex are relayed through the descending reticular system. The impulses transmitted through these fibers have both a facilitory and inhibitory effect, and one of the major functions of the descending system is to influence the cell threshold of lower motor neurons. The system is therefore one of the regulating agents of proximal muscle tone. The excitatory influence can be generated within the reticular formation itself, but the inhibitory influence is primarily dependent on input from higher centers—basal ganglia, cerebellum, and frontal cortex. Again, there is an interplay between lower and higher centers to attain an oscillating balance between excitation and inhibition. Another major role of the descending system is the regulation of vital functions through connections with nuclei of the autonomic outflow—respiration rate and rhythm, heart rate, blood pressure. The respiratory regulation is also dependent on connections with motor neurons in the phrenic nucleus and the thoracic cord.[18,19]

Disorders of the Regulatory Mechanism

If the infant has a less intact central nervous system, there may be a disorder of the inner regulatory mechanisms reflected by poorly organized state patterns. Individual physiologic and behavioral parameters fluctuate and are less synchronous with each other. Thus, the parameters are very loosely linked together or do not coalesce into an observable configuration, and there are more periods when the infant's behavior does not meet the criteria for any of the states. In contrast, there are only brief periods of a few minutes when an infant with an intact central nervous system is in an indeterminant state.[20] Periods of quiet sleep may be practically nonexistent if there are very few intervals when the respiration rate is regular. The rate may actually increase in contrast to the normal decline in the newborn period, and the heart rate and respiration rate may not accelerate and decelerate together.[21]

The regulatory disorder may also be expressed by aberrant inhibitory or excitatory influences within and between neuronal subsystems. Each synapse has a threshold at which it will fire. If there is too much inhibition, a low or median level of incoming stimuli is not registered or perceived. A higher level of input has to bombard the cell to liberate presynaptic substances that influence postsynaptic membranes and bridge the gap so to speak. The impulse can then be transmitted from a receptor to a neuron and from one neuron to another; the message gets through. On the other hand, if there is too much excitation, a very low level of input makes the sensitive cell fire off. Too many messages get through which elicit excessive neuronal activity and an overaroused state.

ABERRANT RESPONSE THRESHOLD. If the above aberrant inhibitory and excitatory influences are descriptively related to the behavior of the infant, there are two patterns. At one end of the continuum is the infant with a very high threshold because of too much inhibition. He is termed hyporesponsive or hyporeactive. It is difficult to arouse the infant from a sleep state, and the transition from one state to another is poorly differentiated. He responds slowly to stimulus changes when he is undressed, handled, or even bathed. There is a slow build up of weak, limited extremity and bodily movement and a quick drop off because of a lower level of tone in the muscles. If the infant becomes sufficiently aroused to cry, the sound may be more a wailful reaction to intrusion, and there is lack of vigorous movement. The period of arousal is very brief, and the infant quickly falls back into a drowsy or sleepy state again.

He may evolve to the alert, inactive state when he is awake in response to an increase in the intensity of stimuli. Excitatory influences from the reticular activating system elicit a high enough level of neuronal activity so that the infant can orient to and register a salient stimulus at that point in time. However, there is a qualitative difference in the level of alertness. There is less facial brightening, and the eyes do not open as widely because of decreased activity in the radiating muscles. The period of alertness and focused attention is very brief.

If the infant is at the other end of the continuum and has a very low threshold, he is termed hyperresponsive or hyperreactive. Stimulation may elicit a wide swing from a sleep state to intense crying, and the infant has very little ability to quiet himself. When he is soothed, the infant may swing back to a sleep state again. The transition from one state to another is poorly differentiated because of the erratic shifts. The reticular activating system falls down in its role as a modulator of neuronal excitability. Too many sensory stimuli get through and overarouse the infant, which elicits almost constant movement with a tense quality. The facial expression also becomes tense, and the infant may have a startlelike wide-eyed look that can be misread by his caregiver. There is underlying autonomic instability evidenced by a rapid, marked change in skin color when uncovered.

The infant cannot suppress the phasic motor activity to focus on a stimulus that has more relevance at that moment. Or the infant can remain in the alert, inactivity state only for a very brief period. The erratic shift of internal states may vary the infant's awareness and response to the point that he perceives a stimulus in a very unstable way, which also interferes with focused attention.

If the infant has an immature nervous system related to a less than optimal uterine environment, a premature birth, or other factors, a disorder of the regulatory mechanisms may be a temporary phenomenon. However, if there is pathology, the imbalance will no doubt continue and may be characterized by an aberrant sensory threshold and related behavioral patterns described in the different stages in Chapter 2. The disorder may be characterized by abnormal muscle tone with related compensatory patterns that are also described in the different stages.

ABERRANT LEVEL OF MUSCLE TONE. There are many variables associated with abnormal tone that will be discussed in this chapter as a supplement to the more functional descriptions in Chapter 2. An infant who will later have cerebral palsy, expressed by spastic hypertonicity or fluctuating tone (athetosis), usually has hypotonic muscles during the first one to two years. He may appear normal to the parents during the early infancy period, except that he has a weaker sucking response. However, the experienced intervener recognizes overall diminished muscle tone and more limited movement. Further indications of pathology are usually observable during the months following early infancy. The neck, and then the back and extremities, stiffen when the infant is handled or startled, and this response may occur if the infant is prespastic or preathetoid. If the infant will later have athetosis and fluctuating tone, he may have a high sensory threshold and a response latency. However, the eventual response is exaggerated with a wide swing from one state to another versus the slow build up typically associated with hypotonia.[22] The characteristic patterns related to spasticity and athetosis gradually evolve and are expressed in the following ways.

Spasticity. If the muscles become spastic because of an imbalance of facilitory influences, movement will be limited in range and direction and will be accompanied by excessive effort. The stretch receptors become highly sensitive because of the low threshold, reflected by an exaggerated, contractive response to a passive muscle stretch. The caregiver feels resistance if she attempts to change the position of a body part, for example, extend and outwardly rotate the flexed arm. Other attempted positional changes will probably also be resisted: extension of the wrist and fingers, abduction of the thumb, abduction and outward rotation of the leg, and dorsiflexion of the ankle and toes. There is increased resistance to stretch up to a certain point followed by a collapse of resistance with a clasp-knife effect. There is less resistance when the extremity is moved slowly.[23] When the child attempts to move, the effort can elicit abnormal levels of cocontraction, especially in proximal joints. For example, all the muscles around the shoulder contract and provide resistance to an elevation of the arm or a backward, forward, or outward movement of the arm. There may be excessive reciprocal inhibition of muscular activity; the activated spastic muscle severely inhibits the opposing muscle and prevents any attempted contraction and movement. As an example, the extensors of the wrist are inactivated and the hand remains in a dropped position. Thus, abnormal synergistic patterns limit movement of the proximal joint in any direction and limit movement of a distal part (hand) in the opposite direction. Because the child cannot grade muscular contractions, there can be an abrupt shift from total flexion to total extension. If he tries to raise his head to look up when sitting in a slumped posture, he will fall backward into extension. If the child has a mild form of spasticity, signs of abnormal tone evolve over a longer time frame and may be evident only to the specialized intervener. There is generally resistance only when the muscle is stretched rapidly.[24]

There are different types of involvement. The muscles may be spastic in one extremity only, which is rare (monoplegia). Or the whole body is involved, but the spasticity is more pronounced in the lower extremities (diplegia). Or all parts of the body are affected, but the degree of involvement is usually asymmetric with more tone on one side and/or more tone in the upper extremities (quadriplegia). Rigidity is a severe form of spasticity which involves cocontraction. The agonist is opposed by an equally spastic antagonist, especially in proximal parts. Thus, there is fixation with resistance of the muscles to passive stretch throughout the range of flexion and extension, and the stovepipe effect severely restricts movement.[25]

It may be that the spastic involvement is in one set of muscles throughout the body. If the child has flexor hypertonicity, he assumes a posture with the arms and legs flexed and pulled in close to the body. His back and shoulders are rounded, and the head is flexed forward. He is pulled up in somewhat of a fetal position, and there is resistance when the caregiver attempts to extend body parts and straighten him out. Or if only the extensor muscles are hypertonic, the head and shoulders are pulled back, which creates a sway in the lower back or lordotic curve. The flexed arms are pulled back with the head and shoulders, and the legs are extended and adducted. The pattern also predominates when the child assumes the prone position, but there is less tone in the extensor muscles relative to the supine position. There is resistance if the caregiver attempts to flex body parts. When only one set of muscles is involved there is excessive reciprocal inhibition. As explained earlier, the spastic muscles inhibit contraction of the opposing muscles, which appear to be weak and actually become weak from lack of use. For example, if the head is always retracted or pulled back, the neck flexors are always inactivated.

The nature of the child's movement can affect the hypertonicity by what is called associated reactions. If the child attempts to move one extremity, this can increase spasticity throughout affected parts. Or if a less involved or uninvolved part of the body is moved, there can be an increase in the tone of more involved parts. The distribution and strength of the muscle tone in a part of the body changes as the result of a change in the position of the head in space and the relationship of the head and trunk, which was further discussed in the stages in Chapter 2. There may also be a change in the type of muscle tone in one particular affected part of the body over time.[26] Or as discussed earlier, hypotonic muscles in infancy may become hypertonic muscles one to two years later. The inner emotional state and the level of environmental stimulation also affect muscle tone. Thus, hypertonicity cannot be viewed as a static, unchanging entity.

Fluctuating Tone. Hypotonia may be the initial sign of another form of cerebral palsy called athetosis which is characterized by fluctuating tone. Muscle stretch receptors continually vary in their sensitivity, reflected by alternate resistance to a postural change and complete absence of resistance. There may be a fluctuation between hypertonicity and hypotonicity or between hypotonicity and normal tone, although hypotonicity predominates. The head and upper body parts are generally more involved than the lower body parts, and one side of the body is usually more involved. The child cannot simultaneously contract opposing muscles around the joint and maintain a position because of the fluctuating tone, and he has a sense of postural instability. Another aberration that adds to the lack of background stabilization is excessive reciprocal inhibition. When the child attempts to move, there is immediate inhibition and relaxation of the opposite group of muscles. This is in contrast to the normal, finely graded inhibition and relaxation, which provides a steadying and guiding influence to the contracted muscles. Thus, movements are poorly controlled and extreme in range. For example, the child cannot grade musculature contractions to partially extend an arm and accommodate to the distance of an object. He overshoots the target. The aberrant, uncoordinated movement pattern is expressed in one of three forms: involuntary, uncontrollable, bizarre movements of the body; jerky movements primarily confined to the face and the distal parts of the extremities; or slow writhing movements.[27] The movements become more exaggerated when the child attempts to intentionally engage in purposeful activity.

Because of the lack of a regulatory influence exerted by stabilizer muscles and a related lack of tonic inhibition, the child may withdraw from tactual contact with a surface or an object in a phasic avoidance reaction.[28] His emotional tone may also fluctuate, characterized by rapid and extreme mood shifts. There is autonomic instability, manifested by irregular respirations, overreaction to temperature changes, perspiration. The sympathetic component of the autonomic nervous system is overly active.

Hyperkinesia Unrelated to Abnormal Tone. The infant or child may express hyperkinesia in a different form that is not related to cerebral palsy. There is a similar lack of inhibitory and stabilizing influences, but the infant or child does not move in extreme ranges between flexion and extension or move an extremity in a very abrupt or rather bizarre way as does the child with athetosis. There is a rapid build up of activity in response to stimuli, which feeds itself because of the intermittent somatosensory input and lack of tonic inhibition. The infant or child has a wiggly, restless demeanor, and he thus has difficulty maintaining periods of focused stillness in a certain position. There is a feeling of muscular tension because of postural instability related to less-developed proximal muscles and less reliable equilibrium responses. Protective avoidance reactions may persist because of an immature tactual system and poor inhibition of phasic movements. There may also be mood swings and autonomic instability. The behavioral characteristics are further described throughout the stages in Chapter 2 relative to a low sensory threshold. A brief description was included in this chapter to illustrate the similarities and differences between hyperkinesia associated with athetosis and hyperkinesia often associated with a learning disability in the later preschool and early school years. There are similar needs in terms of stimulation adaptations, which will be discussed in a later section.

Hypotonia. Low muscle tone is not just a precursor to other types of abnormal tone. Hypotonia is an ongoing characteristic of certain disabilities such as Down syndrome. There is diminished resistance to passive stretch of the muscle and the movement of body parts. The joints may be hyperflexible, which allows them to move in ranges that are impossible if an infant or child has normal muscle tone.[29] Reflexive responses are also diminished (hyporeflexia). The weak musculature limits movement that would strengthen the muscles, and a cycle occurs. Again, there are different levels of involvement. All the muscles in the body may be hypotonic, ranging from a very floppy, ragdoll effect to only mild weakness. Or only some muscles may be weaker, because they are used less. As discussed previously, the antagonist of a spastic muscle can become hypotonic, because the contracted agonist inhibits its use. If the child has a myelomeningocele, some of the muscles may be hypotonic and some of the muscles may be hypertonic.[30]

APPROACHES TO MEDIATE THE ATTENTION LEVEL
AND RESPONSE THRESHOLD

All the variables that have been discussed relative to muscle tone alone support the premise that there cannot be a habilitative cookbook approach. The interplay between a background of nonspecific environmental stimuli, more specific animate and inanimate stimuli, and the maturation of the infant's central nervous system is a unique process that cannot be generalized to another infant or child. The expression of this process dynamically varies from hour to hour and day to day, which also negates generalization in terms of an individual infant or child. The response pattern at a certain point in time must serve as the guide in terms of stimulation needs. However, a framework can be provided to help the caregiver experiment with ways to mediate stimuli and influence the infant's or child's level of arousal and state and his response threshold. Interveners in the field and researchers have found that certain forms of stimulation usually have an excitatory effect, and certain forms of stimulation usually have a calming effect, very probably because of the influence exerted on the reticular formation. This old system is easily conditioned, evidenced by the effect of drugs on its regulatory functions.

Most of the descriptions throughout the stages in Chapter 2 related to the infant or child who has a very low or a very high sensory threshold, or very low or very high muscle tone. The polarity emphasizes the difference in patterns. However, in actuality many infants and children fit somewhere between the polarized ends of the continuum. Likewise, the approaches in Chapter 2 and this chapter do not apply just to the infant or child who is at either end of the continuum. If the infant is blind and has mild or moderate hypotonia because of a low activity level rather than pathology, he may respond positively to some of the approaches in this chapter, which increase the arousal and activity level, and some of the approaches outlined in Chapter 2 for the infant or toddler who has hypotonia. If the infant who is hyperreactive has tense muscles rather than pathologic hypertonia, he may respond positively to approaches in this chapter and Chapter 2 that have a calming and relaxing effect and facilitate freer movement. The tense infant, the very damaged infant who has stiff posturing early on, and the child who has spastic muscles and is still in an earlier stage of development may all enjoy and benefit from some of the approaches outlined for the infant with hypertonia in Chapter 2.

As discussed earlier, hypotonia during the first one to two years may signal a preathetoid or prespastic state. The infant should be observed very closely, especially if he does not have a disability commonly related to low muscle tone such as Down syndrome. If there are signs of stiffening, disorganization, or exaggerated reflex reactions in response to handling and other stimuli, excitatory approaches should not be used. Additional precautions are interspersed throughout the stages in Chapter 2 to alert the intervener and caregiver to behaviors that should not be reinforced. The observations will lead to an earlier diagnosis of pathology and involvement in a specialized therapy program.

The infant or child may have mixed involvement with some body parts that are hypotonic and some body parts that are hypertonic (certain forms of myelomeningocele and hydrocephalus) or only one side of the body is hypertonic (hemiplegia). Or there may be another form of complicated pathology: cerebral palsy of a mixed type involving both spasticity and athetosis. There is even a greater need to skillfully intertwine facilitation and inhibition under the direction of a therapist with specialized training. If this specialized resource is not available locally, every effort should be made to obtain consultation and assistance from a regional center or traveling team.

It is important to recognize hemiplegia early, and this disability is easier to detect in infancy because of the asymmetry of postural and movement patterns. The affected hand is more fisted and is not brought to the mouth, the head is usually turned away from the affected side, and the infant may kick with only one leg. He does not progress to the symmetric phase and bring both hands in the midline and reach with both hands; nor does he assume a bilateral support position when on his stomach; the one arm is adducted in close to the body. With early detection and therapy, functional use of the affected side is facilitated.

Inhibitory Forms of Input

The caregiver can experiment with the following approaches to determine which ones most effectively provide an inhibitory influence if the infant or child has a regulatory disorder expressed by one or more of the following characteristics: hyperresponsiveness to sensory stimuli, hypertonicity, hyperkinesis related or unrelated to fluctuating tone.

Wolff's observations led to the notion that a background of nonspecific environmental stimulation helps the normal infant maintain organizational integrity. A certain level of familiar noises in the home serves an inhibitory function, whereas a noisy, chaotic environment can have a disturbing effect. An unfamiliar environment can also enhance excitability because of the exposure to new forms of stimuli. The overall level of stimulation in the home may have to be further adapted if the infant or child has a regulatory disorder. A room that is decorated in more subdued, cool colors and that contains fewer pieces of furniture and fewer objects and pictures on pieces of furniture and walls will be less excitatory. In this arrangement, there is a lower level of brightness, fewer angles, less contour, and a greater sense of distance, which allows more personal space. The infant or child should not be placed by an open cupboard containing toys or other objects or by a window when he is engaged in an activity. A pet or sibling darting in and out can also be distracting. Pleasant odors in the home may be inhibitory, whereas noxious odors are excitatory—bleach, ammonia. Extract of cherry has been found to have a calming and alerting effect if the child has athetosis. If necessary, the level of stimulation in the room can be further reduced by dimming the lights or pulling down the shades. If there are fluorescent lights in a program or hospital setting, the removal of every other light may have a calming effect. However, Wolff found that when the fluorescent lights were turned off in the nursery, sleep became irregular. When the lights were turned back on, the infants moved back to the regular sleep state again.

The above example of the infants' response to a steady light suggests that the monotony of a stimulus is more important than the modality of the stimulus in lowering the arousal level and altering the state of the infant or child. As a general rule, a stimulus that is repetitive, rhythmic, and slower in tempo is inhibitory. A continuous sound meets this criterion and is generally a very effective form of inhibition. Mellow background music may elicit inner stability,[31] and the music can also mask the excitatory, intermittent PA system in a clinic or hospital setting. Vocalization in even tones and a slow tempo is less excitatory, and the caregiver can decrease the level of stimulation even more by not talking at all. The caregiver just naturally uses the steady sound of her voice to calm the infant or child. She begins with a louder sound at a faster tempo to override the infant's or child's distress behavior. The caregiver then slowly decreases the loudness and the tempo of her sound as the infant or child quiets down. The voice acts as a pacemaker. One caregiver found that a long, steady "aaaaa" for approximately ten seconds was very effective. Or the caregiver may repeatedly say "There" or "Quiet down" or some other word(s). This approach may especially be effective if the infant or child is hyperreactive to stimulation but does not have abnormal tone. However, an artificial sound device must be used with real caution. Wolff found that the infant was far less sensitive to stimuli during regular sleep induced by white noise, and visceral excitations were even blocked out. He raised the question of possible harmful effects, since the artificially induced sleep is not identical with the natural, regular sleep state.

Slow, rhythmic movement has a relaxing effect, and the rocking chair is the most natural source of this type of input. A forward and backward movement with the infant or young child supported in a vertical position up to the shoulder is generally most effective. However, a side to side movement with the infant or child nestled in the arms may be more relaxing in some cases. The child can be calmed and relaxed on the spot by having him stand against the caregiver's body. She then rocks both of their bodies in a rhythmic forward and backward or side-to-side plane.

If the infant is hyperreactive and in a highly aroused state, a different type of rocking input may have to be used to override the self-feeding, intermittent stimuli. The infant is placed in a vertical position up to the shoulder, and a faster rocking speed is used with a high amplitude, which causes a greater postural change.[32] This input may not be effective if the infant or child has abnormal muscle tone.

Slow rolling is another relaxing form of input, especially if the infant or child has hypertonic muscles. He is placed in the supine position, and the caregiver kneels beside the infant or child and places her one hand on the pelvis and the other hand on the rib cage so that the arm remains free (Fig. 3-1A). The caregiver rolls the infant or child from the supine to the sidelying position and then back to supine with a slow, continuous motion by rhythmically moving her own body back and forth (Fig. 3-1B). She repeats the movement until the infant or child begins to relax. If the supine position increases the muscle tone, the caregiver initially places the infant or child in the sidelying position. She gently rolls him back and forth, gradually moving him all the way back to the supine position during the excursion when the body becomes more relaxed. The caregiver rolls the infant or child away from her in one direction and then moves over to the other side and rolls him

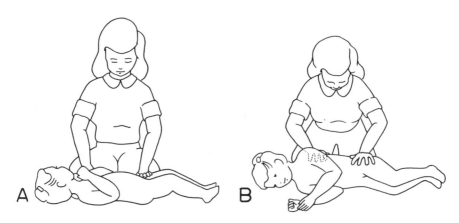

FIGURE 3-1. Slow rolling has a relaxing effect, especially if the child has hypertonia.

in the opposite direction, unless he has involvement only on one side (hemiplegia).[33] The caregiver should also use slow, rhythmic movements when handling the infant or child during care routines.

Neutral warmth has a calming, relaxing effect because of the even body temperature. The infant or child is wrapped mummy fashion preferably in a cotton blanket, because it is less allergenic. He is wrapped in whatever position is comfortable rather than attempting to straighten out hypertonic muscles. The blanket is tucked in well around the feet and neck to prevent drafts. Also, if the infant or child is not snugly swaddled, this can have a disturbing effect, because he is only partially restrained. However, it may be that some infants or children resist confinement. If this is the case, the caregiver can just wrap one or more involved extremities to relax them before an activity. Or the snugness can initially be adjusted somewhat until he gets used to the confinement. The caregiver remains with the infant or child and observes when he is becoming relaxed inside the blanket, which may be after a 10- or 20-minute interval or longer; the time may vary from day to day. The approach can be combined with rhythmic rocking if more inhibition is needed.[34]

This approach is an effective preparatory measure before certain procedures in the clinic or hospital setting. The caregiver or nurse swaddles the infant or child approximately 15 minutes before he is scheduled for an x-ray or another procedure, and he remains swaddled during the procedure, if this is feasible, to maintain the lower arousal state and relaxation. The caregiver or nurse can also swaddle the infant or child approximately 15 minutes before he is scheduled for a session with the therapist, if the initial relaxation will enhance the effect of the approaches.

Neutral warmth can be used as a preparatory measure before dental work is performed, which decreases the need for special restraints and drugs. If the child has hypertonia or fluctuating tone, the following combined approach is often very effective. He is wrapped in the blanket and slowly rolled from supine to side-lying a number of times. The child is lifted from the floor in a flexed position, and he is held in this position in a chair and rocked with a slow and steady movement. The caregiver or intervener curls him up more as he relaxes. The child is carried in a flexed posture and placed in a supine position on the fully reclined dental chair. A pillow is placed under the flexed knees and stabilized with a sandbag. Or he is positioned in a bean bag chair on the dental chair. The swaddled hands do not interfere with the dentist's movements.[35]

Neutral warmth can also be provided by water close to body temperature, which has a calming effect and relaxes hypertonic muscles. If the water is at too high a temperature, the muscles tense up again in two to three hours in a rebound effect, and there may be associated discomfort.[36] The caregiver often plans the bath before bedtime or at a time during the day when the infant or child is more tense.

If the infant or child moves excessively in a disorganized way (hyperkinesis related or unrelated to fluctuating tone), continuous, uninterrupted forms of stimuli have a stabilizing influence. The complete confinement, touch pressure input, and neutral warmth provided by the previously described swaddling procedure may be especially effective. More and more caregivers are also either adapting the commercial carrier or making their own carrier, which places the infant in close physical contact with their body and inhibits diffuse, disorganized activity. Repetitive slow stroking is another effective approach to inhibit excitability and excess movement. The infant or child can lie in a prone or side-lying position, sit leaning over on the caregiver's lap or on a chair, or stand up. The caregiver primarily uses the pads of her finger, excluding the thumb. She slowly strokes down the center of the back from the cervical area to the low lumbar area with a rhythmic alternate movement of the hands. When the one hand reaches the low lumbar area at the end of the stroke, the caregiver places the other hand up on the center of the back in the cervical area before releasing the first hand. Thus, there is continuous contact (Fig. 3-2). The stroke should be firm but not firm enough to stimulate the muscles and increase tension, or too light, which will have a tickling effect. The input is most effective when the fingers are in contact with the skin. The alternate stroking should only be continued for three minutes; the input will become excitable if continued beyond this maximum time. At the end of the last stroke, the caregiver maintains her fingers at the end point for a few seconds to avoid a sudden withdrawal of tactual input. The approach will not have an inhibitory effect

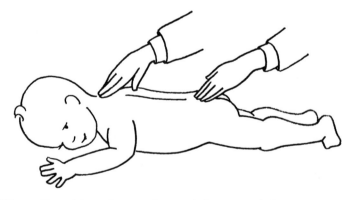

FIGURE 3-2. Repetitive, slow stroking inhibits excitability and excess movement.

if the infant or child is sensitive about being touched in a place he cannot see. The approach is also contraindicated if there is irregular hair growth on the back with a swirl effect, because some of the hairs will be rubbed the wrong way, which is excitatory. Slow stroking is more effective in inhibiting hyperkinesia than decreasing tone in hypertonic muscles.[37]

The following approaches may also dampen excitatory or withdrawal responses. The avoidance reaction is decreased by massaging the feet and hands with a firm, continuous pressure. The infant or child may then be able to assume and maintain a prone, weight-bearing position which develops stabilizing muscles, and feedback from these muscles has an inhibitory effect. If the older infant or child can assume a position with weight on the elbows and knees or the hands and knees (quadruped position), this increases pressure on the carotid sinus. The distension inhibits the excitatory influence of the reticular activating system. If the infant or child has hyperkinesis unrelated to athetosis, activities outlined in the different stages to facilitate the pivot prone posture activate stabilizing muscles and increase postural stability.[38] This posture should not be facilitated if the child has fluctuating tone except under the direction of a therapist consultant.

Other adaptations minimize intermittent forms of stimulation, which elicit or reinforce phasic movements related to hyperkinesis. When the caregiver approaches the excitable infant or child, she can hold his knees or place her hands on his shoulders or another body part for a few seconds, which has a stabilizing effect. Firm pressure above the lip may have the same effect especially if the child has athetosis. The caregiver should maintain firm and continuous contact with the body as much as possible when handling the infant or child. He is not dressed in loose clothing, especially in cooler weather, to avoid a temperature change from a draft, and light, moving tactual input from the clothes. A warm, thick washcloth is placed over nonimmersed parts of the chest and abdomen during the bathing. Warm water is sopped on the washcloth with firm pressure at intervals if necessary.

Disorganized behavior may be an expression of understimulation. The infant or child is attempting to find ways of nourishing his nervous system. If this is the case, inhibitory approaches will increase the disorganization. The focus has to be changed to providing an appropriate level of stimulation in his environment.

When the muscle tone is decreased or excessive movement is inhibited, the infant or child can then move to an alert state and focus on a specific animate or inanimate stimulus either during or following one of the above inhibitory approaches, such as swaddling or rhythmic rocking. The focused attention itself and goal-directed behavior that evolves later in infancy help modulate the cell threshold.[39] The caregiver can experiment with the stimulus dimensions of inanimate objects as another form of modulation. The results of one study[40] suggest that the various dimensions are additive in their effect upon the stimulus intensity. It is the high or low value of the dimensions, rather than the types of dimensions, that determines whether the stimulus is excitatory or inhibitory. An object with fewer angles, less contour, and a lower level of brightness is less intense. If the object is smaller and farther away, this also decreases the level of intensity. Thus, the infant may be most responsive to a mobile that contains fewer objects that are smaller in size. The objects have less complex shapes and fewer designs on them, and they are painted in less bright, cool colors. The objects are not hung too close to the infant but within his visual range. Likewise, a single object may have to be adapted in terms of the above characteristics. The auditory stimulus dimension may also have to be adjusted. The infant or child may not be able to tolerate an intermittent sound (bell), or the sound has to be more muted. A background of continuous instrumental music may help the infant or child tune out distracting stimuli.

If the infant or child is having difficulty manipulating an object because of an increase in muscle tone, the caregiver can reinstate one of the previously described relaxing approaches. She can also gently shake the arm and hand by grasping the top of the shoulder and moving it with a slow, rhythmic, rotary motion. Or if the infant or child is having difficulty because the voluntary effort increases disorganized movement (hyperkinesis), the caregiver reinstates the most effective stabilizing approach. She can also grasp the infant's or child's hands between her hands and maintain the touch pressure contact for an interval, which may have a stabilizing effect. If the infant or child with hyperkinesis can assume the prone, forearm position and bear weight on one arm while he reaches and manipulates an object with the other arm, the weight bearing can have a stabilizing effect.

Because the caregiver can most flexibly mediate her own behavior, animate stimulation will very probably provide the best match, with especially the young infant's threshold level. If the infant is very reactive, the caregiver may not be able to simultaneously look at him, talk to him, and rock him. She may be able to rock him slowly and look at him if she does not vocalize. Or she may be able to slowly rock him and talk to him with a modulated voice while looking away. The infant may have to initially withdraw from animate stimulation. After he has gotten himself together, he turns back and orients to his caregiver.

To exemplify that there is no universal, foolproof recipe, Field[41] found that some infants were more responsive to an inanimate, simple Raggedy Ann doll than to a human face. She reasoned that possibly the doll mirrored the image of the infant more accurately. The doll was more like him with less stimulus information.

With a mediated environment, the infant or child will no doubt gradually begin to tolerate a higher level of stimulation without escalated excitement and without an increase in muscle tone or an increase in disorganized movement. His cell threshold becomes less sensitive. He may remain in a deeper sleep state for longer periods of time. There is a possibility that increased intervals of regular NREM sleep influence the function of a neuronal oscillator, which regulates the sequence and rhythm of movement. Further research will help establish if such an oscillator exists and its functional ramifications.

FACILITORY FORMS OF INPUT

If the infant or child has a regulatory disorder expressed by hyporesponsiveness to sensory stimuli and/or hypotonia, the caregiver can experiment with the following approaches to determine which ones most effectively provide an excitatory influence.

A study of children with Down syndrome[42] indicates that a background of familiar stimuli emanating from the common round of daily events in the home provides a rhythm that has an important organizing effect. It therefore appears that all infants and children have the same need for this type of nonspecific environmental input. The overall level of stimulation in the home may have to be increased somewhat during periods of wakefulness to elicit a higher level of arousal and responsiveness. A room decorated in brighter, warm colors which contains more furniture and more bric-a-brac on pieces of furniture and walls can have an alerting effect. This arrangement provides a higher intensity of brightness, more angles, a higher contour density, and a decreased sense of distance. The intermittent input of a sibling or pet darting in and out and different sights out the window may also have an alerting effect. However, there is the danger of too much busyness, which can be distracting, especially when the infant or child is focusing on a specific stimulus. The level of intensity must be carefully monitored when the infant is younger because of competing physiologic demands.

More distinct odors in the home such as vanilla, peppermint, cloves, certain perfumes, garlic, and mustard have an alerting effect, because the olfactory sense is very old and functional even if the infant or child has a very damaged central nervous system. He should not be intentionally exposed to more noxious odors (paint, ammonia) except under very controlled and well-supervised experimental conditions. There no doubt is a mechanical effect on nonsmelling mucous membranes as well as olfactory receptors, and these types of substances present a safety hazard. Also, the infant or child may begin to view his environment as noxious.

The level of stimulation can be increased by the adaptation of specific forms of input. As a general rule, intermittent, changing, quick stimuli have an excitatory effect. The infant or child may be very responsive to auditory input with the above characteristics, because this sense is also more well developed at birth. He may be jazzed up by music with a louder volume, a fast tempo, and an irregular rhythm. However, Diamond[43] found that a rhythm in some rock music, which is opposite that of the heart/arterial rhythm, can cause muscular weakness. This finding emphasizes the nuances that alter a general rule and the need to closely observe the infant's or child's responses. A variation of the sound pattern from different instruments assuming the foreground or the alternation between instrumentation and lyrics may be excitatory. The music can also be turned on and off to provide intermittency, and the PA system in the clinic or hospital setting may have an alerting effect. In the same vein, the caregiver can try alternating a flickering sound (bell or toy cricket) with a steady sound (prolonged "aaaaaa"). The human voice is a very socially significant stimulus, and a variation of the caregiver's vocal pattern may be the most effective form of input. She can shift from a louder to a softer volume, a faster to a slower tempo, and a higher to a lower pitch in a rather exaggerated way. The caregiver can also experiment with the interspersion of another sensory modality. In studies of normal infants,[44] visual attention to a stimulus was recovered or maintained by the onset of an auditory stimulus (mother's voice or music) or the cessation of an auditory stimulus. Thus, a change of the input in one modality may increase the attention to an unchanging stimulus in another modality.

Light touch receptors are more primitive, and this form of input is transmitted by older tracts which send a lot of collaterals to the reticular formation and heavily influence its function. Tactual input can therefore be adapted to elicit an increased arousal level and phasic movement. The caregiver can rub the skin on the arms, legs, and back with a brisk, light stroke after the infant's bath and before an activity. She experiments with different textures to determine which ones are the most facilitory, being careful not to irritate the skin. The caregiver can also provide light, intermittent touch by nuzzling the infant's or child's neck; lightly rubbing noses with him; lightly clasping his hands, releasing the contact, then lightly clasping the hands again; or lightly stroking the fingers. A light touch input to the palm or sole of the foot may be too intense with a noxious quality, and this form of input should be avoided, unless it is done under the very close supervision of a consultant with an in-depth understanding of facilitory and inhibitory approaches.[45] Likewise, neck nuzzling and other tickling sensations must be used with caution. Contact with the caregiver should be pleasurable rather than being overexcitable.

The infant or child can be left undressed for a period after the bath if this does not elicit autonomic instability, characterized by a color change and lack of recovery. The cooler temperature and the absence of the inhibitory influence provided by clothing and swaddling may elicit increased excitation and movement.

Vestibular input also influences the reticular formation, and movement can be adapted to have a facilitory effect. The caregiver just naturally attempts to arouse the infant by jiggling him and bobbing her head as she talks to him with a varied vocal pattern. Thus, she increases the intensity by combining three modalities with changing qualities. The infant or child can also be aroused by adapting the usual rocking pattern; he is rocked with a more irregular rhythm. If the intensity of the vestibular input needs to be further enhanced, acceleration and deceleration are provided by rather abrupt stops and starts in the rocking movement. The abruptness of the movement must be appropriately adjusted if the infant is very young or if the older infant or child has poor head control to prevent a whiplash effect. The vertical on-shoulder position arouses a sleepy infant, whereas the position soothes a crying infant as discussed earlier.[46]

The following movement adaptation usually increases the arousal level of the younger infant especially. The caregiver stands and holds the infant in her arms. She sways the infant back and forth in a horizontal plane and pauses. She then transfers the infant to a vertical on-shoulder position and moves her body up and down and pauses. There is both a directional change in the movement input and a change in the position of the infant's body. The caregiver repeats the above sequence for one to three minutes. It may be that the infant will be sufficiently alerted if he is swayed back and forth and up and down in the horizontal position without a change to the vertical, on-shoulder position. Or the caregiver can try position changes without the other movement variations; she shifts the infant back and forth between the supine and upright positions a number of times.

The slow rolling approach described earlier can be adapted. The infant or child is rolled from supine to side-lying at a faster tempo, which elicits a more sudden change of position. Again, the speed is adjusted to the degree of head control. The caregiver can also place the infant or child over her lap and tip him forward and backward and from side to side as briskly as he can tolerate. This form of input is provided in both the prone and supine positions if enjoyable. When the head control improves, the caregiver just naturally sways the infant up in the air, lowers him, pauses, and sways him up in the air again. When the protective response evolves in the upper extremities, a new movement can be added to the game; he is supported in the trunk area and tipped forward. The infant or child may react adversely to faster and arrhythmic movement input if he has otitis media.

Proprioceptive input also has a facilitory effect. If resistance is provided to a movement, this elicits increased neuronal activity and tone and more prolonged activity of the working muscle. The caregiver can provide resistance by placing her hand below the occipital bulge when the infant or child raises his head. She can also apply resistance when he flexes or extends an arm or leg. The resistance is applied intermittently: apply, hold, release; apply, hold, release. The force should be graded so that the infant or child can complete the intended movement and not become frustrated.[47] He can also be encouraged to kick against the caregiver's body or the end of the crib with the whole foot.

Kinnealey[48] found that the child with a lower mental age preferred vestibular and vibratory input, whereas the child with a higher mental age preferred visual input. If the infant or child has a very high threshold to sensory input and pain, he may seek intense vibratory input, which can get through and be processed. He places his head against the washer, TV, or piano, because the bones in the head intensify the vibration. If the child is allowed to hold a vibrator, he may even put it on his teeth or on the mastoid bone, the two locations that provide the highest intensity of input. The infant or child should be allowed to control contact with a vibrating household appliance (washer) or the piano. Input via a commercial vibrator should be used only under the direction of a consultant who has in-depth knowledge of the sensory system.

As mentioned previously, the infant may not be very responsive to visual stimuli, especially if there is more severe central nervous system damage. The caregiver can experiment with stimulus dimensions to increase the intensity. A mobile may be more excitatory if the objects are larger and have a more complex shape with more angles. The objects also have a design on them which increases the contour density, and they are painted in warm, bright colors. The mobile is suspended closer to the infant but within his focus range. The brightness can be further increased by adding luminous fish lures or a sphere or cone covered with shiny beads. However, these additions must be firmly attached and the caregiver must respect the need for close monitoring, even when the object is out of reach. Or the very young infant may be attracted to a design on a piece of cardboard which combines contour density and brightness. There is a section that is made up of checkerboard squares and a section that has a white circle on a black background. The combination is based on the premise that brightness may attract attention but does not hold the attention . There has to be a design to focus on.

Individual objects may have to be adapted with the above criteria as a guide when the infant begins to develop manipulative skills. Also, the bottle may elicit heightened interest and proximity seeking when the infant is aroused by hunger sensations. A Mattel talking toy usually increases the alertness of the toddler because of all the pictures on the front, the intermittent sound, and the resistance to the pulling action. A Jack-in-the-box has a similar effect.

Although objects may effectively increase alertness, the jazzed-up effect may have a high energy cost and be shortlived, especially during the early infancy period. The caregiver can more flexibly modulate her behavior to elicit just the right level of excitation. She adapts her voice, facial orientation, and movements in ways that have been described in earlier paragraphs in response to the infant's cues and his arousal and recovery cycles. It may be that a low level of responsiveness is a way of preserving a fragile autonomic regulatory mechanism. If this is the case, an increase in the level of stimulation would enhance the protective, depressed state.

Additional Precautions

The infant's or child's inner regulatory mechanisms may become more functional in response to mediating approaches. However, it is unlikely that his response pattern or muscle tone will qualitatively move within the so-called normal range. Although these approaches can elicit positive effects, there is also the danger of harmful effects. A very open line of communication must exist between professional interveners in varied settings (hospital, clinic, school, specialized center) and the caregiver to recognize signs of too much inhibition or too much excitation, which may be immediately apparent, or there may be a delayed reaction hours later. The caregiver and interveners are alerted by changes in the infant's or child's behavior and emotional tone, breathing, skin color, pupil size unrelated to the level of light, perspiration unrelated to the environmental temperature, loss of appetite, nausea, or any other unusual signs or symptoms. There may also be certain medical contraindications in terms of some forms of input.

Conclusion

The approaches can effectively subserve activities described in the different stages in Chapter 2. The whole purpose of mediating the response threshold and muscle tone is to help the infant or child interact with his environment in an adaptive way. Another equally important payoff of a well modulated environment is increased physiologic stability reflected by a more regular eating and sleeping schedule and more restful sleep. Relative to this is a reminder to not forget the obvious when focusing on the appropriate level of stimulation and a growth-fostering environment. As Wolff observed, a longer duration of alertness most often occurs when the infant is relieved of all distressing circumstances—after he is fed, diapered, and burped.

REFERENCES

1. Wolff, PH: *Observations on newborn infants.* Psychosomatic Med 21:110, 1959.
2. Wolff, PH: *The causes, controls, and organization of behavior in the neonate.* Psychological Issues Vol. 5(1), Monograph No. 17, 1966.
3. Adrian, ED and Matthews, BHC: *The interpretation of potential waves in the cortex.* J Physiol 81:440, 1934.
4. Delcomyn F: *Neural basis of rhythmic behavior in animals.* Science 210: 492, 1980.
5. Dement, WC: *Sleep deprivation and the organization of the behavioral states.* In: Clemente, CD, Purpura, DP, Mayer, FE (eds): *Sleep and the Maturing Nervous System.* Academic Press, New York, 1972.
6. Parmelee, AH and Stern, E: *Development of states in infants.* In: Clemente, CD, Purpura, DP, and Mayer, FE (eds): *Sleep and the Maturing Nervous System.* Academic Press, New York, 1972.
7. Hoffer, BJ, et al: *The development of synapses in the rat cerebellar cortex.* In: Clemente, CD, Purpura, DP, and Mayer, FE (eds): *Sleep and the Maturing Nervous System.* Academic Press, New York, 1972.
8. Scheibel, ME and Scheibel, AB: *Maturing neuronal subsystems: The dendrites of spinal motorneurons.* In: Clemente, CD, Purpura, DP and Mayer, FE (eds): *Sleep and the Maturing Nervous System.* Academic Press, New York, 1972.
9. Purpura, DP and Shofer, RJ: *Principles of synaptogenesis and their application to ontogenetic studies of mammalian cerebral cortex.* In: Clemente, CD, Purpura, DP, and Mayer, FE (eds): *Sleep and the Maturing Nervous System.* Academic Press, New York, 1972.
10. Sterman, MB: *The basic rest-activity cycle and sleep: Developmental considerations in man and cats.* In: Clemente, CD, Purpura, DP, and Mayer, FE (eds): *Sleep and the Maturing Nervous System.* Academic Press, 1972, p. 175.
11. Metcalf, DR: *Invited discussion: Chapter II.* In: Clemente, CD, Purpura, DP, and Mayer, FE (eds): *Sleep and the Maturing Nervous System.* Academic Press, New York, 1972.
12. Barr, ML: *The Human Nervous System.* Harper & Row, New York, 1972.
13. Magoun, HW: *The Waking Brain.* Charles C Thomas, Springfield, Ill, 1963.
14. Ibid.
15. Jasper, HH: *Pathophysiological studies of brain mechanisms in different states of consciousness.* In: Eccles, JC (ed): *Brain and Conscious Experience.* Springer Verlag, New York, 1966.

16. MAGOUN, op. cit.

17. BARR, op. cit.

18. Ibid.

19. FARBER, SD AND HUSS, AJ: Sensorimotor Evaluation and Treatment Procedures for Allied Health Personnel. The Indiana University Foundation, 1974.

20. PRECHTL, HF, WEINMANN, H, AND AKIYAMA, Y: Organization or physiological parameters in normal and neurologically abnormal infants. Neuropadiatrie, 1:101, 1969.

21. PARMELEE AND STERN, op. cit.

22. BOBATH, K AND BOBATH, B: Cerebral palsy. In: PEARSON, PH AND WILLIAMS, CE (EDS): Physical Therapy Services in the Developmental Disabilities. Charles C Thomas, Springfield, Ill, 1972.

23. HARRIS, FA: Muscle stretch receptor hypersensitization in spasticity. Am J Phys Med 57:16, 1978.

24. HARRISON, A: Components of neuromuscular control. In: HOLT, K (ED): Movement and Child Development. JB Lippincott, Philadelphia, 1975.

25. BOBATH AND BOBATH, op. cit.

26. Ibid.

27. BRUMLIK, J: The multiply handicapped patient. Am J Phys Med 46:555, 1967.

28. STOCKMEYER, SA: An interpretation of the approach of Rood to the treatment of neuromuscular dysfunction. Am J Phys Med 46:900, 1967.

29. DRACHMAN, DA: Disorders of tone. Am J Phys Med 46:525, 1967.

30. FIEBER, NM AND KLIEWER, D: Physical therapy in a children's rehabilitation center. In: PEARSON, PH AND WILLIAMS, CE (EDS): Physical Therapy Services in Development Disabilities. Charles C Thomas, Springfield, Ill, 1972.

31. BLANCHARD, BE: The effect of music on pulse-rate, blood pressure and final exam scores of university students. J Sports Med 19:305, 1979.

32. PEDERSON, DR AND TERVRUGT, D: The influence of amplitude and frequency of vestibular stimulation on the activity of two-month-old infants. Child Devel 44:122, 1973.

33. FARBER AND HUSS, op. cit.

34. Ibid.

35. BEEDLE, G AND TUCKER, N: Therapeutic handling techniques for the athetoid or spastic cerebral palsy patient in the dental setting. Presentation Thirtieth Annual Meeting, American Academy for Cerebral Palsy, Los Angeles, September, 1976.

36. FARBER AND HUSS, op. cit.

37. Ibid.

38. STOCKMEYER, op. cit.

39. WOLFF, op. cit., 1966.

40. McGUIRE, I AND TURKEWITZ, G: Visually elicited finger movements in infants. Child Devel 49:362, 1978.

41. Field, TM: *Interaction patterns of pre-term and term infants.* In: Field, TM (ED): *Infants Born at Risk.* SP Medical and Scientific Books, New York, 1979.

42. Piper, MC and Ramsay, MK: *Effect of early home environment on the mental development of Down syndrome infants.* Am J Mental Defic 85:39, 1980.

43. Diamond, J: *Behavioral Kinesiology: The New Science for Positive Health Through Muscle Testing.* Regent House, New York, 1981.

44. Horowitz, FD (ED): *Visual attention, auditory stimulation, and language discrimination in young infants.* Monographs of the Society for Research in Child Development. Serial No. 158, Vol. 39, 1974.

45. Stockmeyer, op. cit.

46. Byrne, JM and Horowitz, FD: *The influence of direction and type of movement on the efficacy of rocking as a soothing technique.* Presentation Biennial Meeting, Society for Research in Child Development, San Francisco, 1979.

47. Farber and Huss, op. cit.

48. Kinnealey, M: *Aversive and nonaversive response to sensory stimulation in mentally retarded children.* Am J Occup The 27:464, 1973.

Chapter 4

HABILITATIVE APPROACHES TO FACILITATE MORE ADAPTIVE ORAL PATTERNS RELATED TO EATING AND EXPRESSIVE LANGUAGE

Athleen B. Coyner and Raeone S. Zelle

Physiologic, anatomic, nutritional, developmental, and interactive parameters of the feeding process have been discussed in Chapters 1 and 2. Aberrations that may occur if the infant or child has a developmental disability have also been described, and many of the habilitative approaches outlined in these two chapters affect the evolvement of feeding and language patterns either directly or indirectly. Several key parameters will be further developed in this chapter as they relate to three stages of functional development. In keeping with the framework throughout the book, the primary emphasis will be on the importance of feeding as a foci of interaction.

FIRST STAGE: BIRTH TO SIX MONTHS FUNCTIONAL LEVEL

Incoordination of the jaw, lips, tongue, palate, pharynx, and larynx is one of the earliest signs of central nervous system damage; thus, significant feeding problems may be evident in the neonatal period. These problems can cause worry and even a feeling of doubt about one's parenting skills, because feeding is a very basic need which any caregiver expects to meet. If the infant does not respond to the usual approaches, the caregiver's anxiety may be expressed by depression and crying. Or she may respond with increased activity, which is asynchronous with the infant's cues. The caregiver frequently interrupts the feeding to look at how much has been taken, to adjust the nipple, burp the infant, or attempt to perk him up or calm him down. The interruptions may actually exaggerate the problem and interfere with a feeble attempt on the part of the infant to express his own suck-pause rhythm. It may be that the infant's cues are confusing. He stiffens, and if his arm is in a certain location, it appears that the infant is pushing his caregiver away; or he arches, which pulls him away from the caregiver's body. These involuntary reflexive movements can be erroneously interpreted as rejection. Or the infant may be lethargic, and it is difficult to tell whether he is awake or asleep during the feeding.

The pair may get off to a wrong start, and the feeding experience becomes task oriented with an overanxious emphasis on an adequate intake. Very little interaction occurs via talking, looking, or touching, and the affect and responsiveness of both the infant and caregiver wane. A mental set may evolve and persist with the caregiver unduly concerned about the infant's nutritional needs, even when there is no longer a real or substantial reason for concern. She is unwilling to let the infant assume a progressively more active role in the feeding process because of the perceived need to guarantee a certain level of intake, even to the point of holding his hands. Under these conditions, the infant may develop a negative mental set about food and mealtime, or he may resign himself to passive dependency.

Although the infant's feeding problems are a source of real concern, the parents may be reluctant to adapt the traditional feeding approaches to the peculiar needs of their infant. It may be that they are not ready to deal with the fact that something may be wrong with their child. The intervener can tune into the parents' concern regarding the nutritional intake because this is a high priority need for all the reasons described in Chapter 1. The focus is centered on ways to help the infant suck more productively and shorten the feeding period rather than his aberrant pattern. Suggested interventions are related to traditional approaches as closely as possible with a gradual introduction of less familiar habilitative adaptations if this is necessary because of more severe problems.

The more comfortable focus on a productive sucking pattern is in keeping with the normal infant's functional development during this first stage. With practice, he more adaptively coordinates his suck, swallow, and breathing; and the nutritive suck becomes stronger and more continuous to meet the infant's increasing nutritional needs. There is an increased length of bursts, a decreased interval between bursts, and a decreased rate of suck with a burst.[1] As the infant develops increased voluntary control of oral muscles, primitive reflexes are inhibited or begin to wane. Facilitative approaches may foster the same outcome if the infant has an aberrant pattern.

Preparation of the Infant for a Feeding

Because the rocking chair is a familiar setting for the feeding, the intervener helps the caregiver adapt the rocking movement per the guidelines in Chapter 3 either to relax the infant or perk him up. The adapted movement facilitates a more natural cuddly feel rather than stiffness or limpness; and the infant is more easily held in the normal position that accompanies sucking, that is, hip, knee, and neck flexion. Snug swaddling can calm the infant and suppress excess activity or promote muscular relaxation, whereas unwrapping the infant may alert him.

The intervener also helps the caregiver observe for hunger cues which may be difficult to read. The normal hungry infant holds his hands close over the abdomen, and the fingers make searching motions. He also fusses and escalates to the crying state, if necessary, to attract attention. During the initial phase of the feeding, the infant's fisted hands are held over the chest. As he begins to sense fullness, the fingers loosen and become fully extended at the end of the feeding. The arms also fully extend in an expression of satiety.[2] The notion that an infant must be fed every three or four hours may not be based on anything but a cultural heritage. Horton, Lubchenco, and Gordon[3] studied infants on a self-regulatory schedule and found that they ate only four times a day; three infants slept for very long intervals between some feedings. Yet, they all gained weight at a satisfactory rate. The activity level is an important factor; a very inactive infant will have less caloric needs. On the other hand, the very tense, overactive infant may express hunger more frequently.

Facilitation of the Reflexive Sucking and Swallowing Response

The above preparatory measures and responsiveness to hunger cues may be sufficient to stimulate a productive reflexive sucking and swallowing response. If not, the intervener helps the mother try additional measures to facilitate adaptation to her breast nipple if she has a desire to breastfeed the infant. A measure as simple as providing upward pressure under a lax jaw to hold it in place may be all that is needed to help the infant close his lips around the nipple. The mother may have to accentuate the tactual stimulation of her nipple by pressing it against the upper lip or the hard palate if this is possible, or by tugging on the nipple at intervals.

If these measures elicit only a fleeting sucking response, the caregiver can experiment with other variations to elicit a reflexive movement of the tongue in response to a tactual stimulus. She can lightly touch the alveolar ridge inside the upper gum and the right and left side of the tongue, which may elicit a movement toward the source of stimulation.[4] The caregiver can also lightly rub the roof of the mouth.

If the infant's hyperactive gag is elicited by the nipple, and he has excessive oral sensitivity, the touch input will have to be introduced in a different manner. The caregiver can rub the gums and roof of the mouth with a firmer stroke, and the infant will possibly also tolerate the age-old custom of washing the tongue with a firmer stroke. The touch input gradually becomes less firm as the sensitivity decreases. It is hoped that the infant will eventually perceive and respond to a light touch on the lips and tongue with a more adaptive, orienting response.

If this more available form of stimulation does not facilitate increased tongue movement, the intervener helps the mother experiment with the following approaches involving a combination of cold and sweet input. A cottonswab is moistened in a sugar and water solution, placed in a plastic bag, and chilled until ice crystals form. The cottonswab is then placed inside the lips in contact with the tongue. Or a sugar tit can be made by wetting a four-by-four sponge in a sterilized sugar and water solution and placing it in a plastic bag to chill in the freezer. One of these forms of input may elicit a sucking response, which can then be adapted to the breast nipple.

If the above facilitative approaches are not effective, it is important to verify if the infant is a nose breather. The mother holds the lips together for five to ten seconds and places the index finger under the nose to feel for exhaled air; or she places a mirror under the nose to check for fogging. If the infant has to partially or fully breathe through his mouth, he cannot close the lips around the nipple. Nor can he handle a larger amount of liquid at one time. The problem should be further investigated by the physician.

APPROACHES TO NORMALIZE TONE. The infant's aberrant pattern may be related to more complex problems. He may have difficulty moving his lips and tongue in a sucking action because of too much or too little tone in the muscles. Additional habilitative measures may be necessary and can be implemented when the oral structures have increased in size. If the cheeks, lips, and tongue are very tense, the following forms of touch input may relax the muscles. The caregiver places the inside surface of the fingers on each cheek and slowly massages the cheeks in a clockwise pattern with continuous pressure until she feels the cheeks soften. She then discontinues the input to prevent too much relaxation. If the lips are also tense, the caregiver places her index finger in a horizontal plane on the skin above the upper lip and massages downward. She then places her thumb inside the upper lip and the index finger on the skin above the upper lip and gently shakes the lip as she pulls downward. Another finger may have to be substituted for the thumb on the younger infant's smaller lip. The caregiver massages upward on the skin below the lower lip with the index finger. She then places the index finger inside the lower lip and the thumb on the skin below the lower lip and gently shakes the lip and pulls it upward. The infant's face may become more expressive in response to these approaches in ways that will promote interaction with his caregiver, which is an equally important benefit. To relax the tongue, the caregiver places one or two fingers on the top of the tongue in the mid-region not far enough back to elicit a gag reflex. She gently shakes the tongue back and forth until she feels the tone decrease, and the input is then discontinued to prevent too much relaxation. The caregiver should apply enough pressure during the shaking to stabilize the tongue and prevent retraction. If the infant has a very sensitive gag reflex, this approach is not usable because the fingers cannot be placed on enough of the tongue surface to produce a shaking movement.

In contrast, if the cheeks, tongue, and lips feel very loose and weak, the caregiver can try the following approaches. She pats the cheeks a number of times with a rather firm tapping pressure by the palmar surface of the fingers, discontinuing the input when the cheeks begin to feel more firm. The caregiver should support the jaw with her little finger if it is lax and remains open. The caregiver then taps down on the tongue, withdraws the contact, and repeats the tapping two or three times, preventing the jaw from opening too widely. She lightly touches the top and bottom lip or lightly brushes her fingers across the lips to facilitate a pursing action and closure.

When the infant is older and there is more surface area under the chin, another approach can be used to increase the stability of a hypotonic tongue or a tongue that is too mobile. The caregiver taps underneath the chin in the soft tissue below the base of the tongue with the back of the index and third finger or the back of just one finger if there is less surface area. The fingers are held at the point of contact for approximately one second and then released, and the tapping movement is repeated two or three additional times.

If the caregiver understands that the mouth remains the dominant source of sensory input to the developing nervous system during the first three months,[5] she may sense more of a need to provide input, especially when the infant has a more limited ability to move the lips, tongue, and jaw, form facial expressions, and bring his hand to his mouth. She will probably come up with her own spontaneous adaptations as she observes and appreciates the power of touch which was deemphasized in infant care for so many years. The caregiver's approaches will no doubt be superior because of her evolving acquaintance with the infant who is the most specialized consultant of all. She can also experiment with suggestions in Stages I and II, Chapter 2, and her own innovations to facilitate the hand-to-mouth schema and progression to oral exploration of objects. This places the infant at the helm in another way. He provides his own tactual input.

APPROACHES TO DECREASE TACTUAL SENSITIVITY. If the infant resists bodily handling, he very possibly will react aversively to more localized tactual contact in the oral area. The focus has to shift to helping him experience more pleasure from physical contact. The caregiver experiments wtih approaches presented in Chapter 3, and the infant may also enjoy an adaptation of the old fashion massage after his bath if he can tolerate being undressed in a warm room. Or the massage can be performed another time during the day even with the clothes on. The caregiver massages the trunk area, applying firm pressure in a hand-hold fashion. She then progresses distally to massage the arms and legs with the same firm hand-holds. If the caregiver feels a need to use a lotion or cream, she must take care to keep the infant warm. Evaporation of the lotion or cream from the skin surface causes a loss of body heat, triggering a drop in body temperature or a shivering response, which in turn can cause increased muscle tone in the extremities as a means of conserving heat.

ADAPTATION OF BOTTLE FEEDING. If the caregiver decides not to breastfeed the infant or concludes that this is not viable following a trial period, she can be helped to experiment with different types of artificial nipples. Each nipple should be given a fair trial instead of rapidly shifting from one to another, because the infant will no doubt lack the ability and flexibility of the normal infant to adapt his sucking action.[6] The advantages and disadvantages of different nipples are discussed in Chapter 1 as well as other modifications and precautions related to bottle feeding. The approaches outlined in this chapter to facilitate a more productive sucking action are also applicable if the infant is fed via a bottle.

Intervention Setting and Overall Focus

The infant's feeding patterns and the interaction between the infant and caregiver can most effectively be observed in the natural home setting. An atypical setting may elicit atypical patterns. Also, the patterns are observed within the context of the total environmental milieu, including the behavior and needs of other family members during feeding time and the physical set up. Such basics as the storage and preparation of the food and the care of utensils influence the feeding experience and the nutritional status of the infant.

The intervener observes the caregiver's nonverbal as well as her verbal responses to suggestions. As mentioned earlier, if approaches are too adrift from her usual practices; if the approaches are presented in a very structured, procedural form with a lot of related "do's" and "don'ts"; or if the approaches elicit adverse reactions from the infant, there is a slim chance that the adaptations will be incorporated in the feeding experience—nor should they, because the goal is to make mealtime a more pleasurable experience. Some of the above suggestions may fit in one or more of the above categories, especially when the infant is very young. The approaches become acceptable to both the caregiver and the infant only later on when he is less fragile and small but still has difficulty coordinating sucking, swallowing, and breathing.

SECOND STAGE: SIX TO TWELVE MONTHS FUNCTIONAL LEVEL

Feeding and mouthing experiences provide copious amounts of input to the oral area. As explained in Stage II, Chapter 2, the receptors become increasingly more discriminative and provide more information about the position of the jaw, tongue, and lips and the nature of food and objects placed in the mouth. The infant compares the feel of a certain food or an utensil (spoon, cup) with past experiences organized in a central map, and he modifies oral movements via a feedback mechanism to make the necessary accommodations. The protective sensitivity of the gag reflex begins to wane as the infant learns to munch and then chew more textured foods. By the time the infant is functionally at the 12-month level, he may be obtaining the bulk of his daily intake from foods and liquids eaten via utensils other than the breast or bottle.

There is a close link between the evolvement of more adaptive oral patterns and the evolvement of more adaptive motor patterns in other parts of the body as discussed in Chapter 2. The infant develops increased midline stability as the stage progresses, and he can sit with his shoulders and trunk aligned and his head in a neutral position, which facilitates good lip closure and a functional position of the tongue and jaw. Trunk rotation is also evolving, which correlates with increased differentiation of the lip, tongue, and jaw movements.

If the infant has a less severe developmental disability and has received a lot of input to the oral area with habilitative assistance, he will reach this functional stage albeit via a different timetable. If he has a more severe disability and a less adequate sensory-motor system, there has to be a more careful, and what can seem like a painstakingly gradual, introduction of new foods and textures. This can become burdensome, and it is understandable that many caregivers cannot deal with the extra demands meal after meal, day after day. This is another example of a habilitative dilemma. Solid foods are often required for growth and optimal nutrition long before the infant gains the neuromotor control, which allows him to adaptively accommodate to the foods and utensils and experiment with self feeding. Also, it is felt that a prolonged liquid diet obtained from a nipple reinforces primitive reflex patterns.

Facilitation of Increased Jaw, Lip, and Tongue Control

Mueller has developed approaches to normalize movements of the lips tongue, and jaw to the extent possible. These approaches and guidelines for positioning are described in a book written for professional interveners[7] and families.[8] There are some key habilitative considerations in this functional stage of development that we would like to emphasize relative to their intervention framework.

IMPORTANCE OF SENSITIVE PACING. Although the jaw control techniques may appear easy when the experienced practitioner is introducing the spoon and cup, the caregiver may feel very awkward when she attempts to apply the demonstrated approaches. The infant senses her awkwardness and uneasiness relative to the experienced practitioner, and he becomes more tense and less responsive. Therefore, it is helpful for the intervener to share her own learning experiences and related feelings so that the caregiver will not expect too much of herself at first. The approaches can also be broken down into simpler steps that require more intervention time, but the outcome is time-cost effective, because there is greater likelihood of follow through and the preservation of an enjoyable mealtime experience. Excessive demands are not placed on either the infant or caregiver. Another outcome has to be considered if the wrong intervention modeling is provided. If during the process of helping the infant acquire basic motions of the lips, tongue, and jaw, he learns that his communicative signals of dislike, discomfort, and frustration are ignored, there can be a mitigating effect in terms of providing a substrate for expressive language. The infant may be able to vocalize, but the important motivational and social aspects of language have been compromised. Also, his inner representation of the interaction with his caregiver and food at mealtime is unpleasant, which has broader ramifications. The intervener must model the importance of not separating out one aspect of development or one set of behaviors in a task-oriented way. The development of feeding and language patterns must remain part of an interrelated whole.

It is important to pace the introduction of new forms of eating within the infant's tolerance level, and his responses should be reinforced with a lot of positive social attention. Some infants are more receptive at the beginning of the meal because of the motivation of hunger. Other infants become frustrated, because they are not obtaining food fast enough, and they might be more responsive later in the feeding after hunger sensations have abated. It is generally best to introduce the new form of input only once per day initially, and the caregiver sensitively observes signals that express when enough is enough. There is gradual substitution of the unfamiliar for the familiar, because too much novelty can be overwhelming.

If the new texture elicits gagging, this can be unpleasant, and the adaptive demands and the desensitization process have to move forward at a slower pace. It may be that the infant can cope if the consistency of the food is adjusted. A thicker liquid is generally easier to manage from the cup and may also reinforce the effect of jaw control in inhibiting a forward movement of the tongue. The lips can be blotted dry with an inward movement before presenting the cup, which enhances the infant's awareness of the rim. The pressure of the rim on the lower lip is increased somewhat to further enhance the sensory awareness if this does not elicit other adverse reactions. Likewise, food that is fairly thick and of uniform consistency (such as pudding) is easier to eat from a spoon. The caregiver can blend food to this consistency or thicken runny commercial baby foods with rice cereal. Plain mashed potatoes (no butter or salt added) can be used to thicken foods for older infants if caloric needs allow this. Salted crackers should not be used because of the possibility of a sodium overload. Foods of a coarser and drier consistency are gradually introduced as the oral sensitivity decreases. The possiblity of a medical reason for the persistent sensitivity of a gag reflex, such as enlarged tonsils brushing against the throat, should not be overlooked.

If the infant with cerebral palsy has a strong tongue thrust, this can present a dilemma. It may seem advisable to wean him from the bottle before he is developmentally ready in order to prevent reinforcing the aberrant pattern. However, all aspects of the infant's development must be considered as well as the parents' feelings. The benefits must be weighed against the changes that weaning may elicit in caregiving practices. The following are examples of questions which must be asked: Will the infant be held as much? Will mealtime become a struggle and change from a positive experience to a negative experience? Will the infant get enough fluid each day?

FACILITATION OF ACTIVE APPROACH BEHAVIORS. In addition to allowing the infant to pace the introduction of habilitative approaches, his participation in the feeding experience can be encouraged in another way typical of this stage. At about seven months, the infant begins to approach the spoon as it comes toward his mouth by leaning his head and trunk a short distance forward (protraction and anterior pelvic tilt). He then moves the head and trunk away from the spoon as he removes the food (retraction and posterior pelvic tilt). He aligns his body back in midline with the pelvis in a neutral position and slightly flexes his head as he swallows.[9] When the disabled infant or child has developed sufficient head and trunk control to sit more erect in a high-chair with appropriate support or in an adapted chair, the above approach and withdrawal movements can be incorporated in the jaw control technique. The caregiver applies jaw control while sitting beside the infant, as described by Mueller, to offer a few spoonfuls of food before returning to the more interactive face-to-face position. She uses her arm and shoulder to help the infant move forward to meet the spoon, move backward to withdraw from the spoon, and return to the midline position.

This approach should be used in conjunction with activities in Stage II, Chapter 2 to foster pelvic flexibility. The infant must have a mobile pelvis to coordinate head, trunk, and pelvic movements as he moves toward the spoon. Otherwise, the head juts forward out of line with the shoulders and hips, which distorts the position of oral structures and interferes with the peristaltic activity during swallowing.

THIRD STAGE: TWELVE TO TWENTY-FOUR MONTHS FUNCTIONAL LEVEL

This period is characterized by further refinement of oral control and feeding skills. The inner representation of the oral structures becomes progressively more coherent, and the movements of the lips, tongue, and jaw become more dissociated as described in Stages IV and V, Chapter 2. Thus, the toddler can chew with a progressively more efficient rotary jaw movement, and his lips become more active when drinking from a cup without an associated pumping movement of the jaw. He can use an intermediary tool as a means to an end including a spoon and cup; and he develops the capacity to feed himself.

If the toddler has a severe disability, he may not develop the necessary coordination of movements to perform the chewing action independently. Mueller has developed a procedure to facilitate the evolvement of chewing, which is outlined in the two sources cited earlier. Even with the implementation of these approaches, the very involved child may never fully inhibit primitive oral reflexes, and he may always need some assistance from his caregiver to perform a rudimentary semblance of the more mature rotary chewing movement. He cannot adapt to multitextured food (vegetable soup) and foods that do not dissolve (raw carrot). The child misses more enhanced and varied forms of sensory input from the ingestion of foods that strengthen muscles, provide fiber, and stimulate the gums. Because of the necessary slower pace, he usually ends up eating lukewarm or fairly cool foods, thus missing the stimulation of temperature variations. Or it may be that he cannot tolerate the variations if the oral area is very sensitive. If he cannot fully adapt to the family menu and eating patterns, this can interfere with his acceptance as a full-fledged member of the family at mealtime.

Deterrents to Facilitation of Independent Feeding Skills

There may be a tendency to stall the facilitation of more independent and less infantile feeding skills for a number of reasons. The weaning process is postponed because of a persistent concern regarding the toddler's intake, a concern that had its origin in infancy. The concern is reinforced by the eating jags typical of this stage. Also, the bottle may be an effective soother, which is especially important if the toddler is hyperreactive or irritable. The caregiver may need extra support to initiate weaning. The authors have found that the following approaches minimize the trauma to both the infant and the caregiver. A schedule is developed to gradually reduce the amount and kinds of fluids taken by bottle. The least important bottle is eliminated first—the one that is not associated with nap or bedtime. The second bottle to be eliminated is the one associated with a daytime sleep period, and the last bottle taken away is the one associated with preparation for night sleeping. The caregiver sits with the toddler and offers him the same fluid formerly given by bottle at the same time of day and in the same context, for example, after eating solid foods, just before naptime and bedtime. Again, change occurs within a supportive matrix of familiarity.

Another problem that may stall facilitation of independent feeding and inclusion as a member of the family at mealtime is excessive messiness, which may be especially upsetting to a family that enjoys neat surroundings. If the toddler is fed before or after the family meal, he is denied the opportunity to socialize and observe more adaptive eating patterns. However, the needs of all family members are important. It may be that the toddler is excluded from meals with the family only on special occasions, for example, meal at a restaurant, a dinner engagement with another family, or when guests are invited to the home. If the other members have an enjoyable evening together on a special occasion, they may feel refreshed and better able to cope with all the stresses and demands of being a family. If they are pressured to include the disabled member or made to feel guilty about his exclusion, this can interfere with his acceptance as a part of the family in ways that are comfortable to the members. Likewise, if their appreciation of a neat environment is devalued, this is weighting the needs of one family member, which can create resentment. Many families respond positively to a suggestion that represents a compromise. For example, the caregiver may be able to tolerate allowing the toddler to experiment with self feeding for a short period during one meal of the day with the help of plastic or newspaper under the highchair.

Conclusions

Within the matrix of a sensitive support system, the catalyst that keeps the caregiver motivated to implement habilitative approaches is the forseeable and observable payoff in terms of the infant's increased adaptiveness and independence. Another sustaining force is the ability to pace the intertwining of habilitative approaches with the family's traditional caregiving practices related to feeding. The caregiver does not fall into the trap of taking on a program that is too ambitious and broad in scope. Instead, she focuses on consistency and the required intensity of a selected number of approaches within the comfort and tolerance level of both herself and the infant. The ultimate habilitative goal is a pleasurable feeding experience for the most part all along the continuum of development.

REFERENCES

1. Brown, JV: *Non-nutritive sucking in great ape and human newborns: Some phylogenetic and ontogenetic characteristics.* In: Bosma, JF (ed): *Fourth Symposium on Oral Sensation and Perception.* US Department of Health, Education, and Welfare, Bethesda, Maryland, 1973, p 118.

2. Givens, D: *Social expressivity during the first year of life.* Sign Language Studies 20:251, 1978.

3. Horton, FH, Lubchenco, LO, and Gordon, HH: *Self-regulating feeding in a premature nursery.* Yale J Biol Med 24:263, 1952.

4. Stark, RE and Nathanson, SN: *Spontaneous cry in the newborn infant: Sounds and facial gestures.* In: Bosma, JF (ed): *Fourth Symposium on Oral Sensation and Perception.* US Department of Health, Education, and Welfare, Maryland, 1973, p 323.

5. Wyke, B: *The neurological basis of movement—A developmental review.* In: Holt, K (ed): *Movement and Child Development.* JB Lippincott, Philadelphia, 1975, p 19.

6. Sameroff, A: *Reflexive and operant aspects of sucking behavior in early infancy.* In: Bosma, JF (ed): *Fourth Symposium on Oral Sensation and Perception.* US Department of Health, Education, and Welfare, Bethesda, Maryland, 1973, p 135.

7. MUELLER, HA: *Facilitating feeding and prespeech.* In: PEARSON, PH AND WIL-LIAMS, CE (EDS): *Physical Therapy Services in the Developmental Disabilities.* Charles C Thomas, Springfield, Ill, 1972, p 283.

8. MUELLER, H: *Feeding.* In: FINNIE, NR: *Handling the Young Cerebral Palsied Child at Home.* EP Dutton, New York, 1975, p 113.

9. DAVIS, L: *Regaining oral functions following CNS insult.* Presentation Workshop, Santa Clara Valley Chapter, Occupational Therapy Assn. of California, Los Gatos, California, June, 1979.

Chapter 5

HIGH-RISK INFANT: FRAMEWORK FOR ASSESSMENT AND INTERVENTION

Joyce Shigekawa and Raeone S. Zelle

FRAMEWORK FOR ASSESSING FETAL DEVELOPMENT

The source of a child's developmental problems can be numerous, and the interaction of biologic, environmental, and social factors influences their expression and resolution. Heretofore the reader has been asked to focus on the infant and child with problems of either pathophysiologic or genetic origin. In this chapter the reader is asked to focus on immaturity as an impediment to optimal development.

With the assistance of rapidly developing technology and medical knowledge, intervention with the immature infant often means extrauterine viability. However, the course toward this viability taxes the immature organism. There is a struggle to achieve homeostasis between the demands of the extrauterine environment and a developing system. Although disabling pathophysiology may be thwarted by technology, research indicates that the consequences of premature birth are most apparent in behavioral differences between the full-term and preterm infant. The responses of the preterm infant often fail to validate the early efforts and expectations of parents. This initial lack of reciprocity seems to have a deregulating effect so that by the time the infant has matured sufficiently for mutual interaction, the parents' quota of responsiveness may be depleted. To help keep parents in synchrony with their preterm infant they must learn to interpret and guide their infant's behavior in a manner that will foster his growth and adaptability.

To understand the behavioral maturation of the preterm infant it is important to review development in the intrauterine environment as we know it. The evolution of early behavior is a continuous process that begins in this environment and continues to unfold after birth. Even a rudimentary understanding of this evolutionary process and the well-modulated environment in which it occurs may increase our sensitivity to the immature organism and enable us to facilitate adaptive responses that enhance interaction with caregivers.

FIRST TRIMESTER

The first sign of life in the uterine environment occurs as early as the fifth week. At this time striated muscle fibers become sufficiently differentiated to respond to direct contact or cellular electrolyte changes. This response occurs even though the motor neurons that innervate the muscle fibers are not as yet functional. Innervation begins during the seventh week and initially occurs in the cephalic and axial-cervical muscles, and the orofacial region is the first to respond to stimulation at eight weeks.[1] This initial reflexive response is generalized, with flexion away from the stimulus involving the cervical and first thoracic levels of the upper trunk. This flexion response progresses to the remaining thoracic and lumbosacral levels so that the head, trunk, and pelvis deviate to the side opposite the stimulus.[2] As flexion is developing, movement of the extremities is also evolving. Extension of the arms appears first, followed by participation of the lower extremities seen in the slight separation of the soles of the feet, which face each other.[3] The contralateral flexion seen during this period pulls the hands away from the mouth, which also opens as part of the reflex pattern.[4] In addition to the differentiation and innervation of muscles, a rudimentary structural framework is also complete at seven weeks in the form of a cartilaginous skeleton.[5]

By the ninth week, flexion toward the stimulus is beginning to emerge. Compared with contralateral flexion, which is brisk and avoiding, ipsilateral flexion is much slower and potentially orienting in nature. However, it is a far less frequent pattern. As Humphrey[6] points out, it is the avoiding reflexes that appear more rapidly than the orienting reflexes related to feeding. The overall flexed or bowed position of the embryo places the hands in close proximity to the face. The hands are, therefore, in a vantage position to stimulate the orofacial area.

By the 10th week, total flexion responses begin to wane. As this occurs, the reflexive response in the upper parts of the body including the head, upper trunk, and arms becomes predominant. Stimulation to the orofacial region elicits arm and hand movements, and stimulation of the hand elicits head turning and movements of the lips and tongue. There is now a substrate for the evolvement of the hand-to-mouth schema. By the 12th week, movement of the throat can be observed, and the fetus begins to swallow amniotic fluid.[7]

More localized reflexive movements of the other parts of the body reflect the distal-proximal direction of sensory maturation. The receptors in the foot and hand become differentiated and more sensitive to stimulation before proximal areas. A plantar toe and palmar digital reflexive response can be elicited at around 11 weeks, and the sensitivity gradually proceeds proximally.[8]

Summary

The mechanical stressors of the intrauterine environment emanating from maternal functions such as aortic pulsations, respirations, periodic gastrointestinal activity, and the mother's movement[9] provide the stimulation necessary to propagate development. In response to these intrauterine forces, developing receptors sensitive to touch and movement in the distal parts and oral facial area are the first to elicit global fetal behavior.[10] By the end of the first trimester, there is evidence of early inhibitory influences, beginning localization of responses, and differentiation of fetal movements. The significance of the primitive behavioral patterns during this trimester is the emerging distinction between protective and orienting responses. These responses form a beginning functional substrate for activity sequences that will be repeated prenatally and postnatally, albeit with more variety and complexity as higher centers evolve.[11]

SECOND TRIMESTER

During the second trimester, there is an increase in fetal movement, and the impact is felt as quickening by the mother at around 16 weeks. Spontaneous movement is evolving but is slow and poor in quality at the beginning of this period, and reflexive responses still predominate.[12] Stimulation of the more distant auditory receptor is felt to elicit fetal movement in this trimester, but there is controversy as to the kinds of sound that are perceptible in the amniotic sac.[13]

The movement of the extremities is still slow, with a long response latency because of the lack of myelinization. Comparatively, the upper extremities are more active than the lower extremities. The distal ends are still more sensitive, evidenced by the highly localized, beginning grasp reflex without tonic spread up the arm. Reflecting structural growth and sensory maturation in the lower extremities, plantar stimulation now elicits a response: plantarflexion or dorsiflexion of the stimulated foot. There is also flexion at the knee and hip, which withdraws the stimulated foot. The response is not accompanied by other bodily activity. Toward the end of the second trimester, the legs become more active with alternate flexion and extension pedaling.[14]

The orofacial area, innervated by the three branches of the trigeminal nerve, remains the most sensitive and active part of the fetus. The reflexive responses are weak and irregular; but in contrast with the first trimester, they are beginning to show some selectivity. Protrusion and puckering of the lips, opening and closing of the jaw in a chewinglike movement, and tongue protrusion appear; and reflexive sucking has been reported at 22 and 24 weeks.[15] There is also an incomplete rooting response, which represents a beginning orientation toward a stimulus. However, the quality of the sucking and rooting responses are poor, characterized by a response latency, weakness, and arrhythmicity.[16]

Respiratory movements become evident, and diaphragmatic contractions result in fetal hiccups at the 22nd week.[17] A faint cry can be provoked during which the eyelids contract tightly and the tongue elevates as it does in the full-term infant. There is also a generally distressed facial appearance. Because crying depends on the expulsion of air and the ability to maintain adequate chest contractions, it will not normally occur in utero.[18] These early components of affective expression and feeding patterns represent increased functional complexity of earlier fetal behaviors. The response patterns are now more clearly orienting or more clearly adversive as well as protective.

In spite of the evidence of early functional activity, there is a complete or almost complete dissociation of state behaviors in the nonviable fetus, and the criteria for either quiet or active sleep are not met during the brief period that he is observed in the extrauterine environment. There is almost continuous bodily movement, respirations are irregular or semi-irregular, and there are very infrequent eye movements. Thus the sleep state must be termed atypical.

Summary

During the second trimester, there is an elaboration and coordination of the primitive patterns seen in the first trimester. There is a beginning coordination of functional activity, but it is incomplete and unevenly distributed. As an example, sucking can be elicited and now includes participation of the lips and tongue, but the immature respiratory apparatus precludes the completion of a functional response. This early but incomplete coordination of function underlies the dissociation of state behaviors and contributes to the disorganization and fragility of this period.

THIRD TRIMESTER

During the last trimester, the fetus is viable, and his continued maturation is observable in the extrauterine environment. The maturational process has been documented by Dargassies,[19] and it is from her work that many of the following descriptions have been derived. There are changes in the quality of movement characterized by increased strength, localization, coordination, and spontaneity. Accompanying these changes is the developing distinction between behavioral states. Fetal activity begins to assume some semblance of organization as certain behaviors coalesce in cycles of activity and quiescence.

Characteristic of the changes in the organization and quality of fetal movement are those evident in the orofacial area. Sucking, swallowing, and breathing become more synchronized at 30 to 31 weeks, and the infant may be able to take some formula from a nipple. He is developing the ability to modify one response to interact with another. During the 32nd week, the infant can bring his hand to his face in an awkward sweeping movement. He is more successful at inserting his fingers in his mouth, because rooting has become a more rapid, complete, and easily elicited response and the sucking reflex has become further refined, with active participation of the lips and pressure of the tongue against the palate. Collectively, these phenomena reflect the neurologic organization and functional changes that occur during the third trimester.

Qualitative changes are also evident in global movement patterns. At the 32nd week, there is more active and varied movement of the whole body, particularly incurvation and twisting of the trunk with participation of the upper limbs and neck muscles. The infant may turn from supine to sidelying and arch his back to propel himself along a surface. However, there is a change in the quality of spontaneous mobility by the 37th week. The preterm infant can no longer stretch, flex, and twist the trunk with the same degree of flexibility because of the rudimentary evolvement of axial stability. There is also a change in the character of localized movements reflected by more vigorous reflexive responses.

Concomitant with this qualitative change in mobility during the last trimester is the spread of muscle tone, which evolves in a caudal-cephalic direction in contrast to the cephalocaudal direction of muscle innervation. At 28 weeks there is a flexor posture imparted by intra-uterine constraint, which does not persist in the extrauterine environment. However, by the 32nd week, there is a beginning distal-proximal diffusion of tone in the lower extremities characterized by some observable flexion in the knees. The upper extremities still lag behind.

There is paradoxical distal strength in the palmar grasp sufficient to lift the infant off a surface, but there is no spread of tone up the extended arm. Thus, a traction response in the arm musculature cannot be felt, and the head hangs limply. By the 37th week, the distal-proximal progression of tone is evident in the flexed, resting position of all four extremities, with the lower extremities assuming the familiar frog position. There is still relatively less muscle tone in the upper body with the neck flexors the last to develop.

Although neck flexion is late in evolving, earlier development of extension and rotatory muscles allow the infant to both withdraw and orient toward a stimulus in a more definite way in this trimester. At the 32nd week, he can motorically resist gavage feedings with neck extension and upper extremity movements. Affectively, he grimaces. There is progression from a partial to a complete rotation movement of the head in the rooting response, with less global involvement of the body. Neck flexion belatedly becomes a part of the response. With the evolvement of increased strength in the neck extensor muscles at 37 weeks, the infant can protectively turn his head to the side in the prone position, bring his hand to his face, and insert his hand in his mouth.

Maturational changes in the last trimester are also characterized by the beginning evolvement of higher-order orienting behaviors and rhythmic cycles. One of the distance receptors, auditon, appears to be functioning in the extrauterine environment as early as the 28th to 32nd week. Respiratory changes have been observed in response to an auditory stimulus during the first hours of life. Salk[20] reported that auditory input influenced the preterm infant's arousal level, reducing activity and bodily tension, whereas other investigators observed that arousal, using heart rate as a parameter, was dependent on whether or not the infant was quiescent or active when the stimulus was presented. Segall[21] found that infants exposed to a program of an auditory stimulus (human voice) showed greater initial cardiac acceleration in response to a novel stimulus (arousal), followed by a response decrement and greater cardiac deceleration in response to a familiar stimulus (orientation). Segall's findings support the ability of the preterm infant to respond to auditory stimuli and suggest that he is able to modify his response adaptively.

The visual sense begins to function in a rudimentary way at 30 weeks, when the eyes briefly open more frequently, which leads to a beginning sleep-wake cycle at the 32nd week. A more intense stimulus elicits a protective response, characterized by head extension, eyelid contraction, and a slow pupillary reaction. A less intense stimulus elicits a semblance of the orienting response; the eyes open more widely. There is controversy concerning the age at which a preterm infant is capable of orienting to a visual stimulus in a more functional way. Mostow and Miranda[22] found evidence of visual attention and fixation in the 31st week, while others have not observed this response in an alert, inactive state until the 36th to 37th week.[23] Dargassies did not observe visual fixation and a lateral pursuit of a moving object until the 41st week. Yet, this same response is observable in the full-term infant a few days after birth. Dargassies hypothesized that the preterm infant cannot process a visual stimulus until the receptors and neural networks have reached a certain maturational level regardless of environmental experiences. A comparative study[24] suggests that the quality of the visual response is different. The preterm infant at 40 weeks gestation fixated on a stimulus for a longer period than the full-term infant, which the investigators postulated may reflect a more immature response pattern. It may take the preterm infant longer to process information because of a longer response latency. Or it may be that his ability to inhibit a response is less well developed; he remains hooked to the stimulus for a longer period.

The emergence of the alert, inactive state reflects a gradual trend from complete dissociation of state behaviors to a beginning coupling of these behaviors and the inhibition of phasic movements. This is also evident in changes that occur in the sleep pattern. The criteria for active sleep can occasionally be seen between 28 to 30 weeks, but there are no components of quiet sleep at this time. Between the 32nd and 36th weeks, there is an observable absence of eye movements and bodily activity during sleep intervals. However, these parameters do not always occur together until the 36th week when the quiet sleep state begins to emerge.[25]

Summary

During the last trimester, functional behaviors seen in the previous trimesters move toward consolidation. Protective as well as orienting characteristics of the premature infant become more distinct and adaptive, and his responsiveness is now augmented by the fact that he can orient to auditory and visual stimulation. He seems more organized and available to his environment. His behaviors during this trimester show beginning coalescence into identifiable states that provide a foundation for continued adaptation in the extrauterine environment.

Qualitatively, however, the premature infant does not become the functional equivalent of his full-term counterpart at 40 weeks. Elicited reflexive responses do not occur with the same strength and predictability that is seen in the full-term infant partly because of lower muscle tone and poor toleration of respiratory loads. There is a smaller proportion of fatigue resistant muscle fibers in the diaphragm and intercostal muscles.[26] Rhythmic regulation of reflexive patterns such as breathing, sucking, and swallowing during feeding is still tenuous, and asynchrony of these patterns poses a greater threat of aspiration for the preterm than the full-term infant.[27]

Although discrete states can now be identified, they are still less stable in their expression and thus less readable. Compared with the full-term infant, state behaviors of the premature infant are more often indeterminate. These differences suggest that the premature infant deals with the extrauterine environment with a substrate which, although functional, is still more fragile than that of the full-term infant. As a result, his behaviors are more precarious and vulnerable. They are more difficult to predict and more easily attenuate interaction with the caregiver.

INTERVENTION FOCUS

The impact of the preterm infant's fragile appearance can be understandably intimidating. The small size, lack of muscle bulk and tone, low level of responsiveness, and sensitivity to environmental input (color change, tremors), are in marked contrast to the parents' image of the expected infant. They very probably will need a lot of support over the months to cope with stresses related to the preterm infant's precarious struggle to live and his unique caregiving needs.

There is also the unexpected relinquishment of the primary caregiving role to nurses in the intensive care nursery because of the preterm infant's dependence on technologic and medical support measures. Given continuity of care over time, the nurse often develops a preference for one infant, which seems to be reciprocated by the infant in that he is more responsive to her caregiving approaches. Such a rapport probably has its roots in the particular nurse's ability to read and respond to his cues sensitively. This intimate communication between nurse and infant describes no other than the acquaintance process. Parents sense this rapport and generally respond in one of two ways. They feel somewhat like outsiders, or they likewise become attached to the nurse. This close relationship allows her to pass on insights and nuances of caregiving to foster the most important acquaintance process of all—that which underlies the attachment of the parents to their infant.

It makes sense to place the infant at the helm and let his behavioral responses modulate the level of stimulation in the new extrauterine environment. This is really the only choice at this point in time, because we know very little about his sensory threshold and processing capacities or the optimal level and pattern of stimulation that will nourish his rapidly developing systems; nor do we understand

the sensitive and safe periods for various forms of stimulati
on the documented effect of higher concentrations of oxygen,
bly recognize the preterm infant's vulnerability and the
danger in the premise that more of something is better.

Tracing the trends in embryonic and fetal development di
earlier, we have some notions regarding a habilitative focus, albe.. in a
provisional vein at this point in time. It is felt that the emphasis should
be on facilitating adaptiveness to extrauterine life rather than developmental gains per se. Caregiving approaches are then judged in terms
of whether they help the preterm infant become more organized in a
behavioral and physiologic sense or more disorganized. In essence, this
is the framework that the sensitive nurse uses. The ultimate goal is to
facilitate progression from almost complete dissociation of state behaviors to some coalescence of these behaviors typical of the term infant as described in the beginning of Chapter 3. He is becoming the
infant that the parents expected; his behaviors are increasingly more
readable and understandable.

The progression reflects the development of inhibitory and excitatory influences and controlling feedback mechanisms as the result
of the evolvement of neuronal networks and neurochemical functions.
Just one example of the immaturity of regulatory mechanisms illustrates the complexity of the process. In the very premature infant, it is
postulated that more inhibitory axosomatic connections control cell
activity in respiratory neurons because of minimal branching of dendrites and the lack of excitatory axodendritic synaptic connections. As
a result of this imbalance, there is the lack of rhythmic excitation of
respiratory neurons and excitation is not maintained for an interval
sufficient to allow a full inspiration. Thus, respirations are irregular
and apnea occurs.[28] Muscular fatigue is also a contributing factor in
apneic episodes as discussed earlier.

Based on Sterman's research findings,[29] a regulatory influence
emanates from the mother in the intrauterine environment. There is an
extension of her physiology, which imposes an 80 or 90 minute rest/
activity cycle on the fetus as early as the fifth month, and the cycle
remains the same until he is born. It is felt that the rest/activity cycle is a
phylogenetic antecedent to the sleep/awake cycle and continues to
exert a temporal influence on the cortex. This raises a question concerning the effect of being deprived of the mother's regulatory influence during the latter months of what should be fetal life. Related to
this are important habilitative questions. What forms of input facilitate
the development of regulatory mechanisms or compensate for the lack
of these influences until they evolve according to a maturational timetable?

Spatial Dimension

Going back to observations of the preterm infant himself, his propensity toward the flexed posture and a confined area may point to the significance of the spatial dimension. When he is freed from restraints and has strength to wiggle around in the incubator, the preterm infant gravitates to a corner and curls up as if he is creating a nestlike enclosure. Following his cues, it is probably important to determine periodically if the infant can tolerate a flexed position, even for a very short period. The fetallike position helps inhibit disorganized phasic activity, and medialward movements in this position further develop flexor muscles. The upper extremities are directed toward the face, which allows the infant to stimulate this precociously developing area and elicit oral reflexive responses; including sucking, which is part of a flexor pattern. The infant can also modulate jerky startlelike movements by folding his hands under his chin.

If the preterm infant is placed in a flexed position even for a brief period, this may help facilitate the development of flexor tone and the evolvement of a molding, cuddly posture more similar to that of the full-term infant, which has social significance. Nurses have devised a hammock that can be suspended in the incubator when the preterm infant cannot tolerate being held in room air. The hammock is designed so that it can be quickly dismantled if there are signs of distress. Interveners observe that the flexed position and movement input calms the hyperreactive infant, increasing periods of quiescence and sleep, which conserves energy. The input can also serve as a substrate for evolvement to an alert, attentive state in response to visual and auditory stimulation. The effects are no doubt related to the influence of the input on the reticular formation as discussed in Chapter 3. The nurse can also help the preterm infant assume a flexed position in a snuggly nest by placing stuffed animals over in a corner to provide touch pressure input and related confinement.

Movement Dimension

The effect of the hammock points to another seemingly important dimension—movement. As explained at the beginning of this chapter, movement can be elicited during the eighth week of intrauterine life, and the vestibular system becomes functional very early on in fetal development. The buoyant amniotic fluid decreases fetal inertia, which is strikingly evident when the activity level inside and outside the fluid medium is contrasted. Richards and Newberry[30] found a significant correlation between the level of fetal activity during the last trimester and postnatal development. Researchers have simulated the intrauterine vestibular input with a rocker bed, hammock, and water bed and reported physiologic and developmental benefits compared with control groups.[31,32,33] For example, the water bed provided gentle, head-to-foot oscillations in a rhythm simulating maternal respirations. The input sharply reduced apnea associated with severe bradycardia, especially if the preterm infant was placed on the water bed before the fifth day. It was felt that the movement increased the afferent sensory input to the reticular formation, which in turn had an excitatory influence on respiratory neurons. The combination of two modalities—horizontal rocker bed and a heartbeat—facilitated a more prolonged period of quiet sleep and a trend toward greater maturation and weight gain.

The staff members in some intensive care nurseries have devised versions of the research equipment mentioned above, but there has to be a precautionary attitude in less controlled situations because of the marked individual differences in the response to vestibular input observed by Korner[34] and all the variables that must be carefully monitored, such as temperature, rate of movement, and bacterial growth. However, a precautionary attitude should not detract from the need for further research of approaches that are effective substitutes for more invasive treatment procedures.

It is also important to develop approaches that support fledgling adaptive capacities. Equipment that reinforces the infant's own breathing efforts and biologic rhythms is an encouraging trend. If the respiratory aide completely breathes for the infant, the diaphragmatic muscle may atrophy. This outcome is in contrast to the increase in fetal breathing movements during the last trimester, which is felt to prepare the muscles for the extrauterine respiratory demands.[35]

In the practical, less-controlled setting, the nurse can experiment to determine what forms of more accessible movement can be processed and enjoyed by the preterm infant. When he is still restricted in the supine position, he may respond positively to an alternate lifing of each side of the mattress, which has a gentle rocking effect. The preterm infant may gradually tolerate being disconnected from lifesaving equipment for even a brief period so that he can be held and gently swayed back and forth and/or up and down in the incubator. There is also a question regarding the significance of the inverted posture that the fetus assumes during the latter months that should be investigated. Of course, there is the rocking chair when the preterm infant can adjust to room air; and the nurse and parents can experiment to determine his preference in terms of the speed, amplitude, and body position when being rocked.

Tactual Dimension

The preference for a confined area discussed earlier emphasizes the importance of touch-pressure input. The fetus receives a lot of this form of input in the confined uterine space, especially as he grows larger and the quarters become more crowded. Swaddling is an age-old approach that lost its appeal in industrial nations when the focus shifted to personal freedom. We are now re-examining the benefits of this type of input as discussed in Chapter 3. From observations of full-term Navajo infants,[36] the confinement has a calming effect, induces sleep, and extends sleep by inhibiting spontaneous startles. The infant may initially resist the confinement for a few minutes, which points to the importance of not making snap judgments in terms of the predominant effect of an approach. It is felt that the inhibition is brought about by decreasing afferent proprioceptive input to the reticular formation. There can also be an opposite alerting effect if the cradleboard is placed in an upright position. The reticular formation then receives input from the vestibular system, which has an excitatory influence. The swaddling also inhibits phasic motor activity, which supports the evolvement to an alert, inactive state. There is the possibility that swaddling helps regulate breathing by decreasing startles. Based on Prechtl's observations reported by Chisholm,[37] there appears to be a correlation between startles and apneic episodes.

This age-old, nonmedicinal practice of mediating the arousal level especially of the hyperreactive infant can be used in the hospital nursery and when he goes home. The infant is wrapped snugly in a blanket or an adaptation of the cradleboard can be devised. A combination of touch-pressure and movement input is provided by the commercial carriers or a homemade version attached to the caregiver's body.

Other forms of tactual input were provided in various studies[38] and related to positive physiologic and developmental outcomes—cuddling, stroking, patting, gentle massaging, hair combing. However, the position of the infant can be important when providing this form of stimulation. Als, Lester, and Brazelton[39] emphasize that tactile stimulation coupled with ventral openness (supine position) may overtax the infant's regulatory state and motor system and elicit disorganized movement and physiologic stress.

Auditory Dimension

The premature infant was exposed to sound in the intrauterine environment, and research findings indicate that this form of input positively influences physiologic functions reflected by an accelerated weight gain.[40] As discussed earlier, it appears that auditory input can have either an excitatory or inhibitory effect evidenced by an increase or decrease in the activity level. There are two points of view in terms of the type of sound that should be provided. If the intervener senses a need to simulate the uterine environment, the sound will be of the mother's heartbeat, respirations, or intestinal sounds. If it is felt that the preterm infant's sensory functions change as does his respiratory and digestive functions, the auditory input is more likely to be a periodic exposure to a tape recording of the mother's voice, taped music, or other sounds found in the extrauterine environment. At this point, the individual infant will have to serve as the guide. If the sound helps him become more adaptive in terms of physiologic and behavioral responses, then it is no doubt right for him. When the preterm infant can tolerate room air, the nurse and parents can experiment with vocal sounds to determine his preference. It may be that he will be more responsive to a softer, flutelike, higher vocal pitch.

A cautionary attitude has to be associated with auditory input because of the increased incidence of a high frequency hearing loss in premature infants unrelated to signs of anoxia or kernicterus.[41] This raises the question of whether the sound level especially in the older incubators or in other equipment—respirator or humidifier—is high enough to damage the cochlea. In the study cited above, young guinea pigs experienced cochlear damage in an incubator, whereas the older guinea pigs did not. A significant increase in hearing defects was related to long periods in an incubator in another study.[42] Or as Lenhardt[43] emphasizes the effects may be evident later in the form of auditory perceptual deficits.

The environmental noise level must also be closely monitored when the infant is in the open warmer bed with no muffling incubator walls and when he is discharged to the home. A gas lawnmower and other pieces of equipment have a high decibel noise level. It may be that sounds are muffled by middle ear effusion because there is a higher incidence of bacterial otitis media in perterm infants, especially if there is prolonged nasotracheal intubation.[44] This may explain a low level of responsiveness to auditory input in some preterm infants.

Visual Dimension

There is one point of agreement: the other distance receptor does not receive light and form visual input in the dark uterine cavity. However, there is scant information that can serve as a guide for providing this form of sensory input when the infant is born prematurely. His response to a visual stimulus may be different as described earlier, but the reasons for the difference are suppositional at this point in time. The development of the vestibular system and possibly other near sensory systems subserve the function of the visual sense. In one study,[45] there was more eye opening if the mother used touch input when interacting with the preterm infant at the 28th to 35th week gestational age. The older touch system sends collaterals to the reticular formation as explained in Chapter 3, and the influence possibly increases the infant's arousal level.

The caregiver's face very possibly is the most salient stimulus when the infant can visually orient if his preference is the same as the term infant. However, the nurse and parents will have to mediate the intensity of animate stimulation as discussed in Stage I, Chapter 2 and in Chapter 3. There is an innate propensity to respond to another person, and the preterm infant may invest too much energy in his orienting and searching behaviors. If so, he throws himself into a state of physiologic stress expressed by a change in his breathing, color, and a fading of the eye brightness. The parents are overjoyed by the infant's beginning attempt to look at them, which may overshadow their sensitivity to his distress signals.

The younger or the more ill infant may especially have a low threshold to social stimuli. He appears relatively unresponsive, which can elicit overactivity on the part of his parents. This in turn increases the infant's protective inattentiveness. The nurse can help parents read this sign of stress and mediate their interactive intensity and forms of stimulation. With support the parents diminish their activity level, imitate the infant's behaviors, and remain still when the infant averts his gaze. The parents' behavior becomes slower and more simplified and thus more similar to the behaviors in the infant's repertoire.[46]

There may be the danger of an overload if the infant is exposed to inanimate forms of visual stimuli. Even the full-term infant flexes his fingers when exposed to a more intense visual stimulus, which is interpreted as withdrawal by the researchers.[47] He extends his fingers toward a weaker stimulus, which is interpreted as an approach behavior. Other investigators[48] report that the full-term infant prefers an intermediate intensity level. Guidelines are provided in Chapter 3 to adjust the intensity of visual stimulus dimensions. The intensity level seems to be an important variable with both inanimate and animate forms of stimulation. Field[49] found that some preterm infants looked longer at a simple Raggedy Ann doll than to the caregiver's face. She reasoned that possibly the inanimate face contained less stimulus information.

Basic Needs

The emphasis on the different stimulus dimensions is not meant to detract from the importance of very basic needs such as nutrition, which is so closely related to growth including the head measurement.[50] There is a trend toward a feeding schedule in the intensive care nursery that corroborates with Dargassies' observation that the preterm infant begins to express a hunger/satiety rhythm. In one study,[51] premature infants on a self-demand schedule signaled a need for a feeding only four or five times a day; and three premature infants went 15, 11, and 9 hours, respectively, between some feedings. Yet they all gained weight. Contingent stimulation and care give the infant some control, which probably generates an environment more suited to his individual needs.

After the preterm infant is out of the woods and makes the transition to a grower status, his needs are very similar to those of the newborn infant in many ways. Thus, suggestions in the section on growth-fostering environment, Stage I, Chapter 2 are very applicable. If there are habilitative needs relative to an aberrant sensory threshold or movement and feeding patterns, some of the suggestions in the habilitative section, Stage I, Chapter 2 and also in Chapters 1, 3, and 4 are relevant.

Conclusions

The uterine environment provides the ultimate sense of oneness with the mother symbolized by the umbilical cord. This nurturing medium supports and influences the fetus' development and prepares him for birth and adaptation to a new environment, symbolized by a severance of the umbilical cord. The newborn infant is equipped with reflexive responses that have survival significance both in terms of physiologic and interactive parameters. Behaviors are becoming organized in configurations that shape caregiving and the affective relationship with another human. In turn, caregiving approaches mediate the expression of state behaviors and the movement from one state to another.

If the infant is born too soon, there are more questions than answers regarding the effect of his early severance from an environment that provides regulation and stimulation within a protective range. The infant may have to be isolated in an incubator, which is a contrast to the intrauterine environment. There is minimal maternal contact and vestibular input, and auditory, tactile, and proprioceptive input are different from those experienced in the fluid medium.

There is a real challenge to answer at least some of the questions through research and empiric observations. The recordings of the sensitive nurse are an invaluable source of information which can be passed on to other nurses caring for the infant and his parents. The documented observations of all the nurses in the unit can be collated to examine the effects of different caregiving approaches and forms of stimulation.

Out of these efforts will come innovative ways to minimize more effectively the dissonance between the extrauterine and intrauterine environments and to preserve and nurture the preterm infant's evolving functional capacities. If he goes home with the ability to hook his family, all will probably go well. However, if he goes home with behaviors that are disorganized and unstable and with a low adaptability to stress, all may not go well. His behaviors precipitate tension within the caregiver, which exacerbates the infant's aberrant response patterns, and a spiral evolves that may ultimately lead to abuse.[52]

REFERENCES

1. HOOKER, D: *Early human fetal behavior, with a preliminary note on double simultaneous fetal stimulation.* Res Publ Ass Res Nerv Ment Dis 33:98, 1954.
2. HUMPHREY, T: *Function of the nervous system during prenatal life.* In: STAVE, U (ED): *Physiology of the Perinatal Period, Vol. 2.* Appleton-Century-Crofts, New York, 1970, p 751.
3. Ibid.
4. BARCROFT, J AND BARRON, DH: *Movement in the mammalian fetus.* Ergebn Physiol 42:107, 1939.
5. WYKE, B: *The neurological basis of movement—A developmental review.* In: HOLT, K (ED): *Movement and Child Development.* JB Lippincott, Philadelphia, 1975, p 19.
6. HUMPHREY, op. cit.
7. HUMPHREY, T: *The development of mouth opening and related reflexes involving the oral area of human fetuses.* Alabama J Med Sci 5:126, 1968.
8. HUMPHREY, op. cit., 1970.
9. WYKE, op. cit.
10. WEEKS, ZR: *Effects of the vestibular system on human development, part I. Overview of functions and effects of stimulation.* Am J Occup Ther 33:376, 1979.
11. HUMPHREY, op. cit., 1970.
12. Ibid.
13. ARMITAGE, SE, BALDWIN, BA, AND VINCE, MA: *The fetal sound environment of sheep.* Science 208:1173, 1980.
14. DARGASSIES, S: *Neurological Development in the Full-Term and Premature Neonate.* Elsevier/North-Holland, Amsterdam, 1974, p 179.
15. HUMPHREY, T: *Some correlations between the appearance of human fetal reflexes and the development of the nervous system.* Profr Brain Res 4:93, 1964.

16. Dargassies, op. cit.

17. Norman, HN: *Fetal hiccups.* J Comp Psychol 34:65, 1942.

18. Humphrey, op. cit., 1970.

19. Dargassies, op. cit., p 197.

20. Salk, L: *Effects of the normal heartbeat sound on the behavior of the new-born infant: Implications for mental health.* World Mental Health 12:168, 1960.

21. Segall, M: *Cardiac responsivity to auditory stimulation in premature infants.* Nurs Res 21:15, 1972.

22. Hack, M, Mostow, A, and Miranda, S: *Development of attention in preterm infants.* Pediatrics 58:669, 1976.

23. Emde, R and Koenig, K: *Neonatal smiling and rapid eye movement states.* J Am Acad Child Psychiatry 8:637, 1969.

24. Sigman, M, et al: *Infant visual attentiveness in relation to birth condition.* Devel Physchol 13:431, 1977.

25. Parmelee, AH and Stern, E: *Development of states in infants.* In: Clements, CD, Purpura, DP and Mayer, FE (eds): *Sleep and the Maturing Nervous System.* Academic Press, New York, 1972, p 199.

26. Keens, TG and Ianuzzo, DC: *Development of fatigue-resistant muscle fibers in human ventilatory muscles.* Am Rev Resp Dis 119:139, 1979.

27. Dargassies, op. cit.

28. Gabriel, M., Albani, M, and Schulte, FJ: *Apneic spells and sleep states in preterm infants.* Pediatrics 57:142, 1976.

29. Sterman, MB: *The basic rest-activity cycle and sleep: Developmental considerations in man and cats.* In: Clemente, CD, Purpura, DP, and Mayer, FE (eds): *Sleep and the Maturing Nervous System.* Academic Press, 1972, p 175.

30. Richards, TW and Newbery H: *Studies in fetal behavior III. Can performance in test items at six months postnatally be predicted on the basis of fetal activity.* Child Devel 9:79, 1938.

31. Barnard, KE: *The Effect of Stimulation on the Duration and Amount of Sleep and Wakefulness in the Premature Infant.* University Microfilms, Ann Arbor, 1972.

32. Neal, MV: *Vestibular stimulation and developmental behavior of the small premature infant.* Nurs Res Report 3:2, 1968.

33. Korner, AF: *Reduction of sleep apnea and bradycardia in preterm infants on oscillating water beds: A controlled polygraphic study.* Pediatrics 61:528, 1978.

34. Ibid.

35. Keens and Ianuzzo, op. cit.

36. Chisholm, JS: *Swaddling, cradleboards and the development of children.* Early Human Devel 2:255, 1978.

37. Ibid.

38. MASI, W: *Supplemental stimulation of the premature infant.* In: FIELD, TM (ED): *Infants Born at Risk.* SP Medical and Scientific Books, New York, 1979, p 367.

39. ALS, H, LESTER, BM, AND BRAZELTON, TB: *Dynamics of the behavioral organization of the premature infant: A theoretical perspective.* In: FIELD, TM (ED): *Infants Born at Risk.* SP Medical and Scientific Books, New York, 1979, p 173.

40. CHAPMAN, JS: *The Relationship Between Auditory Stimulation of Short Gestation Infants and Their Gross Motor Limb Activity.* University Microfilms, Ann Arbor, 1975.

41. DOUEK, E, ET AL: *Effects of incubator noise on the chochlea of the newborn.* Lancet 1110, November 20, 1976.

42. STENNERT, E, SCHULTE, FJ, AND VOLLRATH, M: *Incubator noise and hearing loss.* Early Human Devel 1:113, 1977.

43. LENHARAT, ML: *Incubator noise and hearing loss.* Early Human Devel 2:89, 1978.

44. BERMAN, SA, BALKANY, TJ, AND SIMMONS, MA: *Otitis media in the neonatal intensive care unit.* Pediatrics 62:198, 1978.

45. MINDA, K, ET AL: *Mother-child relationships in the premature nursery: An observational study.* Pediatrics 61:373, 1978.

46. FIELD, TM: *Interactive patterns of pre-term and term infants.* In: FIELD, TM (ED): *Infants Born at Risk.* SP Medical and Scientific Books, New York, 1979, p 333.

47. MCGUIRE, I AND TURKEWITZ, G: *Visually elicited finger movements in infants.* Child Devel 49:362, 1978.

48. HERSHENSON, M, MUNSINGER, H AND KESSEN, W: *Preference for shapes of intermediate variability in the newborn human.* Science 147:630, 1965.

49. FIELD, TM, op. cit.

50. *Stimulation of the newborn.* Lancet 1232, December 4, 1976.

51. HORTON, FH, LUBCHENCO, LO, AND GORDON, HH: *Self regulatory feeding in a premature nursery.* Yale J Biol Med 24:263, 1952.

52. PASAMANICK, B: *Ill-health and child abuse.* Lancet 550, September 20, 1975.

BIBLIOGRAPHY

1. FIROINTINO, MB: *Reflexive Testing Methods for Evaluating C.N.S. Development.* Charles C Thomas, Springfield, Ill, 1970.

2. HOOKER, D: *The Prenatal Origin of Behavior.* University of Kansas Press, Lawrence, 1952.

3. KATZ, V: *Auditory stimulation and developmental behavior of the premature infant.* Nurs Res 20:196, 1971.

4. NILSSON, L, INGELMAN-SUNDBERG, A, WIRSEN, C: *Ett Barn Blir Till.* Bonniers, Stockholm, 1971.

5. PEIPER, A: *Cerebral function in infancy and childhood.* Plenum Publishing, New York, 1963.

INDEX

Arm(s)
    in disabled Stage III infant, protective extension response of, 239–240, *240*
    in disabled Stage V toddler, bilateral coordination of, 386
    strengthening of, 385–386
    in Stage IV toddler, refinement of movements of, 263
    in Stage V toddler, complex manipulative skills of, 324, 326–327
        hypertonia in, effect of on throwing and catching, 362–363
        fluctuating tone in, 370
        hypotonia in, 367
Arm extension
    habilitative approaches for
        in disabled neonate, 97, 111
        in Stage II infant, 167–168
        weight propping and, 173
Articulator(s),
    in Stage II infant, variation of adjustment in, 130
    in Stage III infant, increased neuromuscular control of, 189–190
    in Stage IV toddler, 265–266
    in Stage V toddler, increased ability to dissociate, 330
Associated reactions, in hypertonia, 425
Asymmetric tonic neck reflex, 69
    abnormal, in supine neonate, 96
    waning of, 72
Athetosis, effects of, 425–426
    form of cerebral palsy, 425
    impediment of antigravity response by, 97–98
    in Stage I infant, aberrant weight bearing in, *99*
    in Stage II infant, prone position in, compensatory patterns in, 147–148
        sitting position in, compensatory patterns in, 152, *153*, *171*, 171–172

supine to prone rolling in, compensatory patterns in, 149–150, *150*
    in Stage III infant, kneeling position in, compensatory patterns in, 221, *222*
    quadruped position in, compensatory patterns in, 218, 220, *220*
    sitting position in, compensatory patterns in, 216, *217*
    standing position in, compensatory patterns in, 225–226, *226*
    in Stage IV toddler, object displacement in, facilitation of, 319
    walking in, compensatory patterns in, 294, *295*
    in Stage V toddler,
        effect of
            on jumping, *369*, 370
            on kicking, *369*, 370
            on throwing and catching, 370, *371*
            on walking, *368*, 368, 370
        swaddling for, 431
Attachment process, in neonate, 88
    in Stage II infant, 138
        effect of aberrant stimulation threshold on, 143–144, 145
    in Stage III infant, 199
    in Stage IV toddler, 274, 276, 320
    in Stage V toddler, 342–343
Attention, sustained, of disabled Stage I infant, habilitative approach for, 114–115
Auditory deficit, in Stage I infant, 95
    in Stage II infant
        effect of
            on developmental and interactive patterns, 145–146
            on vestibular system, 146
    in Stage III infant, effect of, 212–213
    vocalization in, habilitative approaches for, 246
    in Stage IV toddler, 288–289

early diagnosis and treatment of, 312

in Stage V toddler, effect of, 357

on caregiver, 357

vestibular dysfunction and, 358

Auditory dysfunction, effect of, on Stage V toddler, 358

Auditory stimulus(i), for decreasing arousal level, 429

for increasing arousal level, 435–436

for preterm infant, 468–469

response to, 462

Auditory system, development of, in Stage II infant, 131

Automobile restraint, for disabled infant or child, 9–10

Avoidance response, remnants of, in Stage V toddler, 329

massaging to decrease, 433

Axial stability, beginning of, in neonate, 73

BABY-PROOFING, of home

for Stage IV toddler, 279

for Stage V toddler, 348–349

Backward protective response, in Stage III infant, 180

Ball play

athetosis and

effect of

in Stage V toddler, 370, *371*

hypertonia and

effect of

in Stage V toddler, 363–364, *364*

hypotonia and

effects of

in Stage V toddler, 367–368, *367*

Bathing, for relaxation of hypertonia, 430–431

Behavior

effects of health problems on, 23–24

goal-directed, in Stage III infant, 193–194

of infant

effect of central nervous system maturation on, 419

proximity seeking, in neonate, 85, 86

state

description of, 416–417

effect of high and low response threshold on, 422–423

effect of regulatory mechanism disorders on, 421–422

effect of reticular activating system on, 419–420

maturational changes in, 418–419

Bilateral coordination, facilitation of, in Stage V toddler, 386

Biorhythm(s), in infants, 34

Bipedal position, equilibrium reactions in disabled Stage IV toddler, 315–316, *315*

Bladder pressure sensation, greater localization of, in Stage V toddler, 344

Blindness. See also Visual dysfunction and Visual impairment.

cortical, 42

in Stage I infant, habilitative techniques for communication in, 114

in Stage II infant

effect of

on developmental and interactive patterns, 145

on vestibular system, 146

vestibular and tactual input in, habilitative approaches for, 176

in Stage III infant, effect of, 211

in Stage V toddler

adaptive tactual search behavior in, facilitation of, 389

running in, habilitative approaches for, 384

Body awareness

habilitative approaches for

in disabled Stage III infant, 244

in disabled Stage V toddler, 393

Drug(s)
  anticonvulsant
    common problems with, 8
    effects of on oral health, 32
    nursing responsibilities in, 7

Ear(s)
  evaluation of
    in disabled children, 26
  problems with
    in disabled children, 25–26
    in Down syndrome, 25–26
    nurse's role in, 26–27
Early intervention program,
    nurse's role in, 50–51
Echolalia, in Stage V toddler, 332
Efficacy-phenomenalism, in Stage
    II infant, 134
Elimination. See also Constipa-
    tion and Toilet training.
  management of, in children with
    paralytic disorders, 28–29
  problems with, in handicapped
    infant, 27–28
Emotional tone, effect of athetosis
    on, 425–426
Encoding, in normal Stage III in-
    fant, 191–192
Environment
  baby-proofing of, at Stage V,
    348–349
  daily activities in, involvement
    of Stage V toddler in, 349–
    350
  effect of, 320
  excitatory effect of, 435
  for feeding of disabled infant,
    448
  fostering of language develop-
    ment in, at Stage V, 347–
    348
  growth-fostering
    for neonate
      contingency in, 90
      physical characteristics of,
        91–92
    interaction of neonate and
      caregiver in, 89–90

inhibitory effect of, 428–429
interaction of infant with, 415–
  416
  interaction of neonate and care-
    giver in, 89–90
noise level in
  preterm infant and, 469
optimal, for development of
  Stage IV toddler, 284
overintrusive,
  at Stage V, 355
overstimulation in
  effect of, on disabled neonate,
    102
  monitoring of, for Stage II in-
    fant, 142
responsiveness to, level of consciousness and, 80–81
safe, for Stage II infant, 141–142
stimulation in, adjustment of for
  individual child, 415
understimulating, effect of, 102
Equilibrium reactions
  evolvement of
    in Stage II infant, 118–119
    in Stage III infant, 180–183
    in Stage IV toddler, 261
    in Stage V toddler, 323
  facilitation of
    in disabled Stage II infant, 174
    in disabled Stage III infant,
      234, 245, 249
    in disabled Stage IV toddler,
      306, .307, 308, 315–316,
      315
    in disabled Stage V toddler,
      382, 382
  maturation of
    in disabled Stage V toddler,
      habilitative approach for,
      382, 382
    in normal Stage III infant, 180
    in normal Stage IV toddler,
      261
Equipment for fostering mobility
  for disabled Stage IV toddler,
    316–317
  for disabled Stage V toddler, 385

movement of
 in third trimester, 461
muscle tone in
 in third trimester, 461–462
neck flexion in,
 in third trimester, 462
palmar grasp in, in third trimester, 462
Finger(s)
 movement of
  in Stage III infant, 186–187
 refinement of
  in Stage IV toddler, 263
Flexibility, increased, of ankles,
  in Stage V toddler, 383, 383
 of lower limbs
  in Stage V toddler, 382–383, 383
 of pelvic movement,
  in disabled Stage V toddler, 381, 381
Flexion, facilitation of, in disabled neonate, in supine position, 103, 104
Flexor muscles
 antigravity
  development of, in Stage II infant, 119
  strengthening of, in disabled Stage V toddler, 378, 380, 380
 of neck
  strengthening of
   in Stage I infant, 104, 105
  strengthening of,
   in Stage II infant, 158
Fluctuating tone. See Athetosis.
Fluoride, prevention of caries with, 31–32

GENDER differences, primitive sense of, in Stage V toddler, 344–345, 346
Genital pressure, greater localization of, in Stage V toddler, 344
Good Start program, 10

Grasp, evolvement of
 in Stage I infant, 74
 in Stage II infant, 125, 126, 126t
 in Stage III infant, 186–187
 in Stage IV toddler, 263–264
 in third trimester fetus, 462
Growth
 assessment of,
  in disabled infant, 21–22
 reduced rates of, 20

HALF-KNEEL position
 habilitative approaches for,
  in hypertonic Stage III infant, 248–249
  in hypotonic Stage III infant, 249
  in normal Stage III infant, 181–182
Hammock, for preterm infant, 466
Hand
 movement of,
  in Stage III infant, 186–187
 refinement of
  in Stage IV toddler, 263
 radial-palmar orientation in, beginning, 327
Hand-to-mouth schema
 evolvement of, fetal substrate of, 458
 habilitative approaches for, in neonate, 105–106
Head
 control of
  development of
   in neonate, 70–71
 raising of
  habilitative approach to
   in hypertonic neonate, 108, 109
   in hypotonic neonate, 108–109
 righting of, in neonate, 71, 72
 support of, visual facilitation and,
  in neonate, 113
Health problem(s)
 effects of
  in disabled infant, 11
  on behavior, 23–24
Health services model(s)
 pathophysiologic/medical, 6
 well child, 5–6

Hearing dysfunction, effect of, on Stage V toddler, 358
Hearing impairment
  in Stage I infant, 95
  in Stage II infant
    effect on developmental and interactive patterns, 145–146
    vestibular system effects, 146
  in Stage III infant
    effect of, 212–213
    vocalization in, habilitative approaches for, 246
  in Stage IV toddler, 288–289
    early diagnosis and treatment of, 312
  in Stage V toddler
    effect on caregiver of, 357
    vestibular dysfunction and, effect of, 358
Hematologic system, of normal infant, 2
Hemiplegia, early recognition of, importance of, 428
Hiding games, caregiver's role in
  at Stage II, 140
  at Stage III, 205
  at Stage IV, 282–283
  at Stage V, 350
Homolateral creeping, in Stage III infant, 180–181
Hydrocephalus
  diagnostic procedures in, parent education concerning, 46
  nursing responsibilities in, 44–45
Hyperkinesis. See also Hyperreactivity and Sensory threshold, low.
  in Stage IV toddler, object displacement by, facilitation of, 319
  inhibitory environment for, 428–429
  phasic movements of, techniques to minimize, 433
  rocking for, 429–430
  stroking for, 432–433, 432
  swaddling for, 431, 432

unrelated to abnormal muscle tone, 426
Hyperreactivity. See also Hyperkinesis, Hypertonia, and Response threshold, low.
  auditory stimulus for, 429
  in infant
    effect of on behavioral state, 422–423
    inhibitory environment for, 428–429
    rocking to inhibit, 430
Hypertonia. See also Hyperreactivity and Response threshold, low.
  effect of movement on, 425
  in neonate
    flexion exercises for, 104–105
    head raising in, habilitative approaches for, 108, 109
    slanted, extended arm position in, facilitation of, 112
    in supine position, 96
    weight bearing in, aberrant patterns in, 99
  inhibitory environment for, 428–429
  manipulation in, difficulty with, 434
  mild, effect of on throwing and catching, 362–363
  mixed with hypotonia,
    need for specialized therapy in, 428
  one-sided, early recognition of, 428
  rocking for, 429–430
  rolling for, 430–431, 430
  in Stage II infant
    body exploration in, habilitative approaches for, 162
    compensatory patterns in mobility in, 151
      prone position in, 147–148, 148
      sitting in, habilitative approaches for, 151–152, 153, 172–173, 172

hematologic system of, 2
high-risk. *See also* Preterm infant.
  feeding difficulty in, 12
  role of nurse in care of, 3–5
hydrocephalic, nursing care of, 44–45
length/height measurement of, technique for, 22
lymphatic system of, 2
motor skill development by, phases in, 62
nervous system growth in, 2
occipital frontal circumference of, technique for measuring, 22
physical growth of, in first year, 1
physiology of, differences from adult, 1–2
renal system of, 2
responsiveness of
  in alert inactivity state, 417
  during crying, 417–418
  during irregular sleep, 416–417
  during regular sleep, 416
  effect of stimuli on, 418
  in waking activity state, 417
safety needs of, 9
skeletal growth in, 1
skin of, 2
sleep patterns in, 35–36
spasticity in, effect of on movement, 423–424
tooth growth in, 1
weighing of, technique for, 22
Inhibition
  of excitatory influences
    environment for, 428–429
    neutral warmth for, 431–432
    rocking for, 429–430
    rolling for, 430–431
    swaddling for, 431
Inhibitory stimuli, 429
Intermediary tools, use of, by Stage IV toddler, 263
Internal experimentation, in Stage V toddler, 335–336
Intervener
  assistance by

for caregiver of Stage V disabled toddler, 377
to facilitate adaptation to mother's breast nipple, 445–446
in preparation of infant for feeding, 445
recognition of abnormal muscle tone in neonate by, 423
Invariance, development of concept of, in normal Stage III infant, 196
Invisible displacement, following of
  in disabled Stage V toddler, 389
  in Stage V toddler, 337

JAW, development of, in normal young infant, 129–130
Jaw control techniques, teaching of by intervener, 450
Jumping
  attempts at, by normal Stage V toddler, 321
  improvement in, in normal Stage V toddler, 324
  in Stage V toddler
    effect of athetosis on, *396, 370*
    effect of hypertonia on, *362, 363*
    effect of hypotonia on, *366, 367*

KICKING
  in Stage V toddler
    attempts at, 321–322
    effect of athetosis on, *369, 370*
    effect of hypertonia on, *362, 363*
    effect of hypotonia on, *366, 367*
    improvement in, 323–324
Knee(s)
  exploration of, in disabled infant, facilitation of, 106
  movement on
    in impaired Stage IV toddler, habilitative approach for, 305–306
    in Stage III infant, 181–182
Kneeling
  in athetotic Stage III infant, compensatory patterns in, 221, *222*

in hypertonic Stage III infant
compensatory patterns in, 221, 222
habilitative approaches for, 247, 248, *248*, 249
in hypotonic Stage III infant
compensatory patterns in, 221, 222
habilitative approaches for, 247, *248*
interaction and movement patterns in, at Stage III, 247

LANGUAGE. *See also* Breathing *and* Respiration.
comprehension of
in Stage IV toddler, 267–268
in Stage V toddler, 333
development of
in disabled Stage I infant, 104, 110
in disabled Stage II infant, 166, 170
in disabled Stage III infant, 245
in disabled Stage IV toddler, habilitative approaches for, 311–312
in disabled Stage V toddler, role of caregiver in, 391–392
expansion of, 331
fostering of in environment, 347–348
in Stage IV toddler, 300
in Stage V toddler, effect of motor impairments on, 375
expressive
delayed, in Stage II infant, habilitative approach for, 166
in Stage V toddler
development of relative to receptive language, 333
structure of, 330–331
Language patterns
effect of visual impairment on, in Stage V toddler, 356
of normal Stage IV toddler, facilitation of by caregiver, 283

oral patterns and evolvement of
in neonate, 81*t*
in Stage II infant, 133*t*
in Stage III infant, 193*t*
in Stage IV toddler, 269*t*
in Stage V toddler, 334*t*
in Stage IV toddler, effect of visual impairment on, 288
symbolic, relationship of to cognitive thought, 331
Larynx
descension of, effect of postural tension on, 374
in neonate, 75
Lip(s), development of
in Stage II infant, 129–130
in Stage III infant, 189
in Stage IV toddler, 265–266
in Stage V toddler, 330
Lower limb(s)
adaptive movements of, habilitative approaches for, in Stage V toddler, 383
flexibility of, habilitative approach for, in disabled Stage V toddler 382–383, *383*
weight bearing over, in Stage III infant, 182–183
Lung, disease of, in Stage II infant, effect of on breathing, 155–156
Lymphatic system, of normal infant, 2

MAKE believe play, at Stage V, 338, 350
Manipulation, difficulty with, in hypertonic child, 434
Massage
for blind Stage II infant, 176
to decrease avoidance reaction, 433
Means-end relationship
facilitation of
in disabled Stage III infant, 236, 244, 251, 254–255
in disabled Stage IV toddler, 306, 318

compensatory
  in neonate, compared with
    normal patterns, 99
  in Stage II infant
    compared with normal pat-
      terns, 154
    effect of on muscles, 169
  in Stage III infant
    compared with normal pat-
      terns, 229
    summary of, 227–228
  in Stage IV toddler, compared
    with normal patterns, 299
  in Stage V toddler
    compared with normal motor
      patterns, 372
    effects of, summary of, 370–
      371, 373
  immature, in Stage III infant, im-
    mature sensory patterns
    and, combined effects of,
    228, 230
  in Stage IV toddler, walking in,
    habilitative approaches for,
    goals of, 303
  in Stage V toddler
    strengthening of antigravity
      extensor muscles in, 378,
      379
    strengthening of antigravity
      flexor muscles in, 378, 380,
      380
    upper limbs in, bilateral co-
      ordination of, facilitation of,
      386
    walking in habilitative ap-
      proaches for, goals of, 377
  in Stage I infant, evolvement of,
    72, 73t
  in Stage II infant, evolvement of
    125, 126t
    summary of, 179
  in Stage III infant
    evolvement of, 184, 185t
    summary of, 256–257
  in Stage IV toddler, 260
    evolvement of, 262t–263t

  in Stage V infant
    at beginning and end of stage,
      328
    infant, evolvement of, 325t–326t
    improvement in, 324
Motor skill(s)
  evolution of, phases in, 62
Movement(s)
  adaptive, of lower limb in Stage V
    toddler, habilitative ap-
    proaches for, 383
  effects of athetosis on, 425
  effects of spasticity on, 423–424
  fetal, in third trimester, 461
  in hypertonia, effects of, 425
  in hypotonia, 426
  input for preterm infant, 467
  for increased responsiveness, 437
  limited, sequelae of, 23
  oral, refinement of, in Stage III in-
    fant, 189–190
  pelvic
    in disabled Stage V toddler
      flexibility of, habilitative ap-
        proach for, 381, 381
      thoracic and, dissociation of,
        habilitative approaches for,
        380–381, 381
  for preterm infant, 467
  in prone position, in disabled Stage
    II infant, habilitative ap-
    proaches for, 175–176
Muscles
  antigravity extensor, strength-
    ening of, in disabled Stage
    V toddler, 378, 379
  antigravity flexor
    development of, in neonate, 119
    strengthening of, in disabled
      Stage V toddler, 378, 380,
      380
  of chest
    development of, in normal Stage
      III infant, 187–188
    in disabled Stage III infant, 231
    of disabled Stage II infant, effect

of compensatory motor patterns on, 169

neck, flexor, strengthening of in disabled neonate, 104, *105*

proximal, strengthening of in hypotonic Stage IV toddler, 304

strength and stability of, in hypotonic Stage IV toddler, habilitative approaches for, 313–314, *314*

ventilatory, strengthening of in disabled Stage V toddler, 392

Muscle cell(s), effects of undernutrition on, 22–23

Muscle relaxant drugs, for handicapped infants, 7

Muscle tone

abnormal. *See also* Athetosis, Hypertonia, and Hypotonia.

signs of in early infancy, 423

in Stage II infant

effect of, on breathing and oral movements, 155–157

in preterm infant, 461–462

Myelomeningocele

bowel management in, 28–29, 45

diagnostic procedures in, parent education concerning, 46

handicaps in, 45

management problems in, 45

urine management in, 45–46

Neck

flexion of, in third trimester fetus, 462

flexor muscles of, in disabled neonate, strengthening of, 104, *105*

shoulder girdle and, cocontraction of, in neonate, 71

Negativism, 341–342

Neonate

abnormal muscle tone in, signs of, 423

attachment of to parents, 87–88

body sense in, primitive, 88

feeding problems in, effects of on caregiver, 443–444

proximity seeking behaviors in, 85, 86

recognition of mother by, 87–88

responsiveness of, to stimuli, 81–82

Nerve cells, effects of undernutrition on, 22–23

Nervous system, growth of, in normal infant, 2

Neutral warmth, relaxing effect of, 431–432

Nipple

artificial

adaptation of for disabled infant, 448

selection of, for disabled infant, 14

mother's facilitation of adaptation to, of disabled infant, 445–446

Nonvegetative vocalization, in neonate, 79–80

Nonverbal communication, of neonate, 77

Nose breathing, in infant, verification of, 446

Nurse

assessment of handicapped infant by, 51–52

attachment of to preterm infant, 464

care of hydrocephalic infant by, 44–45

health guidance provided for disabled infant by, 53

observation of preterm infant by, importance of, 471

responsibilities of

in anticonvulsant therapy, 7

in care of disabled infant, 4

role of

in early intervention program for disabled infant, 50–51

in establishing parent-child relationship with disabled infant, 101–102 statement of, by nursing conference, 5

Nursing intervention
  for child abuse, 48
  for inducing normal sleep patterns in infants, 37–38
  for oral health, 32
  for respiratory dysfunction, 26
Nurturance, smothering, disabled Stage IV toddler and, 287
Nutrition
  deficiency in, effects of, 22–23
  definition of, 13
  management of, in disabled infant, basic principles, 18–19
  in oral health, 33

OBJECT
  concept of
    in Stage I, 84
    in Stage II infant, 134
    in Stage III infant, 195–196
    in Stage IV toddler, 272
    in Stage V toddler, 336–337
  displacement of
    interest of normal Stage IV toddler in, facilitation of, 281–282
    invisible, ability to follow in Stage V toddler, 337
    visible, ability to follow, in Stage IV toddler, 272
  facilitation of
    in disabled Stage II infant, 172, 177
    in disabled Stage III infant, 235–236, 244, 255
    in disabled Stage IV toddler, 319
    in disabled Stage V toddler, 388–389
  graphic collection of, in Stage V toddler, 339
  grouping of, habilitative approaches for, in Stage V toddler, 387–388
  stimulus dimension of, 434
    increase in, 438–439

substitution of one for another, facilitation of, by Stage V toddler, 389–390
Occipital frontal circumference, technique for measuring, 22
Oral cavity
  of Stage I infant
    anatomy of, 75
    structural changes in, 79
  of Stage II infant
    development of, 129
    effect of abnormal muscle tone on, 156
  of Stage III infant, 189
  of Stage IV toddler, structural changes in, 265
  of Stage V toddler, changes in correlation of with postural stabilization, 330
Oral control, aberrant motor patterns and
  in Stage I infant, 100
  in Stage II infant, 155
  in Stage III infant, 231–232
  in Stage IV toddler, 301
  in Stage V toddler, 374
Oral health
  of disabled infant, factors influencing, 31
  effects of anticonvulsant medication on, 32
  nursing intervention for, 32
  problems with, in Down syndrome, 32
Oral patterns
  evolvement of, motor patterns and, 449
  language patterns and
    in Stage I infant, 81t
    in Stage II infant, 133t
    in Stage III infant, 193t
    in Stage IV toddler, 269t
    in Stage V toddler, 334t
Oral receptors, effect of feeding on, 449
Orienting response, fetal, in first trimester, 458–459
Ostomy(ies), management of, 29

attachment of nurse to, 464
auditory input for, 468–469
characteristics of, summary of, 463–464
disturbed relationship of with parents, 457
environment of, noise level in, 469
feeding schedule for, 471
flexed position in, facilitation of assumption of, 466
habilitative focus for, 465
movement for, 467
muscle tone in, 461–462
observation of by nurse, importance of, 471
palmar grasp in, 462
regulatory mechanisms in, 465
response of to auditory input, 462
simulation of intrauterine vestibular input for, 467
state behaviors in, beginning coupling of, 463
study of outcome in, 10–11
swaddling for, 468
tactual input for, 468
visual sense in, 462–463
visual stimulation of
by caregiver's face, 470
mediation of, importance of, 470
Primary circular reactions, in Stage I infant, 82, 83
facilitation of
in disabled Stage I infant, 105–107
Primary standing reflex, 70
Primitive reflexes, 67
Primitive reflexive responses, *70*
Procedures, hospital, swaddling as preparation for, 431
Prone position
in disabled Stage I infant, habilitative approach for, 108
in disabled Stage II infant
habilitative approaches for, 175–176
mobility patterns in, compensatory, 151

proximal movement in, habilitative approaches for, 163–164
rolling to supine position from
compensatory patterns in, 149–150
habilitative approaches for, 168–169
unilateral weight bearing in, habilitative approaches for, 164–165, *164*
in disabled Stage III infant, movement to sitting from, habilitative approach for, 238–239, *239*
rolling to supine position from, 121
supine position and, in disabled Stage II infant, effect of habilitative approaches in, 169
Proprioceptive impairment
tactile impairment and
in Stage II infant, 146
in Stage III infant, 213–214
in Stage IV toddler, 290–291
in Stage V toddler, 359–360
Proprioceptive stimuli, to increase responsiveness, 437–438
Protective extension response of arms, in disabled Stage III infant, habilitative approaches for, 239–240, *240*
Protective response
in disabled Stage II infant, habilitative approaches for, 173–174
in disabled Stage III infant, habilitative approaches for, 234–235, *236, 239*
in disabled Stage IV toddler, habilitative approaches for, 173–174
fetal, in first trimester, 458
Proximity seeking behaviors, in neonate, 85, 86

QUADRIPLEGIA, definition of, 424
Quadruped position
in athetotic Stage III infant, com-

habilitative approaches for, precautions for using, 439
motor, 420–421
in preterm infant, 465
sensory, 419–420
Renal solute load, in feeding of handicapped infant, 16–17
Renal system, of normal infant, 2
Representational thinking, fostering of by caregiver, at Stage V, 350
Respiration
in disabled neonate, habilitative approaches to decrease work of, 116
in disabled Stage III infant, 231
in disabled Stage IV toddler, habilitative approaches for, 312–313
effect of motor impairment on, in neonate, 100
in Stage V toddler, 374
intermeshing of with phonation, in Stage V toddler, 329–330
in neonate
developmental changes in pattern of, 77–78
effect of motor impairment on, 100
quiet, in Stage III infant, 188
in Stage II infant, 128–129
effect of lung disease on, 155–156
in Stage IV toddler, 264–265
strengthening of muscles for, in disabled Stage V toddler, 392
work of, decrease in, in Stage III infant, 189
Respiratory dysfunction, nursing interventions for, 26
Respiratory movements, in second trimester fetus, 460
Respiratory patterns, oral patterns and, effect of motor impairments on in Stage IV toddler, 300–301

Response(s). See also Reaction(s) and Reflex(es).
antigravity, 72
hindrance of by athetosis, 97–98
progressive evolvement of, in Stage I infant, 72, 73t
avoidance
adaptation of, in Stage V, 329
massaging to decrease, 433
backward protective, in Stage III infant, 180
equilibrium
beginning, in Stage II infant, habilitative approach for, 174
in bipedal position, in disabled Stage IV toddler, habilitative approaches for, 315–316, 315
in hypotonic Stage IV toddler, habilitative approach for, 306, 307
maturation of, in normal Stage IV toddler, 261
mature, habilitative approach for, in disabled Stage V toddler, 382, 382
weak, in Stage V toddler, 359
pivot prone, in hypotonic Stage IV toddler, habilitative approach for, 304, 304
primitive reflexive, 68, 70
protective
in disabled Stage III infant, habilitative approaches for, 234–235, 236
of fetus, in first trimester, 458–459
protective extension, of arms, in disabled Stage III infant, habilitative approaches for, 239–240, 240
traction, 70
withdrawal, techniques to inhibit, 433
Response patterns, aberrant, in preterm infant, effects of, 472
Response threshold

examination, 194–195, 254
habitual repertoire, 132, 170
hand-clasping, 83, 106
hand-to-mouth, 82, 105–106, 458
hand-watching, 82, 105, 107
recombining, 193
Search behavior, tactual and adaptive, in blind Stage V toddler, 389
Secondary circular reactions
facilitation of
in disabled Stage II infant, 157–160, 170, 177
in normal Stage II infant, 132
Self, differentiation of, beginning of, in Stage IV toddler, 277
Self-feeding. See Feeding, self.
Self-stimulating behavior, in Stage III disabled infant, 210
Semi-standing position, in Stage III infant, 181–182
Sense(s), adaptive substitution of one for another, in disabled Stage V toddler, 387
Sensory impairment(s)
effects of,
in Stage I infant, 94
in Stage II infant, 145
in Stage III infant, 214–215
in Stage IV toddler, 291
in Stage V toddler, 360
Sensory patterns, immature, immature motor patterns and, at Stage III, 228, 230
Sensory system, maturation of, effect of spatial displacement schemas on, in Stage III infant, 244
organization of, effect of advanced exploratory schema on, in disabled Stage V toddler, 386–387
Separateness
oneness and, conflict between, in Stage V toddler, 342–343
sense of, in normal Stage IV toddler, 278
in normal Stage V toddler, 341

Separation
experiences with, effect of on disabled Stage IV toddler, 320–321
maternal-infant, stages of, 41–42
skills for coping with, facilitation of by caregiver, for normal Stage IV toddler, 284
Separation anxiety
in disabled Stage V toddler, coping with, 390
in Stage V toddler, 343
Separation-individuation process
aided by caregiver, at Stage V, 348
effect of auditory impairment on, in Stage III infant, 213
hatching phase of, 136
impeded, in disabled Stage III infant, 210–211
in normal Stage III infant, 199
symbiotic phase of, in neonate, 85
Seriation of events, by Stage IV toddler, 272
Sex differences, primitive sense of, in toddler, 344–345, 346
Shoulder girdle, neck and, cocontraction of, in neonate, 71
Side-lying position, in disabled Stage II infant, habilitative approaches for, 160
Sitting position
in athetotic Stage II infant, habilitative approaches for, 171–172, 171
in athetotic Stage III infant, compensatory patterns in, 216, 217
in disabled Stage II infant
adaptive equipment for, 175
compensatory patterns in, 151–152, 153
habilitative approaches for, effect of, summary of, 174
in disabled Stage III infant
movement in and out of, compensatory patterns in, 217–218

habilitative approaches to, 236–237

movement to from prone position, habilitative approach for, 238–239, *239*

protective and equilibrium response, habilitative approaches for, 234–235, *236*

rotation in, habilitative approaches to, 237, *238*

weight shifting in, 217

in hypertonic Stage II infant, habilitative approaches for, 172–173, *172*

in hypertonic Stage III infant, compensatory patterns in, 215–216, *216*

in hypotonic Stage II infant, habilitative approaches for, 170–171, *171*

in hypotonic Stage III infant, compensatory patterns in 216–217, *217*

in Stage II infant, 121, 123, *124*
movement from to standing position, 123–125

w-shaped
in disabled Stage II infant, 175
in disabled Stage III infant, 215–216, *216*

Skin
care of, in disabled infant, 29–31
disorders of, in disabled infant, prevention of, 30–31
of normal infant, 2

Sleep
irregular, behavior of infant during, 416–417
in neonate, breathing during, 76
nursing interventions for inducing, 37–38
patterns of, assessment of, 36
problems with
criteria defining, 36
in disabled infant, effects of on parents, 37
regular, behavior during, 416
synchronization of with biologic clock, 35–36

Sleep-wake cycles, 34–36

Sociability, in normal Stage IV toddler, 278–279

Solid foods, introduction of to disabled infant, 15, 450–451

Sound(s)
response to, in neonate, 77
vegetative, of neonate, 77

Spasticity. *See also* Cerebral palsy and Hypertonia.
effect of on movement, in infant, 423–424
posture of child with, 424
types of involvement in, 424

Spatial relationship
awareness of
in Stage III infant, 195
in Stage IV toddler, 271
in Stage V toddler, 336
facilitation of
in disabled Stage III infant, 237, 244, 248–249
in disabled Stage IV toddler, 306, 309, 318
in disabled Stage V toddler, 387

Speech. *See also* Language.
child without, 392–393
in Stage V toddler, characteristics of, 332
synchronization of facial movement and, facilitation of, in disabled Stage V toddler, 392

Spina bifida
bowel management in, 45
diagnostic procedures in, parent education concerning, 46
handicaps in, 45
management problems in, 45
urine management in, 45–46

Spoon feeding, introduction of to disabled infant, 450–451

Standing position
extended, difficulty in mastering, in hypertonic Stage IV toddler, 296
in athetotic Stage III infant, compensatory patterns in, 225–226, *226*

in disabled Stage III infant, interactive and movement patterns in, habilitative approaches for, 249–250

in disabled Stage IV toddler, lateral weight shift in, habilitative approach for, 308, *308*

in hypertonic Stage III infant, habilitative approaches for, 251–252, *252*

in hypotonic Stage III infant
  bouncing in, habilitative approaches for, 250–251
  compensatory patterns in, 226–227, *227*
  habilitative approaches for, 250

in moderately hypertonic Stage III infant, compensatory patterns in, 223, 224, *224*, 225

in normal Stage II infant, 123

in normal Stage III infant, 182–183

in normal Stage IV toddler, 257–258

in normal Stage V toddler, movement to from supine position, 323

in severely hypertonic Stage III infant, compensatory patterns in, 223, *224*

State behavior(s)
  description of, 416–417
  dissociation of, in second trimester fetus, 460
  effect of high response threshold on, 422
  effect of low response threshold on, 422–423
  effect of regulatory mechanism disorders on, 421–422
  effect of reticular activating system on, 419–420
  maturational changes in, 418–419
  in preterm infant, beginning coupling of, 463

Stimulus(i)
  auditory, for hypotonia, 435–436
  effect of on infant's responsiveness, 418

environmental, need to adjust for individual child, 415
  facilitory, 435
  inhibitory, 429
  internal and external, interplay between influence of on interactions with environment, 415–416

STNR. *See* Symmetric tonic neck reflex.

Stoma(s), management of, 29

Strabismus, in Stage IV toddler, 288

Stranger(s), reaction to
  of disabled Stage III infant, 209, 210
  of normal Stage III infant, 200
  of Stage V toddler, 343–344

Stress, on parents of disabled Stage V toddler, 375–376

Striking, of ball, in Stage V toddler, 327

Stroking, for hyperkinesis, 432–433, *432*

Substitution, of one object for another, by disabled Stage V toddler, facilitation of, 389–390

Sucking reflex
  facilitation of
    in disabled infant, 445–446
    in hypertonic neonate, 446–447
    in hypotonic neonate, 447–448
    in Stage I infant, 75–76, 79
    in Stage II infant, 130
    in third trimester fetus, 461

Supine position
  in disabled Stage II infant,
    rolling to prone position from, compensatory patterns in, 149–150
    habilitative approaches for, 168–169
  movement to standing from, in normal Stage V toddler, 323
  in normal Stage II infant, development of patterns in, 119, 121, *122*
    rolling to prone position from, 121

growth of infants and children with, study of, 20
oral health problems in, 32
vocalization in
in Stage III infant, 232
voice in, 374

UNDERGROWTH, studies of, in handicapped children, 20
Undernutrition
effects of
on mental alertness, 23
on nerve and muscle cells, 22–23
Upper limb(s)
in disabled neonate, slanted extended position of, 111–112
in disabled Stage II infant, extension of, 167–168
in disabled Stage III infant, protective extension response of, habilitative approaches for, 239–240, *240*
in disabled Stage IV toddler, strengthening of, 304
in disabled Stage V toddler, bilateral coordination of, facilitation of, 386
strengthening of, 385–386
in Stage II infant, weight propping and, habilitative approaches for, 173
in Stage IV toddler, refinement of movement of, 263
in Stage V toddler,
complex manipulative skills of, development of, 324, 326–327
mild hypertonia in, throwing and catching in, 362–363
Urination, management of, in spina bifida, 45–46

VEGETATIVE sounds, in neonate, 77
Ventilatory muscles. See Breathing *and* Respiration.

Verbalization
of caregiver
adjustment of, to Stage IV toddler, 283
spontaneous for Stage III infant, 205
tailored to level of Stage V toddler, 347
Vestibular dysfunction
auditory impairment and
in Stage IV toddler, 289
in Stage V toddler, 358
Vestibular impairment
in Stage I infant, effects of, 95
in Stage II infant, effects of, 146
in Stage III infant, effects of, 213
in Stage V toddler, effects of, 359
Vestibular system
facilitory effect of, 437
inhibitory effect of, 429–430
intrauterine stimulation of, in preterm infant, 467
Vision
abnormalities of, in disabled infants, 42–43
mobile for stimulation of, in disabled neonate, 115
Visual alertness, in disabled neonate, facilitation of, 113–114
Visual-auditory association, in disabled Stage III infant, habilitative approaches for, 246
Visual dysfunction, in Stage V toddler, effect of on exploratory behavior, 356–357
Visual impairment
partial, in Stage III infant, effect of on explorative behavior, 211–212
severe
in Stage III infant
creeping in, habilitative approaches for, 243–244
reaching in, habilitative approach for, 237–238
in Stage II infant, enhanced exploratory schemas in, ha-

improvement in, 259
readiness for, background components for, 292
role of other family members in, 279–280
in Stage V toddler, effect of athetosis on, 368, 368, 370
effect of hypertonia on, 361–362, 361
effect of hypotonia on, 364–365, 365
improvement in, 322–323
in visually impaired Stage IV toddler, habilitative approaches for, 309–310
Water
intake of, in disabled infant, 18
warm, relaxing effect of, 431–432
Water bed, for simulating intra-uterine vestibular input for preterm infant, 467
Weaning
of disabled infant, approach to minimize trauma of, 453
of infant with cerebral palsy, 451
Weight bearing
in disabled Stage I infant, habili-

tative approach for, 109–110, 110
over legs and feet, in Stage III infant, 182–183
unilateral
in disabled Stage II infant, 146–147
in prone position, habilitative approaches for, 164–165, 164
in Stage II infant, 118

Well-child care, importance of for disabled infant, 3
Well child health service model, 5–6
Wellness, for disabled infant, promotion of by nurse, 53
Withdrawal responses, techniques to inhibit, 433
Word(s), comprehension of, in normal stage III infant, 190–191
W-shaped sitting position
in disabled Stage II infant, 175
in disabled Stage III infant, 215–216, 216